Advances in Spinal Stabilization

Progress in Neurological Surgery

Vol. 16

Series Editor

L. Dade Lunsford Pittsburgh, Pa.

KARGER

Advances in Spinal Stabilization

Volume Editors

Regis W. Haid, Jr. Atlanta, Ga.
Brian R. Subach Atlanta, Ga.
Gerald E. Rodts, Jr. Atlanta, Ga.

145 figures, 2 in color, and 17 tables, 2003

KARGER

Basel · Freiburg · Paris · London · New York ·
Bangalore · Bangkok · Singapore · Tokyo · Sydney

Regis W. Haid, Jr., MD
Emory University School of Medicine
Department of Neurosurgery
The Emory Clinic
Atlanta, GA 30322 (USA)

Library of Congress Cataloging-in-Publication Data

Advances in spinal stabilization / volume editors, Regis W. Haid, Jr., Brian R. Subach, Gerald E, Rodts, Jr.
p. ; cm. – (Progress in neurological surgery, ISSN 0079–6492 ; vol. 16)
Includes bibliographical references and index.
ISBN 3–8055–7431–2 (hard cover : alk. paper)
1. Spine–Surgery. 2. Spinal implants. I. Haid, Regis W. II. Subach, Brian R. III. Rodts, Gerald E. IV. Series.
[DNLM: 1. Spine–surgery. 2. Orthopedic Procedures–methods. 3. Spinal Fusion–methods. WE 725 A2447 2003]
RD533 A285 2003
617.5′6059–dc21 2003047736

Bibliographic Indices. This publication is listed in bibliographic services, including Current Contents® and Index Medicus.

Drug Dosage. The authors and the publisher have exerted every effort to ensure that drug selection and dosage set forth in this text are in accord with current recommendations and practice at the time of publication. However, in view of ongoing research, changes in government regulations, and the constant flow of information relating to drug therapy and drug reactions, the reader is urged to check the package insert for each drug for any change in indications and dosage and for added warnings and precautions. This is particularly important when the recommended agent is a new and/or infrequently employed drug.

www.karger.com
Printed in Switzerland on acid-free paper by Reinhardt Druck, Basel
ISSN 0079–6492
ISBN 3–8055–7431–2

Contents

Neuronavigational Advances

Instrumentation and Technique Update

Series Editor's Note

Three eminent spine surgeons have collaborated as editors for this volume of *Progress in Neurological Surgery*. There is no question that new spinal stabilization techniques, minimally invasive approaches to the spine, and new concepts of biomechanics have revolutionized our understanding of disorders of spinal stability. In this comprehensive volume, the authors describe various techniques and clinically relevant procedures designed to improve the outcomes of spine surgery. Neuronavigational techniques, new bone fusion concepts, and both open and percutaneous spinal stabilization techniques are described. *Progress in Neurological Surgery* is dedicated to providing timely updates of important neurosurgical paradigm shifts. The volume of spinal surgery across the world has dramatically increased. The chapters in volume 16 help to elucidate the role and rationale of these new kinds of spinal stabilization. I am grateful to the editorial efforts of Dr. Haid, Dr. Subach and Dr. Rodts and to all the authors.

L. Dade Lunsford, MD

Foreword

Spinal stabilization has changed dramatically over the last 10 years and the pace of change continues to accelerate. This volume is an excellent mirror of the evolution of spinal stabilization – from the nuts, rods, and bolts first used years ago to the current applications of bilateral fusion using bone morphogenetic protein and gene manipulation or sophisticated bone extenders. Further possibilities for stabilizing the spine, as reflected in this book, include absorbable stabilization devices.

Through the combination of technical advances in minimally invasive spine surgery and neuronavigation, spinal surgery will become less destructive, less painful, and more successful. Most importantly, patient outcomes will improve. The section on instrumentation and technique represents the most up-to-date advances in surgical technique and management of spinal disorders.

The authors have provided a valuable service by compiling the most recent advances in spinal stabilization. This volume is a welcome addition to the personal libraries of spinal surgeons and to institutional libraries.

V.K.H. Sonntag

Haid RW Jr, Subach BR, Rodts GE Jr (eds): Advances in Spinal Stabilization.
Prog Neurol Surg. Basel, Karger, 2003, vol 16, pp 1–13

Bone Morphogenetic Protein (rhBMP-2): Experimental Review and Clinical Update

Brian R. Subach, Regis W. Haid, Jr., Gerald E. Rodts, Jr., Carmen A. Petraglia

The NeuroSpine Institute, Department of Neurological Surgery,
Emory University, Atlanta, Ga., USA

Over 30 years ago, Urist et al. [67, 68] identified a group of protein extracts, derived from the ground substance of mature bovine bone, capable of inducing both cartilage and bone formation when implanted into the soft tissues of study animals. Aptly named, bone morphogenetic proteins (BMPs) by Urist, these glycoproteins comprise a subset of the transforming growth factor-β family of related growth and differentiation factors. Of the more than 20 BMPs isolated to date, 6 appear to be structurally related to each other and capable of initiating the process of endochondral bone formation. The presence of such factors within the matrix of mature bone indicates a likely role in the regeneration and remodeling of bony structures after injury or repetitive stresses [4, 9, 18, 24, 43, 44].

The Basics of BMP Biology

Each of the six known osteoinductive BMPs shares significant similarities on a molecular level. Synthesized within the cell in precursor form, each molecule has a hydrophobic leader or secretory sequence with the mature portion of the protein at the carboxy terminus marked by a highly conserved, seven-cysteine repeat. Each mature BMP begins as 2 monomers of 120 amino acids each, which undergo disulfide linkage dimerization to form either a homologous or a heterologous protein chain. In the case of BMP-2 and BMP-7, the specific structure was first identified by isolating the bovine protein from bone extracts.

Oligonucleotide probes were used to obtain the human complementary DNA (cDNA) sequence. The cDNA clones were then spliced into a viral expression vector and transfected into a carrier cell in a process called recombination. In the case of BMP-2, the cells used were Chinese hamster ovary cells. Such cells produce the pure recombinant differentiation factor rhBMP-2 in large quantities in a process similar to fermentation. This process avoids potential complications related to the transmission of infectious materials from human donor bone tissue and eliminates the possibility of xenograft interactions with human recipients of BMP derived from bovine sources.

An Osteoinductive Role for BMP

In order to function as a suitable graft for bridging bone defects or fusing fracture lines and unstable motion segments, the prospective material would ideally possess three characteristics. The material would provide a source of primitive osteoprogenitor cells, which, under the appropriate influence, would form osteoblasts and osteocytes (osteopromotive). Such precursor cells are unfortunately relatively scarce. Bone marrow, for example, contains a ratio of only one osteprogenitor cell to approximately 50,000 nucleated cells in a young adult. This ratio may dip to 1:200,000 cells in an elderly individual afflicted by degenerative spinal disease [21]. Despite techniques to concentrate marrow extracts, successful efforts have only resulted in a maximum of 5-fold improvement of the unfavorable cellular ratio. Second, the graft material would produce local growth factors to stimulate bone growth and vascularity in the area (osteoinductive). There are numerous reports in the literature detailing the complex interaction of various autocrine and paracrine growth factors released from fibroblasts, platelets, and even the local hematoma that forms at the site of injury [1, 7, 16, 37, 46]. Finally, the third property of the graft material ideally would be its ability to act as a scaffold for bony ingrowth. Such ability is known as osteoconduction.

There are a number of possible reasons, which may account for the osteoinductive role of BMP. BMP acts as a chemotactic agent, a growth factor, and a differentiation factor. BMP acts as a chemotactic factor and initiates the recruitment of progenitor and stem cells toward the area of bone injury. In vivo studies of the local effects of BMP indicate an initial migration of mesenchymal stem cells to the area of implantation far in excess of that supplied by bone marrow grafting [12]. BMP acts as a growth factor and stimulates both angiogenesis and the proliferation of stem cells from surrounding mesenchymal tissues. BMP also acts as a differentiation factor by promoting the maturation of stem cells into chondrocytes, osteoblasts, and osteocytes.

Some cells respond to the growth factor aspect of BMP by altering their rates of proliferation. Yamaguchi et al. [71] demonstrated this in vitro by quantifying cellular proliferation of the rat C26 calvarial osteoprogenitor cells after treatment with BMP-2. This BMP-2 effect, however, appears to maintain specificity for certain cell types. For example, although BMP-7 has been shown to be mitogenic for a human osteosarcoma cell line (TE-85), treatment with BMP-2 showed no measurable effect on proliferation. In contrast, treatment of an osteoblast cell line (MC3T3-E1) with BMP-4 results in an inhibition of growth and a globally diminished proliferative index. By the effects on both mature and immature cell types, it seems reasonable that BMPs must be involved in the regulation of bone growth and maintenance of bone structure.

BMPs may also initiate the differentiation of stem cells into a specific phenotype. For example, the rat calvarial stem cell line (C26) is considered multipotential, in that such cells may be precursors for adipocytes, muscle cells, or osteoblasts. When BMP-2 is added to the culture medium, such cells become mature osteoblasts with increased surface expression of receptors for parathyroid hormone, alkaline phosphatase, and calcitonin [71]. This effect may also be observed in bone marrow cells. For example, the mouse line of marrow cells (W-20-17) may differentiate into either adipocytes or osteoblasts, depending upon the specific hormonal influence. The BMP-2 treatment of such cells results in both the differentiation of the cells into osteoblasts and the surface expression of receptors normally seen on mature cells.

Sources of BMP

At present there are three ways to obtain bone growth and differentiation factors: extraction of the factors from animal or human bone matrix, production of a single factor by cellular hosts using recombinant technology, and direct delivery of the DNA encoding for the factor to cells at the site of desired bone formation.

The first of these was initially employed by Urist et al. [67, 68]. From massive quantities of bovine bone, the group was able to extract a mixture of proteins found to stimulate bone growth in vivo. Under clinical evaluation in Europe as NeOsteo™ (Sulzer Spinetech, Wheat Ridge, Colo., USA), this mixture of BMPs and other associated proteins is derived through a well-engineered isolation process. The precise combination of factors comprising this substance has not yet been fully characterized, but appears to be reproducible through the manufacturer's process. This substance has shown experimental promise in bridging both segment skeletal defects in dogs and in bringing about spinal fusion in animal models of posterolateral arthrodesis. [12, 14, 17, 26, 27]. Like other growth and differentiation factors, a carrier substance is necessary to maintain adequate concentrations at the site of fusion. Substances such as natural coral (hydroxyapatite), collagen, and calcium sulfate have each been investigated [26, 27].

The second method of obtaining bone growth and differentiation factors has previously been discussed (see Molecular Biology). The process of obtaining recombinant human BMPs such as rhBMP-2 (Medtronic Sofamor Danek, Memphis, Tenn., USA and Genetics Institute, Cambridge, Mass., USA) and rhBMP-7 (Stryker Biotech, Hopkinton, Mass., USA) has been described. Such proteins differ from mixtures of extracted substances, mainly in terms of purity of product. Original studies of these substances focused upon animal models of segmental bone defects in the appendicular skeleton of rats, sheep, and dogs [23, 24, 35]. Cole et al. [23] compared rhBMP in a carrier to autologous grafting in a skeletal defect model with considerable success. Gerhart et al. [35] showed the utility of rhBMP in healing segmental femoral defects in sheep. Shortly thereafter, recombinant BMP was applied to animal models of spinal fusion and later, humans.

The third strategy for engineering bone formation involves gene therapy, or the delivery of the appropriate gene, or cDNA encoding for BMP to the local cells, rather than the actual factor. There are two obvious benefits to the strategy as compared to recombinant technology. First, the cost of genetic manipulation is significantly less than that required to both produce and market the purified rhBMP. Second, the potential for prolonged local production of the factor is greater with gene therapy when compared to the relatively short-lived effect of the rhBMP/carrier complex. Attempts to introduce BMP-2 cDNA into animal models are preliminary, but have met with limited success [1, 17, 29, 70].

From the Laboratory

Early work in the isolation of proteins with osteoinductive activity suggested that BMP-2 and BMP-7 were primarily responsible for the effects observed in vivo [3, 22, 23, 53, 59]. As a result, rhBMP-2, produced in a Chinese hamster ovary cell line, was the first of these molecules studied in detail. Implantation of the recombinant factor in a rat model resulted in ectopic bone formation with a dose-effect relationship temporally identical to that of bone-derived extracts; however, the amount of pure rhBMP-2 required to induce formation of a given amount of bone was approximately 10-fold less than that required of the bone extract [5, 12, 13, 51]. Subsequent studies in nonhuman primates show no difference in the dose required to effect consistent posterolateral spinal fusions.

The ability to form bone at ectopic sites, however, had little application to current spinal fusion techniques. Realizing the limitations inherent in

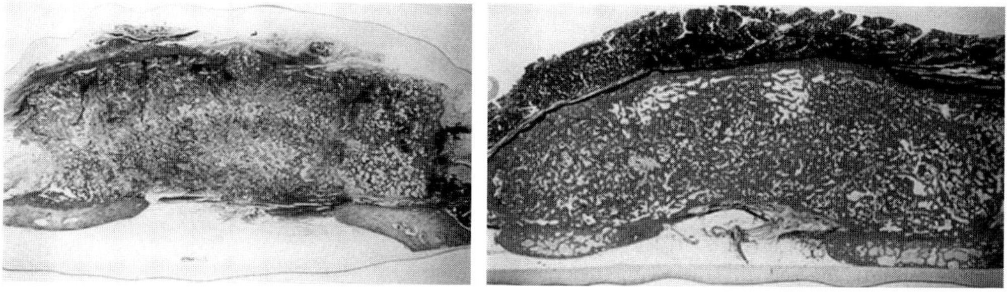

a *b*

Fig. 1. Photomicrograph of intertransverse spinal fusion using carrier matrix alone (***a***) as a control and rhBMP-2/carrier (***b***). Histologic section demonstrates transverse processes at inferior-lateral corners with bridging collagen scar tissue and minimal bone formation (***a***) and abundant new membranous bone formation (***b***).

autogenous and allogeneic bone grafting, investigators began applying BMP technology to animal models of spinal fusion procedures [32, 36, 38, 62]. Multiple studies, involving various concentrations of BMP in a variety of carrier substrates, have shown remarkable results. Early work by Boden et al. [12–15] and Holliger et al. [45] compared rhBMP-2 to autologous bone graft in a rabbit posterolateral lumbar fusion model. Remarkably, all BMP-treated animals (100%) attained solid, bony fusions across the operated level, which were biomechanically stiffer and stronger than the autograft-only fusions observed in 42% of the control group. Similar studies in a canine model also confirmed the efficacy of rhBMP-2 in producing mature fusion masses [28]. The canine study by David et al. [28] demonstrated a dose dependence to the BMP effect, with greater concentrations producing greater effects; however, this contradicts a study by Sandhu et al. [58–60] in a similar canine model, which shows BMP to be more effective than autologous bone graft, but in a dose-independent manner [63]. Most investigators developed the opinion that bone induction was relatively simple in lower species, but was only indirectly applicable to human models. As a result, research focused on developing spinal fusion models in primates. As a developmentally higher species, primates provide a more realistic test environment for evaluating the effectiveness of BMP [40, 41]. Boden et al. [10] applied this belief to a nonhuman primate model of intertransverse spinal fusion and demonstrated effective fusion rates using rhBMP-2 on a ceramic carrier delivered by a minimally invasive approach (fig. 1). Sandhu et al. [60] went a step further to demonstrate clinically, mechanically, and radiographically equivalent spinal arthrodesis using rhBMP-2 without decortication of the prospective fusion bed. Boden et al. [7, 16] and Martin et al. [51], by adding rhBMP-2 to autograft, were able to demonstrate subsequent induction of BMP-6, osteocalcin, and collagen within the graft itself.

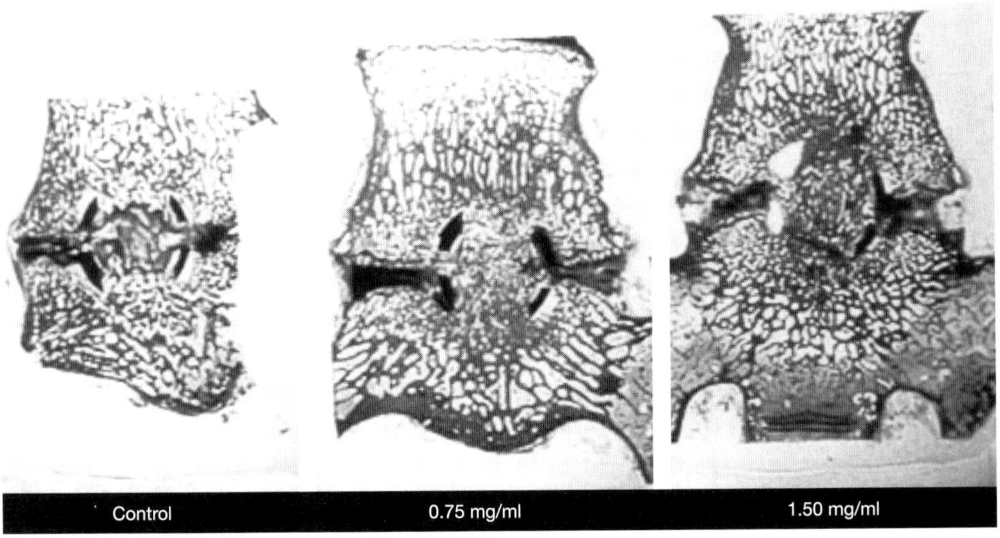

Fig. 2. Threaded titanium interbody cage implanted into the lumbar spine of a primate. Control group is cage alone. Experimental groups are rhBMP-2-impregnated sponges at concentrations of 0.75 and 1.50 mg/ml. Actual spines at 6 months from surgery. Control demonstrates a pseudarthrosis with fibrous scar tissue within the cage. BMP groups both show mature bone bridging the interspace within the cage.

Posterolateral fusion models attempted to replace autograft with a BMP/carrier complex, but still required internal fixation. Attention was then focused upon interbody spinal fusion techniques, which could possibly obviate the need for both autograft and fixation [19, 20, 34, 42, 47, 48, 55, 56, 64, 65]. Zdeblick et al. [73] performed three level anterior cervical fusions in goats using a BAK cage filled with either local autograft or a collagen impregnated rhBMP-2 sponge [49]. Eleven of 21 animals (52%) in the autograft group had histologic evidence of pseudarthrosis, while only 1 (5%) of the BMP group failed to form a solid bony fusion. The biomechanical stiffness of the BMP construct was equal to that of an autograft/cervical-plated level. Boden et al. [8] performed the same procedure in the lumbar spine of primates. Using rhBMP-2 on a collagen carrier in both titanium-threaded interbody cages and threaded bone dowels, both were delivered laparoscopically with a documented improvement of fusion rates over empty cages and autograft-filled cages [8, 57] (fig. 2, 3).

Preliminary results of human clinical studies have been encouraging. In a recent report of a randomized, prospective controlled clinical pilot study, Boden et al. [8] demonstrated solid bony fusions by both clinical and radiographic

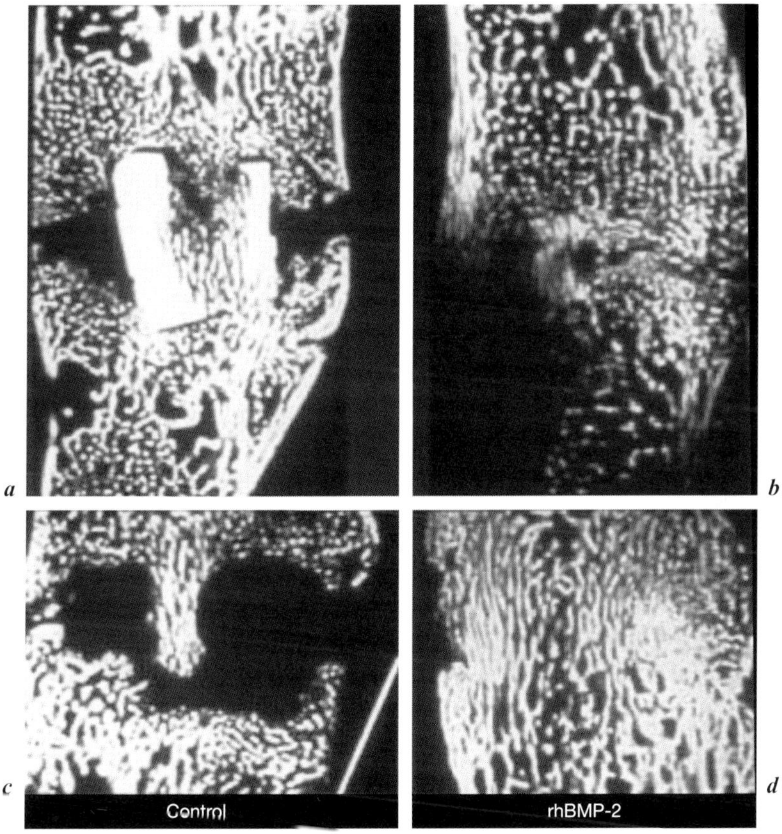

Fig. 3. Bone dowel interbody device implanted into the lumbar spine of a primate. Control group is dowel with autograft. Experimental group is a bone dowel with an rhBMP-2-impregnated sponge inside. Actual spines at 6 months from surgery. Control group demonstrates a solid fusion (***a***) and reabsorption of the bone dowel/autograft construct (***c***). BMP animals (***b***, ***d***) both show mature bone bridging the interspace with resorption of the dowel.

criteria in 11 patients undergoing anterior lumbar interbody fusion procedures with a tapered, threaded titanium cage filled with an rhBMP-2-impregnated collagen sponge (fig. 4). Pain scores, as documented by the Oswestry Disability and the Short Form-36 questionnaires, improved concomitantly as fusion progressed [8, 30, 39, 56, 66, 69].

Based upon the findings in both the primate models and human trials, the United States Food and Drug Administration (FDA) approved rhBMP-2 for limited use in patients with spinal disorders. Specifically, the FDA approved BMP for use as an adjunct to spinal fusion in patients with degenerative disc disease undergoing anterior lumbar interbody fusion using titanium cages (LT cages).

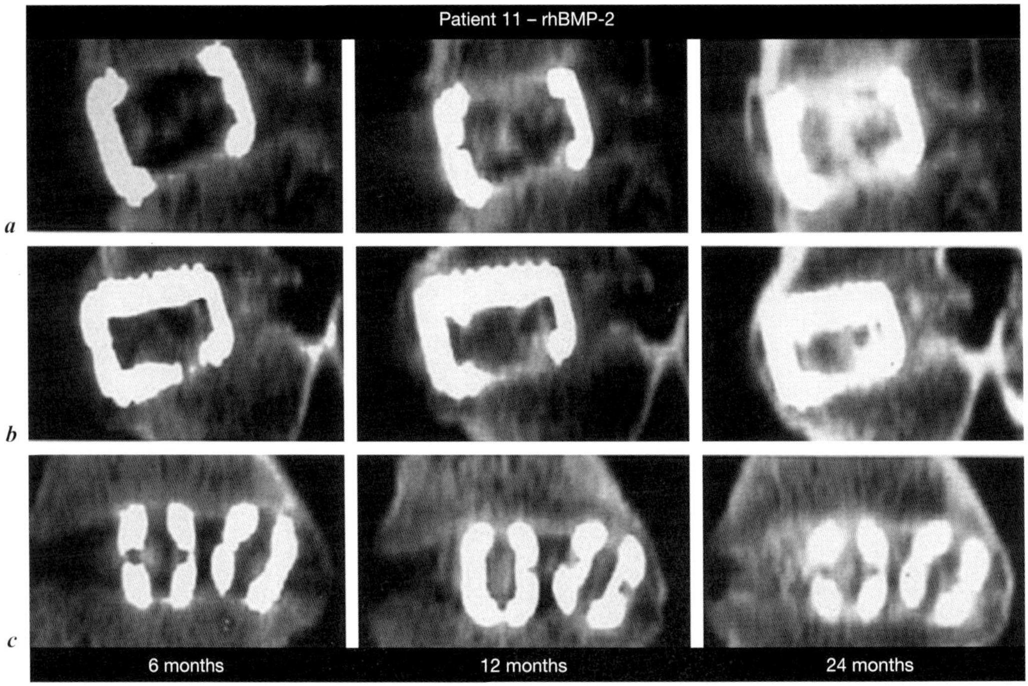

Fig. 4. Computed tomographic reconstructions of a human patient receiving a threaded, titanium cage (Lordotec cage, Medtronic Sofamor Danek, Memphis, Tenn., USA) with rhBMP-2 on a collagen sponge carrier. ***a*** Sagittal view of the left cage at 6, 12 and 24 months. ***b*** Right cage at the same time intervals. ***c*** Coronal views at the same time intervals. All images show fusion with increasing bone density over time.

The cages attempt to both restore and maintain intervertebral height and protect the BMP from exposure to diluting substances such as blood and irrigation fluid. Although approved, BMP has yet to reach the market. Concerns raised by experts include the improper use of the BMP such that vascular and neural elements may come in contact with the protein causing injury, lower fusion rates due to improper or unapproved implantation techniques, and stimulation of infectious or neoplastic processes due to use in patients with such diseases.

Discussion

Research over the past decade has shown the utility of using the growth and differentiation factor, BMP-2, to promote bone formation at the site of bone loss or injury. The in vivo role of BMP-2 and its complex interaction with other growth and differentiation factors remains to be clarified. The use of BMP-2 as a means of replacing harvested autograft and obviating the need for internal fixation, each with its attendant morbidity, appears likely as a result of outcomes from both animal and human studies. Although dose-effect relationships and carrier substrates may provide continued investigational challenges, the use of recombinant technology and gene therapy in the field of bone fusion have been firmly established. In the past 30 years since Marshall Urist first coined the term bone morphogenetic protein, one doubts that he could have envisioned the monumental strides and clinical progress, which researchers in the field have achieved to this point.

Conclusions

The widespread use of spinal fusion procedures in the management of spinal disorders has led investigators to explore the use of growth and differentiation factors in such procedures. Either as an adjunct to allograft bone or as a replacement for harvested autograft, BMPs appear to improve fusion rates after spinal arthrodesis in both animal and human models, while reducing the donor site morbidity previously associated with such procedures [2, 6, 11, 14, 23, 25, 50, 54, 72]. The use of recombinant genetic technology in the production of BMP has improved the efficiency, cost-effectiveness, and safety of producing and using such materials. rhBMP-2, as one of the first factors identified in the process of endochondral bone formation, has been extensively researched over the past decade. The efficacy and dose profile of this differentiation factor in the context of various carrier substrates has been investigated [15, 26, 27, 33, 51, 58, 61]. Based upon the encouraging results of preliminary studies, the future role of rhBMP-2 may lie in the elimination of autologous bone grafting, the reduction of the need for instrumented fixation, and augmentation of accepted fusion rates.

Acknowledgments

The authors wish to thank Medtronic Sofamor Danek for their continued support and assistance in the preparation of the figures.

References

1 Aronow MA, Gerstenfeld LC, Owen TA, Tassinari MS, Stein GS, Lian JB: Factors that promote progressive development of the osteoblast phenotype in cultured rat calvarial cells. J Cell Physiol 1990;143:213–221.

2 Arrington ED, Smith WJ, Chambers HG, Bucknell AL, Davino NA: Complications of iliac crest bone graft harvesting. Clin Orthop 1996;329:300–309.

3 Asahina I, Sampath TK, Nishimura I, Hauschka PV: Human osteogenic protein-1 induces both chondroblastic and osteoblastic differentiation of osteoprogenitor cells derived from newborn rat calvaria. J Cell Biol 1993;123:921–933.

4 Aspenberg P, Jeppsson C, Wang JS, Bostrom M: Transforming growth factor beta and bone morphogenetic protein 2 for bone ingrowth: A comparison using bone chambers in rats. Bone 1996; 19:499–503.

5 Aspenberg P, Turek T: BMP-2 for intramuscular bone induction: Effect in squirrel monkeys is dependent on implantation site. Acta Orthop Scand 1996;67:3–6.

6 Banwart JC, Asher MA, Hassanein RS: Iliac crest bone graft harvest donor site morbidity: A statistical evaluation. Spine 1995;20:1055–1060.

7 Boden SD, Hair G, Titus L, Racine M, McCuaig K, Wozney JM, Nanes MS: Glucocorticoid-induced differentiation of fetal rat calvarial osteoblasts is mediated by BMP-6. Endocrinology 1997;138:2920–2928.

8 Boden SD, Martin GJ, Horton WC, Truss TL, Sandhu HS: Laparoscopic anterior spinal arthrodesis with rhBMP-2 in a titanium interbody threaded cage. J Spinal Disord 1998;11:95–101.

9 Boden SD, McCuaig K, Hair G, Racine M, Titus L, Wozney JM, Nanes MS: Differential effects and glucocorticoid potentiation of bone morphogenetic protein action during rat osteoblast differentiation in vitro. Endocrinology 1996;137:3401–3407.

10 Boden SD, Moskovitz PA, Morone MA, Toribitake Y: Video-assisted lateral intertransverse process arthrodesis: Validation of a new minimally invasive lumbar spinal fusion technique in the rabbit and nonhuman primate (rhesus) models. Spine 1996;21:2689–2697.

11 Boden SD, Schimandle JH: Biologic enhancement of spinal fusion. Spine 1995;20(suppl): S113–S123.

12 Boden SD, Schimandle JH, Hutton WC: 1995 Volvo Award in basic sciences. The use of an osteoinductive growth factor for lumbar spinal fusion. II. Study of dose, carrier, and species. Spine 1995;20:2633–2644.

13 Boden SD, Schimandle JH, Hutton WC: Lumbar intertransverse-process spine arthrodesis using a bovine-derived osteoinductive bone protein. J Bone Joint Surg Am 1995;77:1404–1417.

14 Boden SD, Schimandle JH, Hutton WC: Evaluation of a bovine-derived osteoinductive bone protein in a non-human primate model of lumbar spinal fusion. Trans Orthop Res Soc 1996; 21:118.

15 Boden SD, Schimandle JH, Hutton WC, Damien CJ, Benedict JJ, Baranowski C, Collier S: In vivo evaluation of a resorbable osteoinductive composite as a graft substitute for lumbar spinal fusion. J Spinal Disord 1997;10:1–11.

16 Boden SD, Sumner DR: Biologic factors affecting spinal fusion and bone regeneration. Spine 1995;20(suppl):102S–112S.

17 Boden SD, Titus L, Hair G, Liu Y, Viggeswarapu M, Nanes MS, Baranowski C: 1998 Volvo Award in basic sciences: Lumbar spine fusion by local gene therapy with a cDNA encoding a novel osteoinductive protein (LMP-I). Spine 1998;23:2486–2492.

18 Boonen S, Broos P, Dequeker J, Bouillon R: The prevention or treatment of age-related osteoporosis in the elderly by systemic recombinant growth factor therapy (rhIGF I or rhTGF beta): A perspective. J Intern Med 1997;242:285–290.

19 Burns BH: An operation for spondylolisthesis. Lancet 1933;224:i233.

20 Calandruccio RA, Benton BF: Anterior lumbar fusion. Clin Orthop 1964;35:63–68.

21 Caplan AI: Mesenchymal stem cells. J Orthop Res 1991;9:641–650.

22 Centrella M, McCarthy TL, Canalis E: Current concepts review: Transforming growth factor-beta and remodeling of bone. J Bone Joint Surg Am 1991;73:1418–1428.

23 Cole BJ, Yasko A, Browne MA: The ability of recombinant human bone morphogenetic protein to heal segmental bone defects – A comparison of physiologic carriers to autologous bone graft. J Bone Miner Res 1992;7(suppl):S251.

24 Cook SD, Baffes GC, Wolfe MW, Sampath TK, Rueger DC, Whitecloud TS 3rd: The effect of recombinant human osteogenic protein-1 on healing of large segmental bone defects. J Bone Joint Surg Am 1994;76:827–838.

25 Cook SD, Dalton JE, Tan EH, Whitecloud T, Rueger DC: In vivo evaluation of recombinant human osteogenic protein (rhOP-1) implants as a bone graft substitute for spinal fusions. Spine 1994;19: 1655–1663.

26 Damien CJ, Christel PS, Benedict JJ, Patat J-L, Guillemin G: A composite of natural coral, collagen, bone protein, and basic fibroblast growth factor tested in a rat subcutaneous model. Ann Chir Gynaecol 1993;82:117–128.

27 Damien CJ, Parsons JR, Benedict JJ, Weisman DS: Investigation of a hydroxyapatite and calcium sulfate composite supplemented with an osteoinductive factor. J Biomed Mater Res 1990;24: 639–654.

28 David SM, Murakami T, Tabor OB, Grub HE, Meyer RA Jr, Howard BA, Wozney JM, Hanley EN Jr: Lumbar spinal fusion using recombinant human bone morphogenetic protein-2 (rhBMP-2): A randomized, blinded and controlled study. Trans In Soc Study Lumbar Spine 1995;22:14.

29 Delloye C, Verhelpen M, D'Hemricourt J, Govaerts B, Bourgois R: Morphometric and physical investigations of segmental cortical bone autografts and allografts in canine ulnar defects. Clin Orthop 1992;282:273–292.

30 Fairbank JCT, Davies JB, Mbaot JC, O'Brien JP: The Oswestry low back pain disability questionnaire. Physiotherapy 1980;66:271–273.

31 Fang J, Zhu YY, Smiley E, Bonadio J, Rouleau JP, Goldstein SA, McCauley LK, Davidson BL, Roessler BJ: Stimulation of new bone formation by direct transfer of osteogenic plasmid genes. Proc Natl Acad Sci USA 1996;93:5753–5758.

32 Fernyhough JC, Schimandle JH, Weigel MC, Edwards CC, Levine AM: Chronic donor site pain complicating bone graft harvesting from the posterior iliac crest for spinal fusion. Spine 1992; 17:1474–1480.

33 Fischgrund JS, James SB, Chabot MC, Hankin R, Herkowitz HN, Wozney JM, Shirkhoda A: Augmentation of autograft using rhBMP-2 and different carrier media in the canine spine fusion model. J Spinal Disord 1997;10:467–472.

34 Fraser RD: Interbody, posterior, and combined lumbar fusions. Spine 1995;20(suppl): S167–S177.

35 Gerhart TN, Kirker-Head CA, Kriz MJ, Holtrop ME, Hennig GE, Hipp J, Schelling SH, Wang E: Healing segmental femoral defects in sheep using recombinant human bone morphogenetic protein. Clin Orthop 1993;293:317–326.

36 Goldberg VM, Stevenson S: Natural history of autografts and allografts. Clin Orthop 1987;225: 7–16.

37 Goldberg VM, Stevenson S, Shaffer JW: Biology of autografts and allografts; in Friedlaender GE, Goldberg VM (eds): Bone and Cartilage Allografts. Park Ridge, American Academy of Orthopaedic Surgeons, 1991, pp 3–12.

38 Goulet JA, Senunas LE, DeSilva GL, Greenfield MLVH: Autogenous iliac crest bone graft. Clin Orthop 1997;339:76–81.

39 Grevitt M, Khazim R, Webb J, Mulholland R, Shepperd J: The short form-36 health survey questionnaire in spine surgery. J Bone Joint Surg Br 1997;79:48–52.

40 Hanisch O, Tatakis DN, Boskovic MM, Rohrer MD, Wikesjo UM: Bone formation and reosseointegration in peri-implantitis defects following surgical implantation of rhBMP-2. Int J Oral Maxillofac Implants 1997;12:604–610.

41 Hanisch O, Tatakis DN, Rohrer MD, Wohrle PS, Wozney JM, Wikesjo UM: Bone formation and osseointegration stimulated by rhBMP-2 following subantral augmentation procedures in nonhuman primates. Int J Oral Maxillofac Implants 1997;12:785–792.

42 Harmon PH: Anterior extraperitoneal lumbar disk excision and vertebral fusion. Clin Orthop 1960;18:169–198.

43 Heiple KG, Chase SW, Herndon CH: A comparative study of the healing process following different types of bone transplantation. J Bone Joint Surg Am 1963;45:1593–1616.

44 Hogan BLM: Bone morphogenetic proteins: Multi-functional regulators of vertebrate development. Genes Dev 1996;10:1580–1594.

45 Holliger EH, Trawick RH, Boden SD, Hutton WC: Morphology of the lumbar intertransverse process fusion mass in the rabbit model: A comparison between two bone graft materials – rhBMP-2 and autograft. J Spinal Disord 1996;9:125–128.

46 Kim SS, Denis F, Lonstein JE, Winter RB: Factors affecting fusion rate in spondylolisthesis. Spine 1990;15:977–984.
47 Kozak JA, Heilman AE, O'Brien JP: Anterior lumbar fusion operations: Technique and graft materials. Clin Orthop 1994;300:45–51.
48 Kumar A, Kozak JA, Doherty BJ, Dickson JH: Interspace distraction and graft subsidence after anterior lumbar fusion with femoral strut allograft. Spine 1993;18:2393–2400.
49 Kuslich SD, Ulstrom CL, Griffith SL, Ahern JW, Dowdle JD: The Bagby and Kuslich method of lumbar interbody fusion. Spine 1998;23:1267–1279.
50 Laurie SWS, Kaban LB, Mulliken JB, Murray JE: Donor-site morbidity after harvesting rib and iliac bone. Plast Reconstr Surg 1984;73:933–938.
51 Martin GJ, Boden SD, Morone MA, Moskovitz PA: Posterolateral intertransverse process spinal fusion arthrodesis with rhBMP-2 in a non-human primate: Important lessons learned regarding dose, carrier, and safety. J Spinal Disord 1999;12:179–186.
52 McHorney CA, Ware JE, Lu R, Sherbourne CD: The MOS 36-item short form health survey (SF-36). III. Tests of data quality, scaling assumptions, and reliability across diverse groups. Med Care 1994;32:40–66.
53 Muschler GF, Hyodo A, Manning T, Kambic H, Easley K: Evaluation of human bone morphogenetic protein 2 in a canine spinal fusion model. Clin Orthop 1994;308:229–240.
54 Rawlinson N: Morbidity after anterior cervical decompression and fusion: The influence of the donor site on recovery, and the results of a trial of surgibone compared to autologous bone. Acta Neurochir 1994;131:106–118.
55 Ray CD: Threaded titanium cages for lumbar interbody fusions. Spine 1997;22:667–680.
56 Sacks S: Anterior interbody fusion of the lumbar spine: Indications and results in 200 cases. Clin Orthop 1966;44:163–170.
57 Sandhu HS, Kabo IM, Turner AS, Liu D, Kanim LEA, Toth IM: RhBMP-2 augmentation of titanium fusion cages for experimental anterior lumbar fusion. Proceedings of the 11th Annual Meeting of the North American Spine Society. Rosemont, North American Spine Society, 1996, p 47.
58 Sandhu HS, Kanim LE, Kabo JM, Toth JM, Zeegen EN, Liu D, Delamarter RB, Dawson EG: Effective doses of recombinant bone morphogenetic protein-2 in experimental spinal fusion. Spine 1996;21:2115–2122.
59 Sandhu HS, Kanim LE, Kabo JM, Toth JM, Zeegan EN, Liu D, Seeger LL, Dawson EG: Evaluation of rhBMP-2 with an OPLA carrier in a canine posterolateral (transverse process) spinal fusion model. Spine 1995;20:2669–2682.
60 Sandhu HS, Kanim LE, Toth JM, Kabo JM, Liu D, Delamarter RB, Dawson EG: Experimental spinal fusion with recombinant human bone morphogenetic protein-2 without decortication of osseous elements. Spine 1997;22:1171–1180.
61 Shimandle JH, Boden SO, Hutton WC: Experimental spinal fusion with recombinant human bone morphogenetic protein-2 (rhBMP-2). Spine 1995;20:1326–1337.
62 Scene CL, Freeze A, Weil RJ, Marquette PJ: Analysis of harvest morbidity and radiographic outcome using autograft for anterior cervical fusion. Spine 1997;22:2222–2227.
63 Schuster JJ: CRC Handbook of Sample Size: Guidelines for Clinical Trial. Boca Raton, CRC Press, 1990.
64 Sorenson KH: Anterior interbody lumbar spine fusion for incapacitating disc degeneration and spondylolisthesis. Acta Orthop Scand 1978;49:269–277.
65 Stauffer RN, Coventry MB: Anterior interbody lumbar spine fusion. J Bone Joint Surg Am 1972;54:756–768.
66 Stewart AL, Hays RD, Ware JE: The MOS short form general health survey (SF-36). Med Care 1988;26:724–732.
67 Urist MR: Bone. Formation by autoinduction. Science 1965;150:893–899.
68 Urist MR, Strates BS: Bone morphogenetic protein. J Dent Res 1971;50:1392–1406.
69 Ware JE, Sherbourne CD: The MOS 36-item short form health survey (SF-36). I. Conceptual framework and item selection. Med Care 1992;30:473–483.
70 Wozney JM: Bone morphogenetic proteins and their gene expression; in Noda M (ed): Cellular and Molecular Biology of Bone. Boston, Academic Press, 1993, pp 131–167.

71 Yamaguchi A, Katagiri T, Ikeda T, Wozney JM, Rosen V, Wang EA, Kahn AJ, Suda T, Yoshiki S: Recombinant human bone morphogenetic protein stimulates osteoblastic maturation and inhibits myogenic differentiation in vitro. J Cell Biol 1991;113:681–687.
72 Younger EM, Chapman MW: Morbidity at bone graft donor sites. J Orthop Trauma 1989;3: 192–195.
73 Zdeblick TA, Ghanayem AJ, Rapoff AJ, Swain C, Bassett T, Cooke ME, Markel M: Cervical interbody fusion cages: An animal model with and without bone morphogenetic protein. Spine 1998;23:758–766.

Brian R. Subach, MD, Neurosurgery
550 Peachtree Street/ Suite 806, Atlanta, GA 30308-2247 (USA)
Tel. +1 404 686 8101, Fax +1 404 686 4805

Haid RW Jr, Subach BR, Rodts GE Jr (eds): Advances in Spinal Stabilization.
Prog Neurol Surg. Basel, Karger, 2003, vol 16, pp 14–28

Cellular and Genetic Approaches for Spinal Fusions

Gregory A. Helm[a, b], *D. Greg Anderson*[c]

Departments of [a]Neurosurgery, [b]Biomedical Engineering and [c]Orthopedic Surgery, University of Virginia Health System, Charlottesville, Va., USA

A variety of evolving technologies are currently being evaluated in preclinical studies to promote tissue repair and/or regeneration in the spinal region. Cellular and genetic techniques to induce bone formation for interbody or posterolateral spinal arthrodesis are an attractive approach, since this technology could be employed through a minimally invasive approach with decreased morbidity and potentially higher fusion rates compared to traditional open procedures. Tissue engineering techniques are also being evaluated for disc repair and regeneration using various growth and differentiation factors, mesenchymal stem cells (MSCs) and genetic therapies. Percutaneous soft tissue stabilization techniques are also within the scope of current technologies, potentially allowing stabilization of the spine by the induction of ligamentous tissues, thus avoiding extensive spinal arthrodesis procedures. Clearly, tissue-engineering techniques will continue to evolve and certainly lead to more effective, and less invasive, procedures for the treatment of traumatic, neoplastic and degenerative spine problems.

Stem Cell Technologies

The direct application of osteoinductive stem cells on a bioresorbable matrix, or scaffold, may be a useful strategy for engineering bone and soft tissues in the paraspinal region. Stem cells have several advantages for inducing osteogenesis compared with the application of bone growth factors alone. Pluripotent stem cells have the capacity to differentiate into the desired cell type and form appropriate matrix elements under the control of various growth and differentiation factors. By supplying stem cells to the site, the growth factor response is not dependent solely on the availability of local stem cell populations, which may be diminished due to senility, radiation, medical factors, or medications which might alter the intrinsic stem cell population. Therefore, direct implantation of pluripotent cells with or without growth factors has the potential to yield more rapid and uniform bony healing. Osteoprogenitor cells have been isolated from the bone marrow of rats, rabbits, dogs, and humans, as well as nonmarrow locations such as adipose tissue. These cells can be isolated and expanded in tissue culture, prior to implantation into a target location. Stem cells also have the potential to be genetically altered to express various growth factors or other therapeutic genes prior to implantation.

A variety of studies have demonstrated the utility of using stem cells to achieve bone formation. Bruder et al. [1] placed autologous canine MSCs obtained from bone marrow onto porous cylinders composed of hydroxyapatite and tricalcium phosphate. The implant was subsequently grafted into critical-sized femoral defects. Implants without MSCs produced atrophic nonunions in all treated animals. Implants containing the MSCs produced lamellar and woven bone within the carrier and resulted in a solid union at the site of the defect. Bruder et al. [2] also successfully achieved bone induction using human MSCs on a ceramic carrier in athymic nude rats. Using radiography, biomechanical testing, and histologic analysis, the human MSCs were capable of healing critical-sized femoral defects. Quarto et al. [3] studied the use of autologous bone marrow stromal cells delivered on a macroporous hydroxyapatite carrier for the healing of large bony defects (>4.0 cm) in a small human clinical series. The implant was placed within the defect, and the fracture was stabilized with external fixation. In each instance, the composite implant was able to achieve successful union of the bony defect, thus producing the first direct evidence that tissue engineering of bone can be successfully applied to humans in a clinical setting.

Bone Morphogenetic Protein Gene Therapy

Bone Morphogenetic Protein Overview

Bone morphogenetic proteins (BMPs) are a group of secreted proteins that are members of the transforming growth factor-β (TGF-β) superfamily based on their high degree of homology within the C-terminal seven-cysteine region [4–7]. These proteins were originally recognized for their ability to form ectopic bone by inducing primitive mesenchymal cell chemotaxis, proliferation, and differentiation into chondrocytes and osteoblasts [8–13]. The ectopic bone is formed primarily through endochondral mechanisms, recapitulating many of the events seen during embryonic development [7, 10, 11, 13–15]. However, when delivered in high concentrations, direct or intramembranous bone formation can also be induced at the treatment site. Other BMPs have been found experimentally to induce the formation of various other tissue types, including cartilage, tendon, and ligament [16–24]. Molecular cloning techniques have allowed the production of certain BMPs in large quantities, which has contributed to the rapid advancement of our collective understanding of BMP biology and potential for clinical applications [7].

BMPs are initially synthesized as monomeric precursors that, after proteolytic cleavage, undergo dimerization through disulfide bonding [15, 25]. These dimers, which can be either homologous or heterologous, are released extracellularly and act by binding to type I and II receptors [26–34]. Receptor binding and subsequent transphosphorylation leads to the phosphorylation and activation of various cytoplasmic Smad proteins [35–40]. These activated Smad proteins then translocate to the nucleus and initiate cellular responses, including chemotaxis, proliferation, and differentiation.

Gene Therapy Overview

Gene-based therapies attempt to deliver specific genes, known as the transgene, to target cells to change the existing physiologic state or disease process [41, 42]. Delivery of the genetic material to the target cell can be accomplished by both nonviral and viral vectors. Nonviral or synthetic delivery techniques include the use of molecular conjugates, liposomes, naked DNA, plasmids, electroporation, or the incorporation of the transgenes with viral proteins. To date, the majority of these techniques are limited by their relatively low cellular transduction rates. In contrast, viral vectors can be highly efficient in their delivery of genetic material. Some of the more common viruses used for gene therapy include the adenovirus, herpes virus, retrovirus, and adeno-associated viruses (AAV). These vectors are often genetically modified so that they are replication-deficient, through the removal of specific portions of the viral genome, which allow for the insertion of a therapeutic transgene. Although gene therapy as a concept continues to capture the imagination of basic scientists and clinical researchers, the advancement of the techniques toward human use has proven difficult [41–44]. Technical hurdles such as insufficient transgene expression, an inability to circumvent the host immune system, and a failure to achieve long-term transgene expression continue to present a challenge for many clinical applications. Fortunately, bone induction using BMPs may be an ideal application of gene therapy because long-term expression of the BMP is not required to achieve therapeutic bone formation. In fact, the elimination of BMP expression may be advantageous in that tissue overgrowth or toxicity is less likely to be encountered.

Viral Vectors

Adenoviral Vectors. Adenoviruses are double-stranded DNA viruses which bind to specific cell surface receptors, enter the cells by endocytosis, and subsequently release their DNA into the cytoplasm [45, 46]. The viral genome is divided into immediate early genes, early genes, and late genes according to the time in which the genes are expressed. The immediate early genes activate early gene transcription, while the early genes are involved both in subsequent viral replication and host immune evasion. The late genes code for the adenoviruses' structural proteins [46]. Most adenoviral vectors studied to date are derived from the adenovirus serotype-5, which are rendered replication-defective by deletion of the E1 region. The E3 region is often deleted as well to make room for larger transgenes. First generation adenoviral vectors can accommodate up to 8 kb of foreign DNA.

The advantages of adenoviral vectors include their ability to be produced in high titers, their extrachromosomal life cycle, which reduces the risk of insertional mutagenesis, and their ability to transfect numerous cell types [46, 47]. There are several potential disadvantages of the adenoviral vector for gene therapy. Because the virus does not integrate into the cellular genome, the length of gene expression is limited and therapeutic genes are not passed to the progeny of the transduced cells. Perhaps the most problematic issue with adenoviral vectors, however, is the robust humoral and cellular immune response that can occur at the treatment site resulting in reduced transgene expression. Intense research efforts are currently directed at blunting the immune response by alterations to the adenoviral vector such as deleting the viral DNA polymerase gene (Δpol adenoviral vectors) or completely eliminating the viral genome (gutless adenoviral vectors).

AAV Vectors. AAV, which are defective single-stranded DNA parvoviruses, are also attractive vectors for BMP gene therapy studies [48]. AAV vectors have the ability to integrate stably into the target cell's genome, transduce a variety of cell types, maintain high levels of gene expression, transfect both proliferating and quiescent cells, and be generated in high titers. Numerous studies have demonstrated that AAV can efficiently transduce muscle and other cells in vivo with little inflammatory response and no evidence of insertional mutagenesis. The production of AAV vectors was initially fraught with numerous technical difficulties; however, current techniques of vector production lead to a high yield of recombinant AAV, completely free of wild-type AAV.

Retroviral Vectors. Retroviral vectors enter target cells through interactions between the viral envelope proteins and cell surface glycoproteins. Importantly, retroviruses contain single-stranded RNA. Once the viral genome is released into the cytoplasm, retroviral reverse transcriptase produces a double-stranded DNA copy, which subsequently integrates into the host genome during mitosis. One disadvantage to using retroviral vectors is that retroviruses can only integrate their genetic material into proliferating cells [49]. Therefore, it may be difficult to achieve adequate cellular transduction at sites requiring bone induction by direct injection. Other major disadvantages of retroviral vectors are their low infectivity and instability of the virions. The utilization of retroviruses for BMP gene therapy will most likely be limited to ex vivo approaches, such as for the genetic modification of MSC populations.

Herpes Viral Vectors. Herpes viruses are double-stranded DNA viruses which can cause significant human pathology, including cold sores and encephalitis. Gene therapy studies utilizing herpes viral vectors typically utilize genetically modified herpes simplex type 1. In the normal life cycle of these viruses, the virion fuses with the cell membrane and is transported to the nucleus where, after several phases of gene transcription, the cell lyses and releases progeny viral particles. Herpes viruses also have the ability to enter a latency phase, during which time the viral genome is not actively transcribed. This latency phase can be lost during cell division [46]. Herpes viral vectors have the advantage of being able to accommodate up to 40 kb of foreign DNA and can be utilized to insert foreign DNA into a variety of cell populations, including myocytes, with limited toxicity. Herpes viral vectors may, therefore, be a reasonable vector for BMP gene therapy [50].

Nonviral Vectors

Direct Plasmid Injection. Wolff [51] was the first to show that the direct intramuscular injection of plasmid DNA could lead to low level, short-term gene expression. Other researchers have now demonstrated the successful transduction of the myocardium, brain, thyroid, and various tumors using this technique [52–55]. Inadequate cellular transduction rates can be significantly increased by pretreatment of the injected area with hypertonic saline or bupivacaine [56]. Systemic gene expression can also be obtained by the direct intravenous injection of naked DNA in adults, although rapid degradation of the DNA prior to reaching the target cell remains problematic in the absence of a delivery system, such as cationic liposomes [57]. Currently, no published studies have demonstrated successful bone formation using direct injections of osteogenic plasmid into either orthotopic or heterotopic sites.

Electroporation. The diffusion of extracellular DNA into a cell in vitro and in vivo can be significantly increased by permeabilizing the cell's membrane using short, high intense electric pulses. The technique essentially opens small pores in the cell's membrane, through which molecules can diffuse down concentration gradients. When the pores spontaneously close, the DNA is sealed within the cell's cytoplasm, where it can be transported to the nucleus [58]. This technique can increase the transduction rate over a 1,000-fold compared to direct plasmid injection, and has been utilized to transduce liver, melanoma, skin, and muscle cells [59, 60]. The ideal parameters for cellular transduction appear to vary between tissues. In addition, only short-term gene expression has been achieved. The utilization of this approach for the delivery of osteogenic genes has yet to be defined.

Gene Gun. Another interesting technology which is currently under investigation for transducing cells with foreign DNA is the gene gun. The technique involves the coating of gold particles with plasmid DNA, which are subsequently bombarded into the tissue of interest [61]. Under optimal conditions, the gene gun can be utilized to transduce 10–20% of the cells at the treatment site. Although gene expression of up to 60 days has been achieved, the depth of tissue penetration is limited to <0.5 mm [62]. In addition, low levels of gene expression are generally achieved, which is problematic for BMP gene therapy, where relatively high levels of local BMP expression are required for tissue induction.

Liposomes. Liposomes are commonly used to deliver DNA to cells in vitro [63]. Cationic derivatives of diacylglycerol and cholesterol, lipid derivatives of polyamines, and quaternary ammonium detergents are typically used to form the cationic lipid-DNA complexes. The cationic-lipid compounds serve to decrease the negative changes of the DNA plasmids and facilitate entrance of the plasmids through the cell membrane. Liposome preparations also contain neutral or 'helper' lipids, including cholesterol or dioleoylphosphatidylethanolamine, to improve DNA release from the endosome into the cytoplasm [64]. Liposomes can transduce a wide variety of cells and tissues, including vascular endothelium, lung, brain, and skin [65, 66]. The attachment of cell-specific antibodies to the liposomal membrane may improve tissue specificity of this transduction technique. Intense research efforts are currently directed at improving liposome production and delivery, which may render these vectors ideal for BMP gene delivery in the near future.

Polymer-DNA Complexes. High-molecular-weight cationic polymers, such as poly-*L*-lysine, poly-*L*-ornithine, polyethylenimine, and chitosan, can improve DNA delivery to cells via nonspecific absorptive uptake [67, 68]. Various synthetic polymers can also be utilized to improve cellular transduction rates and can be designed to be biodegradable, thermosensitive, and biocompatible [69]. Polymers can also be constructed with targeting ligands, such as antibodies, transferrin, and asialoglycoprotein to improve tissue specificity. Additional modifications to these molecules can also be made to improve cellular uptake and cytoplasmic trafficking of the therapeutic gene.

Direct BMP Gene Therapy

The promotion of osteogenesis through the direct injection of adenoviral vectors in vivo has been successfully achieved in both immunosuppressed and immune-competent animals [70, 71]. All immune-competent animals tested with BMP adenoviral vectors, to date, have demonstrated evidence of an immune response at the treatment site. The immune response appears to be both humoral and cellular, and is directed against both the injected adenoviral particles and cells transduced by the adenoviral vector. It remains unclear whether there is a major immune response directed against the foreign BMP (i.e. human BMP gene in animal models) expressed using gene therapy techniques. A variety of different BMP adenoviral vectors have been shown to induce bone formation in athymic nude rodents, including Ad-BMP-2, Ad-BMP-4, Ad-BMP-6, Ad-BMP-7 and Ad-BMP-9. In immune-competent rodents, Ad-BMP-6 and Ad-BMP-9 are able to overcome the host immune response and induce significant bone formation. Figure 1 demonstrates the mechanisms involved in osteogenesis using direct BMP gene therapy with an adenoviral vector.

In the paraspinal region, direct injection of adenoviral vectors, including Ad-BMP-2 and Ad-BMP-9, have been shown to induce spinal fusion in athymic nude rodents, without producing central or lateral stenosis caused by exuberant bone formation [71, 72]. The fusion mass completely integrates with the adjacent laminae and spinal processes, without evidence of pseudoarthrosis, suggesting that decortication of cortical bone is not required for bony fusion when BMPs are applied in the paraspinal region. Stereotactically injected BMP vectors into the paraspinal musculature is a compelling approach, since multiple, percutaneous injections could be performed to produce a fusion mass with a predetermined three-dimensional shape and in locations specific for each pathological process. Postprocedural pain would be minimal since the technique would not require muscular dissection. Patients requiring neural decompression could be taken to surgery following successful bony fusion, where extensive laminectomies, facetectomies, and foraminotomies could be performed without leading to spinal instability. Figure 2 demonstrates a posterolateral spinal fusion in the lumbar region of a rabbit using percutaneous, direct gene therapy of a BMP-6 adenoviral vector, demonstrating significant bone formation with excellent union with the host transverse processes.

Ex vivo BMP Gene Therapy

Another approach that is currently being investigated by several research groups is ex vivo gene therapy, a technique in which osteogenic genes are inserted into cells in tissue culture, and the genetically altered cells are subsequently implanted into regions requiring bone formation in experimental animals [73]. The cellular implants express and secrete bone morphogens, which in turn induce the osteogenic response. Lieberman et al. [74, 75] demonstrated that a murine bone marrow stromal cell line, which had been transduced with BMP-2 cDNA using an adenoviral vector, could induce both heterotopic and orthotopic bone formation in severe combined immune-deficient (SCID) mice.

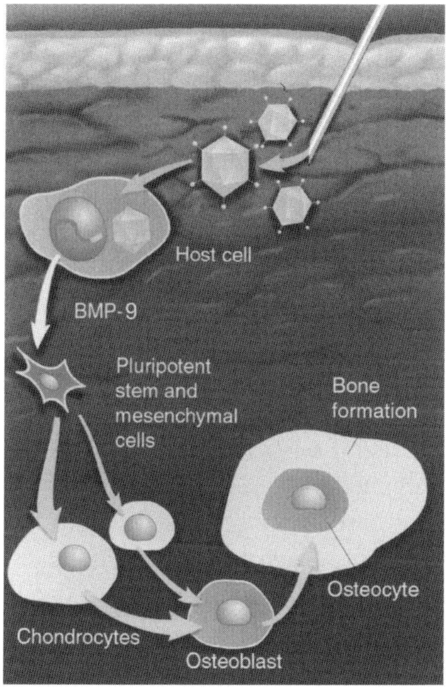

Fig. 1. Diagram showing mechanisms of bone formation using direct, percutaneous injection of an adenoviral vector containing the BMP-9 gene. Expression of BMP-9 by the transduced cells leads to migration, proliferation, and differentiation of MSCs, ultimately leading to successful osteogenesis.

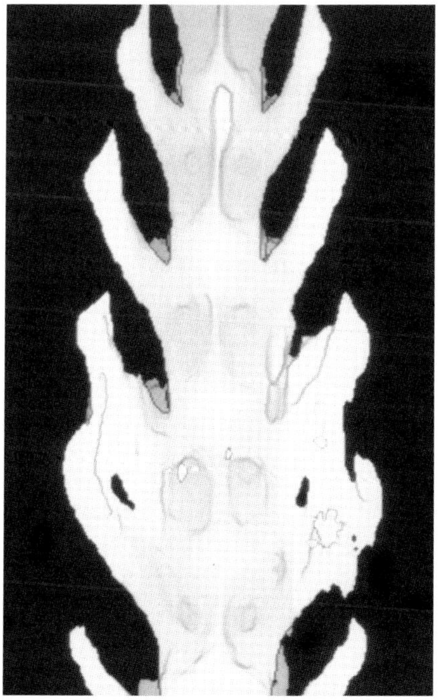

Fig. 2. Three-dimensional CT reconstruction of rabbit lumbar spine treated with bilateral, percutaneous injections of a BMP-6 adenoviral vector using a posterolateral approach, demonstrating significant bone induction and a successful transverse process spinal fusion. The data demonstrates that successful osteogenesis can be achieved in immune-competent rabbits using current gene therapy technologies.

In a similar study, Riew et al. [76] transduced marrow-derived MSCs with the BMP-2 gene and autologously reimplanted the genetically modified cells in the paraspinal region in rabbits. One of the five treated rabbits demonstrated as successful intertransverse process spinal fusion, which was assessed radiographically and histologically. Although only 20% of the treated animals showed significant bone formation, this study clearly demonstrated the potential of ex vivo gene therapy techniques. This group subsequently demonstrated that the rate of bone formation could be increased to 100% in the treated region by implanting the cells 7 days following viral transfection [77].

Musgrave [78] transduced mesenchymal cell populations obtained from human muscle with the BMP-2 gene using an adenoviral vector. The transduced cells were implanted into SCID mice and demonstrated successful ectopic bone formation. Lee et al. [79] inserted the BMP-2 gene into muscle-derived mesenchymal cells in mice and implanted the cells into mouse critical-sized cranial defects. The transduced cells significantly increased the healing rate of defects compared to control cells. In addition, fluorescent in situ hybridization was utilized to demonstrate incorporation of the transduced cells into the induced bone. In another compelling study, Turgeman [80] isolated human MSCs from the bone marrow of normal patients, as well as patients suffering from osteoporosis. The cells were transduced with the BMP-2 gene and subsequently grafted into ectopic and orthotopic locations, leading to successful osteogenesis. Utilizing a retroviral BMP-2 vector, Laurencin et al. [81] demonstrated successful heterotopic bone induction by BMP-2-transduced cells delivered on a PLAGA-HA scaffold in a SCID mouse model. The expression of the human bone morphogenetic protein-7 gene by periosteal-derived rabbit mesenchymal cells has also been shown to induce bone and articular cartilage repair in a rabbit knee osteochondral defect model [82]. In an elegant study, Moutsatsos et al. [83] genetically engineered a murine MSC line to secrete BMP-2 in a regulated fashion. The BMP-2 gene was under control of a doxycycline-responsive promoter, such that the presence of doxycycline in vitro and in vivo would downregulate BMP-2 expression. In vivo implantation of this cell line led to both orthotopic and ectopic bone formation in a regulated fashion, suggesting that long-term regulation of bone induction may be possible.

Our lab has recently demonstrated that human MSCs transduced with the BMP-9 gene can induce robust bone formation in athymic nude animals. In an ectopic model, the implanted cells survive long-term, as assessed by an anti-human mitochondrial stain, and contribute to the cellular composition of the ectopic bone. Local host stem cells at the injection site are also stimulated by the secreted BMP, and differentiate into chondrocytes and osteoblasts at the treatment site. The genetically modified cells were also capable of forming significant bone formation in the paraspinal region following percutaneous injection. The fusion mass integrated completely with the adjacent host spine, similar to the direct BMP adenoviral vector treatment sites, without evidence of posttreatment neural compression (unpubl. data).

In another set of interesting studies, Boden et al. [84, 85] have reported a novel ex vivo gene therapy technique which utilizes the insertion of the osteogenic LMP-1 gene into allogenic bone marrow cells. These investigators demonstrated significant bone formation by the transduced cells in the paraspinal region of rodents, in spite of relatively low transduction rates. LMP-1 gene therapy is unique in that it is thought to induce the secretion of a variety of osteogenic growth factors, which in turn stimulate bone formation.

These ex vivo techniques have the advantage of not only expressing osteogenic morphogens, but also supplying the treated region with bone precursor cells, which may be of limited supply at the treatment site. For example, it is unclear whether pluripotent stem cells are uniformly present throughout the body in the adult human, which could make direct BMP or BMP gene therapy treatments ineffective. Also, the number of MSCs may decrease with age, which might decrease the physiologic activity of BMPs. The introduction of stem cells, which are genetically modified to secrete bone morphogens, is, therefore, a compelling approach. The harvest and expansion of autologous stem cells for widespread human use may be hampered by high costs, cellular contamination, and other technical difficulties. Therefore, other approaches such as the genetic modification of traditional bone grafts (which contain cellular precursors such as stem cells and osteoblasts) at the time of surgery may be a more reasonable near-term approach.

Future Research and Development

Recent studies have clearly demonstrated the potential utility of MSCs and BMP gene therapy for the promotion of bone formation for spinal applications. However, the field of molecular spine surgery is certainly in its infancy. Many of the techniques are under continuing development and may require refinement prior to clinical application. The establishment of an allogenic or xenogeneic source of stem cells, which could be modified to attenuate potential host immune responses, would have significant advantages compared to autologous cells for clinical application. Various groups are currently studying the use of genetically modified porcine cells, which are genetically altered to decrease their expression of foreign antigens. In addition, ex vivo gene therapy approaches are currently being developed to induce local immunosuppression around the transplanted cells. The efficacy of BMP gene therapy might also be improved

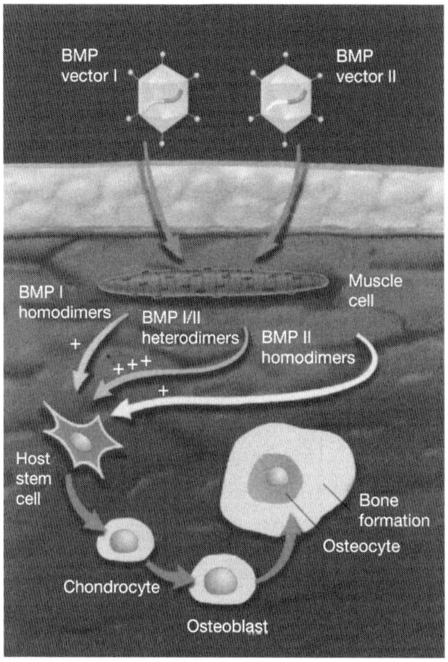

Fig. 3. Diagram demonstrating the local production of potent BMP heterodimers using combinational gene therapy techniques with two BMP adenoviral vectors. Two homodimeric and one heterodimeric species are produced, which may be more effective at promoting bone formation than treatment with a single BMP vector.

by achieving the expression of a cocktail of different growth factors at the treatment site. Several growth factors, including BMP-6 and TGF-β3, have been shown to have synergistic effects on stem cells in vitro. In addition, the generation of potent BMP heterodimers could be produced using a combination of vectors, which may have improved osteogenic effects compared to their respective BMP homodimers alone (fig. 3). Finally, the optimal gene delivery system for osteogenic genes has certainly not been firmly established for human use. Although viral vectors have clearly been the most effective approach in animal studies, their use in humans may be limited by their antigenicity. Therefore, the development of novel nonviral approaches which are able to achieve short-term, high-level transgene expression would be ideal for human use. It is anticipated that many of these issues will be addressed in the near future and that cutting edge tissue engineering technologies can be successfully applied to treat human spine pathology.

Acknowledgment

This work was supported by an NIH grant (1 RO1 AR/AI46488–01A2) and Medtronic-Sofamor Danek; we thank Mona Banton for her editorial support.

References

1 Bruder SP, Kurth AA, Shea M, Hayes WC, Jaiswal N, Kadiyala S: Bone regeneration by implantation of purified, culture-expanded human mesenchymal stem cells. J Orthop Res 1998;16:155–162.
2 Bruder SP, Kraus KH, Goldberg VM, Kadiyala S: The effect of implants loaded with autologous mesenchymal stem cells on the healing of canine segmental bone defects. J Bone Joint Surg Am 1998;80:985–996.
3 Quarto R, Mastrogiacomo M, Cancedda R, Kutepov SM, Mukhachev V, Lavroukov A, Kon E, Marcacci M: Repair of large bone defects with the use of autologous bone marrow stromal cells. N Engl J Med 2001;344:385–386.
4 Celeste AJ, Iannazzi JA, Taylor RC, Hewick RM, Rosen V, Wang EA, Wozney JM: Identification of transforming growth factor beta family members present in bone-inductive protein purified from bovine bone. Proc Natl Acad Sci USA 1990;87:9843–9847.
5 Sampath TK, Reddi AH: Homology of bone-inductive proteins from human, monkey, bovine, and rat extracellular matrix. Proc Natl Acad Sci USA 1983;80:6591–6595.
6 Sampath TK, Nathanson MA, Reddi AH: In vitro transformation of mesenchymal cells derived from embryonic muscle into cartilage in response to extracellular matrix components of bone. Proc Natl Acad Sci USA 1984;81:3419–3423.
7 Wozney JM, Rosen V, Celeste AJ, Mitsock LM, Whitters MJ, Kriz RW, Hewick RM, Wang EA: Novel regulators of bone formation: Molecular clones and activities. Science 1988;242:1528–1534.
8 Urist MR: Bone: Formation by autoinduction. Science 1965;150:893–899.
9 Urist MR, Silverman BF, Buring K, Dubuc FL, Rosenberg JM: The bone induction principle. Clin Orthop 1967;53:243–283.
10 Urist MR, Dowell TA, Hay PH, Strates BS: Inductive substrates for bone formation. Clin Orthop 1968;59:59–96.
11 Urist MR: A morphogenetic matrix for differentiation of bone tissue. Calcif Tissue Res 1970 (suppl):98–101.
12 Urist MR, Strates BS: Bone morphogenetic protein. J Dent Res 1971;50:1392–1406.
13 Urist MR, Sato K, Brownell AG, Malinin TI, Lietze A, Huo YK, Prolo DJ, Oklund S, Finerman GA, DeLange RJ: Human bone morphogenetic protein (hBMP). Proc Soc Exp Biol Med 1983; 173:194–199.
14 Yamaguchi A, Katagiri T, Ikeda T, Wozney JM, Rosen V, Wang EA, Kahn AJ, Suda T, Yoshiki S: Recombinant human bone morphogenetic protein-2 stimulates osteoblastic maturation and inhibits myogenic differentiation in vitro. J Cell Biol 1991;113:681–687.
15 Reddi AH, Wientroub S, Muthukumaran N: Biologic principles of bone induction. Orthop Clin North Am 1987;18:207–212.
16 Helm GA, Li JZ, Alden TD, Hudson SB, Beres EJ, Cunningham M, Mikkelsen MM, Pittman DD, Kerns KM, Kallmes DF: A light and electron microscopic study of ectopic tendon and ligament formation induced by bone morphogenetic protein-13 adenoviral gene therapy. J Neurosurg 2001; 95:298–301.
17 Aspenberg P, Forslund C: Enhanced tendon healing with GDF 5 and 6. Acta Orthop Scand 1999; 70:51–54.
18 Chang SC, Hoang B, Thomas JT, Vukicevic S, Luyten FP, Ryba NJ, Kozak CA, Reddi AH, Moos M Jr: Cartilage-derived morphogenetic proteins. New members of the transforming growth factor-beta superfamily predominantly expressed in long bones during human embryonic development. J Biol Chem 1994;269:28227–28234.
19 Chen P, Carrington JL, Hammonds RG, Reddi AH: Stimulation of chondrogenesis in limb bud mesoderm cells by recombinant human bone morphogenetic protein 2B (BMP-2B) and modulation by transforming growth factor beta 1 and beta 2. Exp Cell Res 1991;195:509–515.
20 Evans CHPD, Robbins PDP: Genetically augmented tissue engineering of the musculoskeletal system. Clin Orthop 1999;367S:S410–S418.
21 Grande DAP, Breitbart ASMD, Mason JP, Paulino CMD, Laser JBS, Schwartz REMD: Cartilage tissue engineering: Current limitations and solutions. Clin Orthop 1999;367S:S176–S185.
22 Kapur SP, Reddi AH: Chondrogenic potential of mesenchymal cells elicited by bone matrix in vitro. Differentiation 1986;32:252–259.

23 Reddi AH: Extracellular bone matrix dependent local induction of cartilage and bone. J Rheumatol Suppl 1983;11:67–69.
24 Sampath TK, Reddi AH: Distribution of bone inductive proteins in mineralized and demineralized extracellular matrix. Biochem Biophys Res Commun 1984;119:949–954.
25 Reddi AH: Bone morphogenetic proteins: An unconventional approach to isolation of first mammalian morphogens. Cytokine Growth Factor Rev 1997;8:11–20.
26 Feng XH, Derynck R: Ligand-independent activation of transforming growth factor (TGF) beta signaling pathways by heteromeric cytoplasmic domains of TGF-beta receptors. J Biol Chem 1996;271:13123–13129.
27 Feng XH, Filvaroff EH, Derynck R: Transforming growth factor-beta (TGF-beta)-induced down-regulation of cyclin A expression requires a functional TGF-beta receptor complex. Characterization of chimeric and truncated type I and type II receptors. J Biol Chem 1995;270: 24237–24245.
28 Chen RH, Moses HL, Maruoka EM, Derynck R, Kawabata M: Phosphorylation-dependent interaction of the cytoplasmic domains of the type I and type II transforming growth factor-beta receptors. J Biol Chem 1995;270:12235–12241.
29 Chen RH, Derynck R: Homomeric interactions between type II transforming growth factor-beta receptors. J Biol Chem 1994;269:22868–22874.
30 Derynck R: TGF-beta-receptor-mediated signaling. Trends Biochem Sci 1994;19:548–553.
31 Lawler S, Candia AF, Ebner R, Shum L, Lopez AR, Moses HL, Wright CV, Derynck R: The murine type II TGF-beta receptor has a coincident embryonic expression and binding preference for TGF-beta 1. Development 1994;120:165–175.
32 Ebner R, Chen RH, Lawler S, Zioncheck T, Derynck R: Determination of type I receptor specificity by the type II receptors for TGF beta or activin. Science 1993;262:900–902.
33 Ebner R, Chen RH, Shum L, Lawler S, Zioncheck TF, Lee A, Lopez AR, Derynck R: Cloning of a type I TGF-beta receptor and its effect on TGF-beta binding to the type II receptor. Science 1993;260:1344–1348.
34 Chen RH, Ebner R, Derynck R: Inactivation of the type II receptor reveals two receptor pathways for the diverse TGF-beta activities. Science 1993;260:1335–1338.
35 Zhang Y, Derynck R: Regulation of Smad signalling by protein associations and signalling crosstalk. Trends Cell Biol 1999;9:274–279.
36 Feng XH, Lin X, Derynck R: Smad2, Smad3 and Smad4 cooperate with Sp1 to induce p15(Ink4B) transcription in response to TGF-beta. EMBO J 2000;19:5178–5193.
37 Derynck R, Zhang Y, Feng XH: Smads: Transcriptional activators of TGF-beta responses. Cell 1998;95:737–740.
38 Derynck R: SMAD proteins and mammalian anatomy. Nature 1998;393:737–739.
39 Lawler S, Feng XH, Chen RH, Maruoka EM, Turck CW, Griswold-Prenner I, Derynck R: The type II transforming growth factor-beta receptor autophosphorylates not only on serine and threonine but also on tyrosine residues. J Biol Chem 1997;272:14850–14859.
40 Filvaroff E, Erlebacher A, Ye J, Gitelman SE, Lotz J, Heillman M, Derynck R: Inhibition of TGF-beta receptor signaling in osteoblasts leads to decreased bone remodeling and increased trabecular bone mass. Development 1999;126:4267–4279.
41 Miller AD: Human gene therapy comes of age. Nature 1992;357:455–460.
42 Trapnell BC, Gorziglia M: Gene therapy using adenoviral vectors. Curr Opin Biotechnol 1994;5: 617–625.
43 Marcel T, Grausz JD: The TMC Worldwide Gene Therapy Enrollment Report, end 1996. Hum Gene Ther 1997;8:775–800.
44 Anderson WF: Gene therapy. Sci Am 1995;273:124–128.
45 Seth P, Willingham MC, Pastan I: Adenovirus-dependent release of ^{51}Cr from KB cells at an acidic pH. J Biol Chem 1984;259:14350–14353.
46 Kramm C, Sena-Esteves M, Barnett FH, et al: Gene therapy for brain tumors. Brain Pathol 1995;5: 345–381.
47 Le Gal La Salle G, Robert JJ, Berrard S, Ridoux V, Stratford-Perricaudet LD, Perricaudet M, Mallet J: An adenovirus vector for gene transfer into neurons and glia in the brain. Science 1993; 259:988–990.

48 Fisher KJ, Jooss K, Alston J, Yang Y, Haecker SE, High K, Pathak R, Raper SE, Wilson JM: Recombinant adeno-associated virus for muscle directed gene therapy. Nat Med 1997;3: 306–312.
49 Culver KW: Gene therapy for malignant neoplasms of the CNS. Bone Marrow Transplant 1996; 18(suppl 3):S6–S9.
50 Coffin RS, Howard MK, Cumming DV, Dollery CM, McEwan J, Yellon DM, Marber MS, MacLean AR, Brown SM, Latchman DS: Gene delivery to the heart in vivo and to cardiac myocytes and vascular smooth muscle cells in vitro using herpes virus vectors. Gene Ther 1996;3: 560–566.
51 Wolff JA: Direct gene transfer into mouse muscle in vivo. Science 1990;247:1465–1468.
52 Nomura T: Gene expression and antitumor effects following direct interferon (IFN)-gamma gene transfer with naked plasmid DNA and DC-chol liposome complexes in mice. Gene Ther 1999;6: 121–129.
53 Ardehali A: Direct gene transfer into donor hearts at the time of harvest. J Thorac Cardiovasc Surg 1995;109:716–720.
54 Schwartz B: Gene transfer by naked DNA into adult mouse brain. Protein Sci 1996;5:488–494.
55 Sikes ML: In vivo gene transfer into rabbit thyroid follicular cells by direct DNA injection. Hum Gene Ther 1994;5:837–844.
56 Davis HL: Direct gene transfer into skeletal muscle in vivo: Factors affecting efficiency of transfer and stability of expression. Hum Gene Ther 1993;4:151–159.
57 Zhang G: High levels of foreign gene expression in hepatocytes after tail vein injections of naked plasmid DNA. Hum Gene Ther 1999;10:1735–1737.
58 Mir LM: Introduction of definite amounts of nonpermeant molecules into living cells after electropermeabilization: Direct access to the cytosol. Exp Cell Res 1988;175:15–25.
59 Titomirov AV: In vivo electroporation and stable transformation of skin cells of newborn mice by plasmid DNA. Biochim Biophys Acta 1991;1088:131–134.
60 Aihara H, Miyazaki J: Gene transfer into muscle by electroporation in vivo. Nat Biotechnol 1998; 16:867–870.
61 Yang NS: In vivo and in vitro gene transfer to mammalian somatic cells by particle bombardment. Proc Natl Acad Sci USA 1990;87:9568–9572.
62 Zelenin AV: Bacterial beta-galactosidase and human dystrophin genes are expressed in mouse skeletal muscle fibers after ballistic transfection. FEBS Lett 1997;414:319–322.
63 Felgner PL: Lipofection: A highly efficient, lipid-mediated DNA-transfection procedure. Proc Natl Acad Sci USA 1987;84:7413–7417.
64 Farhood H: The role of dioleoyl phosphatidylethanolamine in cationic liposome mediated gene transfer. Biochim Biophys Acta 1995;1235:289–295.
65 Ono T: Plasmid DNAs directly injected into mouse brain with lipofectin can be incorporated and expressed by brain cells. Neurosci Lett 1990;117:259–263.
66 Raz E: Intradermal gene immunization: The possible role of DNA uptake in the induction of cellular immunity to viruses. Proc Natl Acad Sci USA 1994;91:9519–9523.
67 Nishikawa M: Nonviral vectors in the new millennium: Delivery barriers in gene transfer. Hum Gene Ther 2001;12:861–870.
68 Boussif O: A versatile vector for gene and oligonucleotide transfer into cells in culture and in vivo: Polyethylenimine. Proc Natl Acad Sci USA 1995;92:7297–7301.
69 Maheshwari A: Soluble biodegradable polymer-based cytokine gene delivery for cancer treatment. Mol Ther 2000;2:121–130.
70 Varady P, Li JZ, Cunningham M, Beres EJ, Das S, Engh J, Alden TD, Pittman DD, Kerns KM, Kallmes DF, Helm GA: Morphologic analysis of BMP-9 gene therapy-induced osteogenesis. Hum Gene Ther 2001;12:697–710.
71 Alden TD, Pittman DD, Beres EJ, Hankins GR, Kallmes DF, Wisotsky BM, Kerns KM, Helm GA: Percutaneous spinal fusion using bone morphogenetic protein-2 gene therapy. J Neurosurg 1999; 90:109–114.
72 Helm GA, Alden TD, Beres EJ, Hudson SB, Das S, Engh JA, Pittman DD, Kerns KM, Kallmes DF: Use of bone morphogenetic protein-9 gene therapy to induce spinal arthrodesis in the rodent. J Neurosurg 2000;92:191–196.

73 Gazit D, Turgeman G, Kelley P, Wang E, Jalenak M, Zilberman Y, Moutsatsos I: Engineered pluripotent mesenchymal cells integrate and differentiate in regenerating bone: A novel cell-mediated gene therapy. J Gene Med 1999;1:121–133.
74 Lieberman JR, Le LQ, Wu L, Finerman GA, Berk A, Witte ON, Stevenson S: Regional gene therapy with a BMP-2-producing murine stromal cell line induces heterotopic and orthotopic bone formation in rodents. J Orthop Res 1998;16:330–339.
75 Lieberman JR, Daluiski A, Stevenson S, Wu L, McAllister P, Lee YP, Kabo JM, Finerman GA, Berk AJ, Witte ON: The effect of regional gene therapy with bone morphogenetic protein-2-producing bone-marrow cells on the repair of segmental femoral defects in rats. J Bone Joint Surg Am 1999;81:905–917.
76 Riew KD, Wright NM, Cheng S, Avioli LV, Lou J: Induction of bone formation using a recombinant adenoviral vector carrying the human BMP-2 gene in a rabbit spinal fusion model. Calcif Tissue Int 1998;63:357–360.
77 Cheng SL, Lou J, Wright NM, Lai CF, Avioli LV, Riew KD: In vitro and in vivo induction of bone formation using a recombinant adenoviral vector carrying the human BMP-2 gene. Calcif Tissue Int 2001;68:87–94.
78 Musgrave DS: Human skeletal muscle cells in ex vivo gene therapy to deliver bone morphogenetic protein-2. J Bone Joint Surg Br 2002;84:120–127.
79 Lee JYMD, Musgrave DMD, Pelinkovic DMD, Fukushima KMDP, Cummins JB, Usas AMD, Robbins PP, Fu FHMD, Huard JP: Effect of bone morphogenetic protein-2-expressing muscle-derived cells on healing of critical-sized bone defects in mice. J Bone Joint Surg Am 2001;83-A: 1032–1039.
80 Turgeman G: Engineered human mesenchymal stem cells: A novel platform for skeletal cell mediated gene therapy. J Gene Med 2001,3.240–251.
81 Laurencin CT: Poly(lactide-co-glycolide)/hydroxyapatite delivery of BMP-2-producing cells: A regional gene therapy approach to bone regeneration. Biomaterials 2001;22:1271–1277.
82 Mason JM, Breitbart AS, Barcia M, Porti D, Pergolizzi RG, Grande DA: Cartilage and bone regeneration using gene-enhanced tissue engineering. Clin Orthop 2000;379(suppl):S171–S178.
83 Moutsatsos IK, Turgeman G, Zhou S, Kurkalli BG, Pelled G, Tzur L, Kelley P, Stumm N, Mi S, Muller R, Zilberman Y, Gazit D: Exogenously regulated stem cell-mediated gene therapy for bone regeneration. Mol Ther 2001;3:449–461.
84 Boden SD, Titus L, Hair G, Liu Y, Viggeswarapu M, Nanes MS, Baranowski C: Lumbar spine fusion by local gene therapy with a cDNA encoding a novel osteoinductive protein (LMP-1). Spine 1998;23:2486–2492.
85 Boden SD, Liu Y, Hair GA, Helms JA, Hu D, Racine M, Nanes MS, Titus L: LMP-1, a LIM-domain protein, mediates BMP-6 effects on bone formation. Endocrinology 1998;139: 5125–5134.

Gregory A. Helm, MD, PhD
Department of Neurosurgery, University of Virginia Health System
PO Box 800212, Charlottesville, VA 22908 (USA)
Tel. +1 434 924 1642, Fax +1 434 924 2994, E-Mail gah9r@virginia.edu

Haid RW Jr, Subach BR, Rodts GE Jr (eds): Advances in Spinal Stabilization.
Prog Neurol Surg. Basel, Karger, 2003, vol 16, pp 29–38

Bone Substitutes

Karin R. Swartz, Gregory R. Trost

University of Wisconsin-Madison, Madison, Wisc., USA

There has long been a need to minimize the morbidity associated with spinal fusions. Bone substitutes are the most recent focus of this process, in an attempt to minimize the morbidities of donor site harvesting without compromising fusion. Autograft bone, consisting primarily of cancellous and some cortical bone, is the current standard for spinal fusion constructs. However, harvesting autograft usually requires a second incision and involves a risk of associated morbidities, such as infection, blood loss, hematoma formation, neurologic and vascular damage, pain, joint destabilization, and fractures. Furthermore there is a limit to the size, shape, and volumes of harvested autograft. Methods for strengthening the spine and improving nonunion/delayed healing rates are actively being pursued.

The ideal graft should be biocompatible, osteoinductive, and resorbable. This allows for incorporation with the surrounding tissues, including vascularization [1, 2]. An ideal graft should be malleable, but once in vivo, should not flow out of the graft bed [3]. It must restore the spine to its functional state [2] with pain relief [4], allowing for decreased disability. Furthermore, an ideal graft must be sterile, to abolish the risk of disease transmission. Finally, it should be easy to use and cost-effective.

Physiology

Bone development occurs via several processes, specifically osteogenesis, osteoinduction, and osteoconduction [2]. Osteogenesis is the creation of bone, primarily occurring through the bone-building capabilities of osteoblasts, the deposition by osteoblasts of rigid extracellular matrix (ECM), and the eventual mineralization of the ECM into bone. The osteoblastic activity is normally balanced by the bone-resorbing function of osteoclasts, which also allows for remodeling. Bone remodeling, a balance between bone formation (osteoblastic) and bone resorption (osteoclastic) functions, is important for skeletal growth as well as maintenance of normal bone structure. Various growth factors (GFs) have been implicated in the function of maintaining/healing bone, including transforming growth factor-β (TGF-β), platelet-derived growth factor, insulin-like growth factors, fibroblast growth factors, and bone morphogenetic proteins (BMPs) [3].

Osteoinduction involves active recruitment of mesenchymal stem cells and facilitation of their differentiation along the osteoblastic lineage [2]. Osteoinduction more commonly occurs in cancellous more so than cortical bone, and appears to be under the control of BMPs, as opposed to the other GFs, which are not osteoinductive. Osteoconduction, which involves the ingrowth of cells to create and support a stable bony environment, is likewise achieved more readily through cancellous than cortical bone.

Bone Allograft

Cadaveric sources of bone graft are available autograft substitutes that have undergone sterilization and processing. Tissue processing can weaken the cadaveric bone graft and affect healing properties. Furthermore, despite processing, there is a small but recognized concern over the possibility of disease transmission. Grafts are typically a combination of both cancellous and cortical bone – cancellous for its osteoinductive and osteoconductive properties, cortical for its load-bearing capacity. Allografts come in many different sizes and shapes. As the number of procedures using allograft continues to rise, the availability will become limited, thus prompting searches for alternatives.

Alternatives to bone banking involve products of tissue engineering, consisting of natural or synthetic scaffolds with GFs, and of GF therapeutic techniques that involve direct implantation of cytokines, transduction of genes encoding cytokines with osteogenic capability, or of transplantation of cultured osteogenic cells [5].

Tissue Engineering

Tissue engineering applications are potential approaches for the future of bone repair strategies. These applications rely on GFs for development of new tissue through chemotaxis, proliferation, differentiation, and new tissue formation [3]. The development of carriers, delivery systems, and specific GFs is underway.

Table 1. Commercially available substitutes [adapted from 2]

OrthoBlast™	Heat-sensitive copolymer with cancellous bone chips and DBM, available as injectable paste or putty; osteoconductive, bioresorbable, limited osteoinduction
DynaGraft®	Heat-sensitive copolymer with DBM, available as injectable gel, matrix, or putty; osteoconductive, bioresorbable, limited osteoinduction
ProOsteon®	Coral HA composite; available in granular or block form; osteoconductive and bioresorbable
Grafton®	DBM combined with glycerol, available as gel; osteoconductive, bioresorbable, limited osteoinduction
OSTEOSET®	Surgical grade calcium sulfate; available as various-sized pellets; osteoconductive, bioresorbable
AlloMatrix™	DBM with surgical grade calcium sulfate powder; available as injectable or formable putty; osteoconductive, bioresorbable, limited osteoinduction
*Colla*graft™	Mixture of HA, tricalcium phosphate, and bovine collagen; available as strip configurations; osteoconductive, bioresorbable, limited osteoinduction when mixed with bone marrow
Vitoss	Surgical grade tricalcium phosphate; available as blocks or morsels; osteoinductive, bioresorbable

DBM = Demineralized bone matrix; HA = hydroxyapatite.

Carriers

Carrier substances can be divided into four major categories: inorganic materials (bioglasses and ceramics), synthetic polymers (especially polymethylmethacrylate), natural polymers (primarily collagen), and composites (various) (table 1) [3]. Collagen combined with hydroxyapatite is one of the most widely used first-generation composite carriers, which is both flexible and able to bond directly with bone [3]. As scaffolds, carriers must act as permissive environments for osteoconduction to be successful [3] (table 2).

Hyaff-11

Hyaff-11 is a new semisynthetic biopolymer that can be fabricated into porous scaffolds for tissue reconstruction. It is a benzyl ester derivative of the polysaccharide hyaluronic acid, a natural component of the ECM. Hyaluronic acid plays a role in proteoglycan organization, cell differentiation, and wound healing. It has well-established biocompatibility, and is biodegradable in 8–12 weeks in vivo [6]. In a study by Kim and Valenti [6], Hyaff-11 was used as scaffolding for the delivery of rhBMP-2, and showed low constitutive levels of release of BMP-2, with good retention of the morphogenetic protein at the site, with success based on the resultant increased expression of osteoblasts with bone formation.

Table 2. Pros and cons of carrier substances [adapted from 3]

Substance	Inorganic materials	Synthetic polymers	Natural polymers	Composites
Pros	Similar structureto bone Resorbable or nonresorbable Affinity for BMPs	Reproducible manufacture Readily tailored Controlled release Ease of sterilization	Excellent biocompatibility May have natural affinity for GFs	Benefits from different materials exploited
Cons	Brittle/difficult to mold May be exothermic	Breakdown products might be inflammatory Solvents or cross-linkers might denature proteins Nonphysiologic material	Pathogen transmission Sterilization Potential immunogenicity	Complex manufacture
Examples	Porous coralline HA B-tricalcium phosphates (B-TCP) Hyaluronic acid Calcium phosphate cements Metals Calcium sulfates	Poly (α-hydroxy acid) Polypropylene fumarate Polyanhydrides Polyphosphazenes Polozamers	Fibrin glue Collagen (type I) Chitosan Hyaluronic acid Gelatin DBM	Collagen-TCP Collagen-HA TCP-cellulose

HA = Hydroxyapatite; DBM = demineralized bone matrix.

PLA-DX-PEG

Saito et al. [5] developed a biodegradable synthetic polymer to deliver BMP-2. PLA-DX-PEG (poly-*D*,*L*-lactic acid-*p*-dioxanone-polyethylene glycol) is available as a block copolymer that is biocompatible and biodegradable. It offers an alternative to bone banking with no disease transmission, no evidence of immunoreaction or foreign body reaction, and is more effective than collagen-BMP-2 systems in regard to calcium content of formed ossicles. Also, it swells a little when in contact with water and thus fills the dead space at the bone-implant interface and provides a layer of scaffolding for new bone [5].

Polymethylmethacrylate

Polymethylmethacrylate is the only available cement with reports of clinical application and experience for vertebroplasty in the treatment of osteoporosis [1].

Polyetheretherketone

Polyetheretherketone (PEEK) is a radiolucent, biocompatible synthetic polymer that purports similar stiffness to cortical bone. It is a polyaromatic semicrystalline thermoplastic which is available as a cage (Stryker Solis®) or in a pellet form for injection molding or machined cage (Invibio™ PEEK-OPTIMA®). When in cage form, it can be packed with either auto- or allograft to facilitate fusion.

Poly(*L*-Lactic Acid)

Poly(*L*-lactic acid) cages are radiolucent bioabsorbable cages that demonstrate higher elasticity and thus less stiffness than metal cages. They have been proven mechanically sufficient and resorb after providing support for an average of 6 months [7].

Demineralized bone matrix products (ex: Osteofil™) are other osteoinductive graft substitutes. No current objective clinical data [8] is available.

Delivery Systems

Techniques for application of GFs are many, with the most commonly cited described next: (1) delivery of DNA encoding a GF or in vivo gene therapy, (2) delivery of a cell to produce the GF or ex vivo gene therapy also called cell therapy, and (3) delivery of the protein itself via some carrier matrix [3].

The latter of these has advanced the furthest, with ongoing attempts to discover optimal carriers for GFs. These carriers would allow controlled release (appropriate kinetics) with therapeutic dosing and would act as sturdy scaffolds [3], thus encouraging cells to migrate and differentiate (osteoconduction and osteoinduction), as well as allow ingrowth of blood vessels, passage of nutrients, and expulsion of waste products [3]. Degradation and breakdown of the carrier matrix should either be inert or beneficial to healing, and should be synchronized with the rate of bone regeneration: too slow, and bone growth/remodeling is retarded and carries a risk of encapsulation, and too fast, and the definition of optimal shape may be lost [3].

Gene therapy, in its most generic terms, can be divided into in vivo or ex vivo techniques to deliver a gene sequence for the osteoinductive factor (rather than the factor itself) [9]. Both involve insertion of foreign cDNA directly into a host (in vivo) or into donor cells (ex vivo) via a vector, ultimately forming cells whose primary purpose is to produce a desired GF [3]. In the in vivo model, also known as in situ therapy, a vector is directly introduced into host cells inside the body, the vector acting as the carrier. In the ex vivo model, also known as cell therapy, the cells can either be harvested from the patient or another donor; that cell then becomes the carrier for the secreted GF (using tissue culture expansion and gene transduction), and then is delivered into the host [3, 10]. The success of gene therapy relies on accurate transduction, transcription, translation, and expression (table 3).

Table 3. Pros and cons of gene therapy techniques

	Pros	Cons
Ex vivo	No viral particle transmission No DNA complexes Higher efficiency of transduction	More technically demanding Cost
In vivo	Easier No harvesting Potentially lower cost	Difficult targeting specific cells Transduction efficiency Vector diffusion from site Host response to viral proteins

Growth Factors

The current trend in osteoinductive bone graft substitutes for minimally invasive spine fusions includes providing GF cytokines in addition to the scaffolding of the carriers. Categories of factors used in these substitutes include purified bone GFs, recombinant bone GFs, and gene therapy-delivered GFs. The working current hypothesis is that a burst followed by sustained factor release is ideal, allowing for cellular migration to the area, with eventual commitment to osteoblastic lineages with propagation of cellular numbers [3]. An example of a GF invested as an osteoinductive bone graft is BMP.

Bone Morphogenetic Proteins

BMPs have been proposed to revolutionize bone surgery. BMPs are members of the TGF-β family, which guides the differentiation of stem cells down specific lineages (i.e., bone, cartilage) [6, 8, 11–17]. Urist [18] initially discovered that devitalized bone could induce ectopic bone in rodents, and then went on to isolate the protein from demineralized bone matrix; others went on to clone these bone-inducing substances, and currently over forty have been identified [19]. They act locally, and thus must be delivered directly to the site needed. BMPs trigger osteoblastic differentiation of marrow mesenchymal stem cells, preosteoblasts, and undifferentiated mesenchymal cells [6, 8, 11–17].

BMP-2 is the most widely studied, and is one of the most potent osteoinductive of the BMPs [6, 8, 11–14, 16, 18, 20, 21]. Other chondrogenic/potentially osteogenic morphogenetic proteins include BMP-4 [13], BMP-6 [17], BMP-7 (aka osteogenic protein-1, OP-1) [15], and BMP-9 [11]. BMPs have many roles besides osteogenesis: BMP-4 has been implicated as proapoptotic in somatic development [22], BMP-9 in fetal and adult liver function [23] as well as in CNS development [24], BMP-2, BMP-7 and BMP-4 in CNS development [25], and BMP-4 and BMP-7 in lung development [26].

Sustained production of high levels of activated BMP-2 using recombinant adenovirus type 5 (Ad5BMP-2) has been achieved by Olmsted et al. [14]. In their research, they were able to elicit BMP synthesis upon infection even by non-osteoprogenitor cells, which was 3-fold more active than equivalent concentrations of rhBMP-2 [14].

The issue of physical containment of BMP still needs to be optimized, such that it remains in place, without causing unwanted bone growth that could potentially cause neurovascular compromise.

Preclinical Data

Animal models, especially small animals, have shown success with treatment of fractures and segmental defects [3]; Murata et al. [27] showed successful rapid bone growth from an onlay over bone without periosteum, using rhBMP-2 and bioabsorbable atelocollagen in rats. Ripamonti et al. [28] used BMP-7 (OP-1) to grow bone over a cranial defect in baboons. Boden [29] developed a rabbit model to characterize the healing process, and sequenced a novel cDNA encoding for LMP-1 (LIM-mineralizing protein-1, an intracellular protein which induces osteoblastic differentiation); when implanted locally in the bone marrow transfected with LMP-1 cDNA, he reported 100% fusion. Majumdar et al. [11, 30] isolated multipotential mesenchymal cells from the bone marrow and cultured them in the presence of TGF-β3 and recombinant human BMPs (rhBMP-2 and rhBMP-9) causing chondrogenic differentiation, a technique that could allow for delivery of chondrogenic GFs to the site of articular cartilage repair. Noshi et al. [16] further advanced the bone-forming capability of a composite using marrow mesenchymal stem cells and porous hydroxyapatite by adding rhBMP-2 to the composite, which resulted in accelerated bone formation.

Clinical Trials

Boden et al. [20] were the first to demonstrate the clinical efficacy of rhBMP-2 for single-level spinal arthrodesis, comparing tapered titanium fusion cages packed with either rhBMP-2 (1.5 mg/ml) soaked onto bovine collagen sponge or with morselized iliac autograft. Success was based on shorter hospital stays, shorter operative time, less blood loss, and improved fusion in the cage-BMP construct.

Sandhu [8] performed anterior lumbar interbody fusions using combined threaded titanium cages filled with autograft and compared with cages filled with rhBMP-2, and found the cages filled with rhBMP-2 had better outcomes, including high fusion rates, shorter operative time, and shorter hospital stays.

Table 4. Comparisons of autograft, allograft, and substitutes

Bone graft	Structure/ strength	Osteoconduction	Osteoinduction	Osteogenesis	Price
Autograft					
Cancellous	No	+++	+++	+++	
Cortical	+++	++	++	++	
Allograft					
Cancellous					
Frozen	No	++	+	No	
Freeze-dry	No	++	+	No	
Cortical					
Frozen	+++	+	No	No	
Freeze-dry	+	+	No	No	
Substitutes					
OrthoBlast™	No	++	+	No	10 cm^3: USD 850/
DynaGraft®	No	++	+	No	5 cm^3 USD 470
ProOsteon® 500R	?	++	No	No	10 cm^3: USD 850/
Grafton®	No	++	+	No	5 cm^3 USD 470
OSTEOSET®	No	++	No	No	10 cm^3: USD 1,150
AlloMatrix™	No	++	+	No	6 strips: USD 1,109/
*Colla*graft™	No	++	+	No	3 strips: USD 683
Vitoss	No	++	No	No	10 cm^3: USD 525

Friedlaender et al. [15] evaluated rhOP-1 (BMP-7), comparing clinical and radiographic results in the treatment of tibial nonunion in a controlled, prospective, randomized, and partially blinded clinical trial. They inserted intramedullary rods packed with either rhOP-1 in a type I collagen carrier or with fresh bone autograft. They determined there were no statistically significant differences in the results at 9 months, with 81 and 85% clinical success (respective) and 75 and 84% radiographic success (respective). Interestingly, postoperative osteomyelitis rates at the nonunion site were greater in the autograft group (21% in autograft patients, 3% in OP-1 patients).

Other Issues

Different anatomical sites may require different substitutes. Special consideration must be given to variables of the involved kinetics with different locations, the effects of medications, the impact of disease processes, and of aging on the efficacy of function [2, 3, 6].

Objective measures determining utility of any bone-stabilizing product must certainly include cost containment issues centered around operating room functions, including time required for the procedure, duration of needed anesthesia, supplies used/needed, and length of stay in recovery and in hospital (table 4).

As always, success of fusion depends on many factors, but is maximized by the basic tenets of properly prepared sites, exposed cancellous bone, mechanical loading and stability.

References

1 Heini PF, Berlemann U: Bone substitutes in vertebroplasty. Eur Spine J 2001;10:S205–S213.

2 Greenwald AS, Boden SD, Goldberg VM, Khan Y, Laurencin CT, Rosier RN, for the Committee on Biological Implants: Bone-graft substitutes: Facts, fictions, and applications. J Bone Joint Surg Am 2001;83:S98–S103.

3 Li RH, Wozney JM: Delivering on the promise of bone morphogenetic proteins. Trends Biotechnol 2001;19:255–265.

4 Jackson DW, Scheer MJ, Simon TM: Cartilage substitutes: Overview of basic science and treatment options. J Am Acad Orthop Surg 2001;9/1:37–52.

5 Saito N, Okada T, Horiuchi H, Murakami N, Takahashi J, Nawata M, Ota H, Nozaki K, Takaoka K: A biodegradable polymer as a cytokine delivery system for inducing bone formation. Nat Biotechnol 2001;19:332–335.

6 Kim HD, Valenti RF: Retention and activity of BMP-2 in hyaluronic acid-based scaffolds in vitro. J Biomed Mater Res 2002;59:573–584.

7 Van Dijk M, Smit TH, Sugihara S, Burger EH, Wuisman PI: The effect of cage stiffness on the rate of lumbar interbody fusion. Spine 2002;27:682–688.

8 Sandhu HS: Anterior lumbar interbody fusion with osteoinductive growth factors. Clin Orthop 2000;371:56–60.

9 Boden SD, Hair GA, Viggeswarapu M, Liu Y, Titus L: Gene therapy for spine fusion. Clin Orthop 2000;379S:S225–S233.

10 Oakes DA, Lieberman JR: Osteoinductive applications of regional gene therapy: Ex vivo gene transfer. Clin Orthop 2000;379S:S101–S112.

11 Majumdar MK, Wang E, Morris EA: BMP-2 and BMP-9 promote chondrogenic differentiation of human multipotential mesenchymal cells and overcome the inhibitory effects of IL-1. J Cell Physiol 2001;189:275–284.

12 Kingsley DM: What do BMPs do in mammals? Clues from the mouse short-ear mutation. Trends Genet 1994;10:16–21.

13 Akiyama H, Shukunami C, Nakamura T, Hiraki Y: Differential expressions of BMP family genes during chondrogenic differentiation in mouse ATDC5 cells. Cell Struct Funct 2000;25:195–204.

14 Olmsted EA, Blum JS, Rill D, Yotnda P, Gugala Z, Lindsey RW, Davis AR: Adenovirus-mediated BMP2 expression in human bone marrow stromal cells. J Cell Biochem 2001;82:11–21.

15 Friedlaender GE, Perry CR, Cole JD, Cook SD, Cierny G, Muschler GF, Zych GA, Calhoun JH, LaForte AJ, Yin S: Osteogenic protein-1 (bone morphogenetic protein-7) in the treatment of tibial nonunions. J Bone Joint Surg Am 2001;83:S151–S158.

16 Noshi T, Yoshikawa T, Dohi Y, Ikeuchi M, Horiuchi K, Ichijima K, Sugimura M, Yonemasu K, Ohgushi H: Recombinant human bone morphogenetic-2 potentiates the in vivo osteogenic ability of marrow/hydroxyapatite composites. Artif Organs 2001;25:201–208.

17 Boskey AL, Paschalis EP, Binderman I, Doty SB: BMP-6 accelerates both chondrogenesis and mineral maturation in differentiating chick limb-bud mesenchymal cell cultures. J Cell Biochem 2002;84:509–519.

18 Urist MR: Bone: Formation by autoinduction. Science 1965;150:893–899.

19 Wang EA, Rosen V, Cordes P, Hewick RM, Kriz MF, Luxenberg DP, Sibley BS, Wozney JM: Purification and characterization of other distinct bone-inducing factors. Proc Natl Acad Sci USA 1988;85:9484–9488.

20 Boden SD, Zdeblick TA, Sandhu HS, Heim SE: The use of rhBMP-2 in interbody fusion cages: Definitive evidence of osteoinduction in humans: A preliminary report. Spine 2000;25: 376–381.

21 Subach BR, Haid RW, Rodts GE, Kaiser MG: Bone morphogenetic protein in spinal fusion: Overview and clinical update. Neurosurg Focus 2001;10/4:1–6.
22 Sanders EJ, Parker E: Ablation of axial structures activates apoptotic pathways in somite cells of the chick embryo. Anat Embryol 2001;204:389–398.
23 Miller AF, Harvey SA, Thies RS, Olson MS: Bone morphogenetic protein-9. An autocrine/paracrine cytokine in the liver. J Biol Chem 2000;275:17937–17945.
24 Lopez-Coviella I, Berse B, Krauss R, Thies RS, Blusztajn JK: Induction and maintenance of the neuronal cholinergic phenotype in the CNS by BMP-9. Science 2000;289:313–316.
25 Jordan J, Bottner M, Schluesener HJ, Unsicker K, Krieglstein K: Bone morphogenetic proteins: Neurotrophic roles for midbrain dopaminergic neurons and implications of astroglial cells. Eur J Neurosci 1997;9:1699–1709.
26 De Caestecker M, Meyrick B: Bone morphogenetic proteins, genetics, and the pathophysiology of primary pulmonary hypertension. Respir Res 2001;2/4:193–197.
27 Murata M, Maki F, Sato D, Shibata T, Arisue M: Bone augmentation by onlay implant using recombinant human BMP-2 and collagen on adult rat skull without periosteum. Clin Oral Impl Res 2000;11:289–295.
28 Ripamonti U, van den Heever B, Sampath TK, Tucker MM, Rueger DC, Redoli AH: Complete regeneration of bone in the baboon by recombinant human osteogenic protein-1 (hOP-1, bone morphogenetic protein-7). Growth Factors 1996;13:273–289.
29 Boden SD: Biology of lumbar spine fusion and use of bone graft substitutes: Present, future, and next generation. Tissue Eng 2000;6:383–399.
30 Majumdar MK, Banks V, Peluso DP, Morris EA: Isolation, characterization, and chondrogenic potential of human bone marrow-derived multipotential stromal cells. J Cell Physiol 2000;185: 98–106.

Gregory R. Trost, MD
Department of Neurological Surgery
University of Wisconsin-Madison
600 Highland Ave, Madison, WI 53792-3232 (USA)
Tel. +1 608 263 1410, E-Mail trost@neurosurg.wisc.edu

Haid RW Jr, Subach BR, Rodts GE Jr (eds): Advances in Spinal Stabilization.
Prog Neurol Surg. Basel, Karger, 2003, vol 16, pp 39–54

Resorbable Technology for Spinal Stabilization

Daniel K. Resnick[a], *Joseph T. Alexander*[b], *William C. Welch*[c]

[a] Department of Neurological Surgery, University of Wisconsin, K4/834 Clinical Science Center, Madison, Wisc.,
[b] Department of Neurological Surgery, Wake Forest University, Winston-Salem, N.C., and
[c] Department of Neurological Surgery, University of Pittsburgh, Pittsburgh, Pa., USA

Incredible advances in the surgeon's ability to restore stability to the unstable spine have been made in the last decade. Using metal implants, surgeons can now effectively stabilize any motion segment of the spine. With the concomitant use of autograft or allograft bone, high fusion rates can be achieved in the vast majority of cases. There are, however, drawbacks to the use of such systems.

Autograft bone is not always available for a given application and autograft harvest is associated with nontrivial morbidity in a substantial fraction of patients [1]. The use of allograft bone is associated with lower fusion rates than autograft bone in most cases. The use of allograft is often limited by both cost and availability. Machining of allograft bone to predetermined shapes is a technology- and labor-intensive process, and processing of the bone for infection control and mechanical consistency is expensive. Finally, the use of metallic implants is associated with late complications related to implant failure, erosion into soft tissue structures, and degradation of the bone/implant interface.

In response to these drawbacks, several companies have developed resorbable biomaterials that can serve as temporary fixation devices, structural supports, and osteoconductive or even osteoinductive conduits for new bone growth. These products offer the potential advantages of unlimited supply, significant cost savings, and a reduction in patient morbidity. This chapter is intended to serve as an overview of some of these new biomaterials and their potential applications. This overview will be incomplete, as the pace of new development in this field is staggering. Many of the substances and devices presented are not FDA approved or are FDA approved for uses outside of the spine. The reader is cautioned to review the FDA-approved indications for the use of any of the described products prior to the experimental or therapeutic use of any of the products described.

Resorbable Synthetic Bone Substitutes

Autograft bone remains the gold standard for spinal fusion procedures, especially lumbar posterolateral fusion. Autograft bone is osteogenic, in that it contains the cellular components responsible for new bone formation. Autograft is osteoinductive, in that it contains diffusible proteins which induce neighboring cells to produce bone. Autograft is also osteoconductive, in that it has a structure which allows for the migration of osteogenic cells which can then form new bone [2]. Depending upon the size, shape, and source of the autograft, mechanical strength may be negligible (cancellous) or substantial (tricortical iliac crest, fibula, rib). Drawbacks to the use of autograft include harvest site morbidity as well as limited availability. The use of allograft bone avoids the problem of graft site morbidity, and allograft humeral, femoral, and patellar grafts are available for use as large load-bearing struts. Allograft bone is osteoconductive, and in some preparations may be somewhat osteoinductive (such as in demineralized bone matrix). Unfortunately, allograft bone is not always readily available. Allograft is expensive to preshape into readily used sizes. Finally, some patients may refuse the use of allograft for religious reasons or because of fear of infection.

Although there are many alternatively prepared allograft products (Grafton™, Dynagraft™, Osteofil™) and xenograft products (Collagraft™, True Bone Ceramics™) available for use which may extend the utility of allograft use, the manufacture of these products still requires the use of processed donor (human or animal) bone. In some cases, the extensive preparation of these products has resulted in unexpected toxicity. For example, Botsman et al. [3] and Wang et al. [4] recently presented evidence to suggest that the glycerol carrier in Grafton (Osteotech, Eatontown, N.J., USA) may be toxic in large doses. This discussion will center on synthetic resorbable bone substitutes.

The use of synthetic bone graft material would negate the risks of harvest site morbidity, disease transmission, and limited donor availability. The ability to machine the material would allow for the creation of multiple shapes and sizes that could be used as 'off-the-shelf' bone substitutes. Substantial cost savings may be realized with reasonably priced implants if the costs of autograft harvest (estimated to be USD 1,500–5,000 for iliac crest [5, 6]) and allograft harvest and preparation (machined allograft bone wedge approximately USD 3,000 per level, allograft femoral ring USD 1,200–2,400 per level;

source: University of Wisconsin operating room) are avoided. Ideally, these synthetic bone grafts would be totally absorbed by the body and replaced by native bone.

Calcium sulfate (plaster of Paris) has been used for bone defect repair since 1892 [7, 8]. Peltier and Jones [9] used calcium sulfate pellets to fill unicameral bone cysts in 26 patients with excellent results, and Coetzee [10] used similar pellets to treat osseous defects in the skull and facial bones in 110 patients. Recently, Kelly et al. [7] reported the use of Osteoset™ (Wright Medical Technology, Tenn., USA) a highly processed form of calcium sulfate for repair of bone defects in a series of 109 patients with various bone lesions. Osteoset was used as a bone graft substitute if the surgeon recommended the use of morsellized graft, the bone void was not intrinsic to the stability of the structure, and the void shape could accommodate the calcium sulfate pellets. Overall results were excellent, with 100% pellet resorption and 94% new bone growth (radiographic criteria) noted at 1 year [7]. No spinal fusions were performed during the study, and other materials were used in addition to the pellets in 65% of cases. Hadjipavlou et al. [11] recently reported excellent results with calcium sulfate-filled titanium cages in an interbody fusion model in adult sheep. These authors obtained roughly equivalent results with cages filled with either autograft iliac crest or with calcium sulfate. There are at present, however, no published reports of the use of calcium sulfate for human spinal fusion.

Processed coralline grafts, including hydroxyapatite, have been used extensively for the repair of bone defects. Additionally, these products have been used for spine surgery with a number of different applications. Hydroxyapatite is a poorly crystalline calcium phosphate compound which is similar in mineral composition to bone [6]. Calcium phosphate and hydroxyapatite are osteoconductive, if the porosity, pore size, and degree of pore interconnectivity are optimized [6]. Substantial research has established that the ideal pore size is between 100 and 500 μm [12]. Calcium hydroxyapatite is most commonly formed through processing of coral, which contains calcium phosphate and calcium carbonate in the form of aragonite. Several natural corals, particularly *Porites* and *Goniopora*, have pore sizes and pore interconnectivity which allow for osteoconduction. These corals have been harvested, cleansed, and then used as graft material (Biocoral™ Inoteb, France), particularly in dental surgery [13]. These corals may also be chemically treated via the 'replamineform' process. This process results in the conversion of aragonite to hydroxyapatite without changing the three-dimensional structure of the coral [6]. ProOsteon™ 200R, 500R, and Interpore porous hydroxyapatite™ (Interpore Cross International, Calif., USA) are produced in this fashion. The numbers 200R and 500R refer to the nominal pore diameter of the crystalline structure, either 200 or 500 μm. The mechanical properties of coralline hydroxyapatite grafts are more similar to cancellous rather than cortical bone. In general, increasing porosity increases the osteoconductivity of the graft and lowers the compressive strength.

Coralline hydroxyapatite has been used as a bone substitute for both cervical interbody as well as lumbar posterolateral fusion in animal, and in some cases human trials. In 1996, Zdeblick et al. [14] studied the use of ProOsteon 500R in a multilevel anterior cervical fusion in a goat model with or without plate fixation. They found that although only 48% of grafts incorporated with the hydroxyapatite alone, 71% incorporated if anterior cervical plate fixation was added. However, none of the implants were completely replaced by host bone at 12 weeks. Biomechanical testing revealed that the hydroxyapatite-fused segments behaved poorly without plate fixation. However the addition of an anterior cervical plate improved performance such that segments fused with hydroxyapatite and a cervical plate behaved similar to segments fused with allograft (but not autograft) bone and cervical plate in torsion. Hydroxyapatite-fused segments were inferior to both autograft and allograft in flexion/extension testing [14]. Boden et al. [15] studied the use of hydroxyapatite in a rabbit model of lumbar posterolateral fusion. They found that the use of coralline hydroxyapatite alone resulted in 0/14 solid fusions. Combination of hydroxyapatite and autograft bone in a 1:1 ratio resulted in a fusion rate of 50% (7/14). Bozic et al. [16] found that the combination of hydroxyapatite and bone marrow aspirate resulted in 25% fusion rate in a rabbit model. Addition of electrical stimulation (100 μA implantable direct current stimulator) significantly improved fusion rates. Similarly, Baramki et al. [17] noted a significantly lower fusion rate for hydroxyapatite-grafted animals (50%) than autograft-grafted animals (100%) in a sheep model of posterolateral fusion.

Despite these rather lukewarm animal results, Thalgott et al. [18] used hydroxyapatite (ProOsteon 200R) in combination with an anterior cervical plate for cervical interbody fusions in a group of 26 patients. In this retrospective series of 26 patients, 41 disc spaces were considered 'incorporated' at 24 months. Radiographic fusion was impossible to judge because the graft material was not resorbed at 24 months and remained more radio-dense than native bone. The criteria used for the determination of 'incorporation' was loss of a radiolucent line around the graft. The validity of this radiographic criterion for the determination of bony fusion is questionable. Iseda et al. [19] found that the appearance or disappearance radiolucent stripe around a hydroxyapatite graft did not correlate with changes in the ^{99m}Tc-HMDP uptake ratio following surgery in a small group of patients.

Tricalcium phosphate is a synthetically produced ceramic which has a porous structure amenable to osteoconduction. It has been used alone and in combination with hydroxyapatite as a bone graft substitute. It is completely resorbed by the body and is gradually replaced by new bone formation [1].

It is virtually identical to bone in terms of its mineral composition, and no reports of systemic toxicity exist. A comparative study by Emery et al. [20] demonstrated that the use of tricalcium phosphate (pore size 400 μm) resulted in superior histological results compared to hydroxyapatite or calcium carbonate in a canine interbody fusion model. Toth et al. [21] studied the use of different β-tricalcium phosphate/hydroxyapatite preparations in a goat cervical interbody fusion model and found that β-tricalcium phosphate performed as well or better than autograft at 3 and 6 months following fusion (radiographic, histological, dual-energy x-ray absorptiometry, and biomechanical testing). There was a definite increase in the bony union rate at 3 months with increasing porosity (0% union rate for autograft and 30% porous ceramic, 67% for 50% porous ceramic, and 83% for 70% porous ceramic). Delecrin et al. [1] used a similar compound (Triosite™ Zimmer, France) in a study of 58 patients undergoing surgery for scoliosis. In a prospective randomized study, these authors found that patients who received the ceramic graft had less blood loss and had no graft site complications. The authors noted that half of the autograft group experienced pain at the donor site 6 months following surgery. There were no significant differences between autograft and ceramic groups in terms of radiographic appearance or functional outcome at a minimum follow-up of 24 months (mean follow-up 48 months) [1].

A pure β-tricalcium phosphate synthetic bone product has been recently introduced (Vitoss™, Orthovita, Pa., USA). Vitoss has a unique crystalline structure, imparted by the manufacturing process, which increases its porosity significantly. The porosity of Vitoss is between 88 and 92%, compared to an approximate 55% porosity of hydroxyapatite-calcium carbonate. The increased porosity of this product allows for the rapid penetration of blood and blood products as well as for the migration of osteoblasts. Animal experiments using a humeral defect model have confirmed that the tricalcium phosphate is rapidly and nearly completely replaced by native bone in a matter of weeks (fig. 1, 2). The formation of bone in the humeral model is more rapid and more complete than that seen with coralline hydroxyapatite bone substitutes (fig. 1). In time, the graft is completely resorbed and replaced by new bone. When combined with autogenous bone marrow, the osteoinductive properties of the tricalcium phosphate are superior to demineralized bone matrix in a rat Urist pouch test [22]. A similar β-tricalcium phosphate compound has been developed (but is not yet FDA approved) that has biomechanical properties similar to cortical bone, can be machined and shaped easily, and can even be delivered in a semiliquid or putty form (Cortoss, Orthovita, Pa., USA).

Several other types of compounds have been used as synthetic bone substitutes. Madawi et al. [23] studied a bioactive osteoconductive polymer made of methyl methacrylate, calcium gluconate, and polyamide fibers. These authors

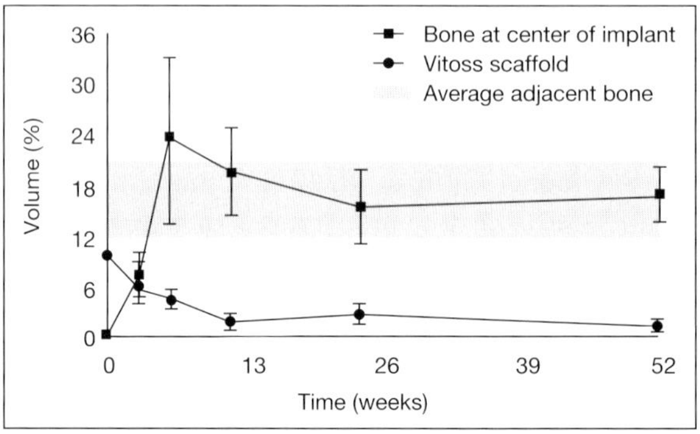

Fig. 1. Rapid absorption of Vitoss with regrowth of new bone within the graft.

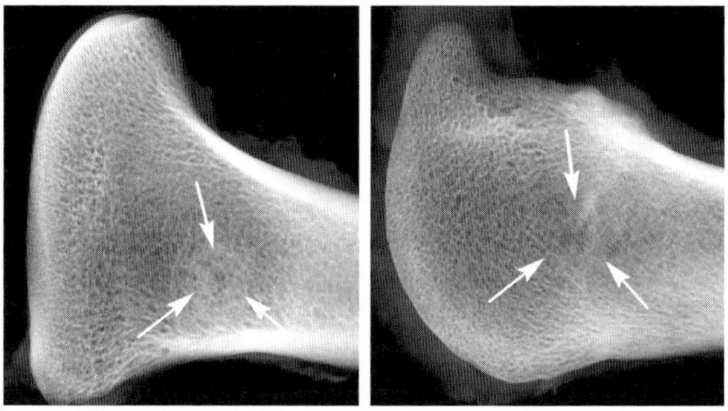

Fig. 2. Vitoss tricalcium phosphate bone substitute in a canine humeral defect model. The implant is almost completely resorbed at 6 weeks postimplant (***a***) and is indistinguishable from normal bone radiographically and histologically at 12 weeks (***b***).

noted favorable clinical results with this compound in trial of cervical interbody fusion; however, the graft never radiographically incorporated into native bone. Schulte et al. [24] used a bioglass-polyurethane composite to replace vertebral bodies following corpectomy for metastatic lesions in 5 patients. All patients also underwent titanium plate fixation. No instances of implant failure were noted. Roessler et al. [25] reported sobering results in their clinical study of a resorbable compound made up of polyethylene oxide and polybutylene terephthalate (Polyactive 70/30™ HC Implants, The Netherlands) for reconstitution of iliac crest bone graft harvest sites. Although this substance had shown very promising results in multiple animal models, human trials failed to show a favorable effect on clinical or radiographic outcome. This study serves as a reminder that there is no substitute for properly designed human clinical trials for the development of bone graft substitutes. Differences in the healing capabilities of the animal species, influences of patient age, and differences in the graft environment all play a role in bone healing [25, 26].

Resorbable Fixation Devices

Implants placed during spinal fusion surgery function in various ways. Screw/rod or screw/plate systems function to provide immediate structural stability, thus allowing early mobilization of the patient, maintaining spinal alignment and promoting the ultimate arthrodesis. Traditionally, these systems were manufactured of stainless steel, which has more recently been largely replaced by titanium alloy. Although both of these metals have performed well in their primary function, there are drawbacks such as stress shielding due to the excessive rigidity and permanence of the constructs that can in turn lead to bone resorption and osteopenia [27, 28]. Corrosion, wear debris and even rare allergic reactions have been seen, more so with stainless steel implants. Metallic artifact on imaging studies can obscure anatomic detail and cause diagnostic dilemmas. Once arthrodesis has occurred, the fixation systems no longer have a purpose [27, 29]. The indications for explantation of spinal fixation hardware are still controversial, but it is commonly performed.

Bioresorbable polymers have been increasingly explored as replacements for metal, bone and nonresorbable synthetic materials in recent years. Obviously, biodegradable implants eliminate the need for explantation. In addition, they can reduce stress shielding, by having a better match of strength and elasticity to bone as well as by gradually reducing load sharing as structural integrity is lost [27, 28, 30]. Lastly, they avoid the problems of metal corrosion, debris, and imaging artifact. This section will explore the properties and potential uses of these polymers in spinal surgery.

Bioresorbable materials and plates have been used to repair orbital and mandibular fractures since 1972 [31, 32]. Polylactic acid (L-isomer) (PLLA) and polyglycolic acid (PGA) and other polyhydroxy acids have been identified in the research to be promising polymers for resorbable implantable devices [33]. PLLA alone is resistant to hydrolytic degradation, which makes implants of this polymer quite strong but takes years for resorption to occur, if it occurs at all. These implants may also result in a foreign body reaction over time and thus require removal [34, 35]. In comparison, pure PGA implants absorb much more quickly when exposed to moisture yet suffer loss of tensile strength and rapid polymer breakdown [36]. Researchers have experimented with combinations of both polymers in order to utilize the favorable characteristics of each. LactoSorb™ (Biomet, Warsaw, Ind., USA) is a resorbable plate system approved for use in

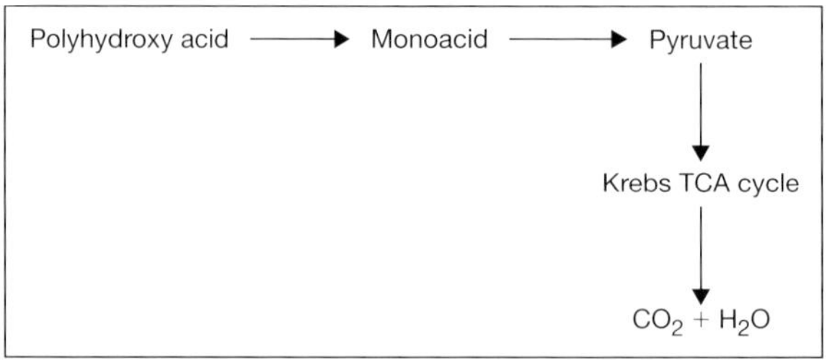

Fig. 3. Schematic illustration of the degradation of a prototypical resorbable polymer. (Certain intermediate products of degradation can also be excreted in the urine.)

craniomaxillofacial surgery. It consists of a combination of synthetic PGA and PLLA. This PGA/PLLA copolymer is manufactured in an 82% PLLA and 18% PGA ratio. The increased amount of PLLA in this copolymer gives it degradation characteristics midway between the predominately PGA products and pure PLLA implants [37]. MacroPore™ (MacroPore., San Diego, Calif., USA), another resorbable product with potential spine applications, is produced by the combination of PLLA and a noncrystalline copolymer mixture of poly(*L*-lactide) and poly(*D,L*-lactide).

The implant resorption time is most strongly affected by the chemical composition of the polymer, but there are many additional variables in this process [29, 38]. Gogolewski [28] has identified the implant's physical structure and mass, polymeric molecular weight, chain orientation, and presence of additives as some of the many factors influencing the rate of degradation, along with the stress on the implant and the characteristics of the implantation site. For example, he notes that an implant placed under significant load in a highly vascularized site will likely degrade at an accelerated rate [28].

The PGA component of the LactoSorb implant is degraded to glycolic acid by hydrolysis and further degraded to glycine, which may be used for protein synthesis or further converted to serine. All other implant (LactoSorb and MacroPore) components are hydrolyzed to lactic acid, which then enters the tricarboxylic acid cycle (fig. 3) [39]. The use of these plates avoids several potential complications associated with metallic fixation devices, such as migration, stress shielding, and interference with imaging techniques [39]. Currently, the most commonly reported side effect is a sterile inflammatory reaction to the implants [35, 40–43].

Local tissue reaction to polyhydroxy acid implants is governed by the chemical nature of the polymer, the physical characteristics of the implant, and by its degradation rate. Towards the latter part of the degradation process, the implant may rapidly lose structural integrity, and the production rate of polymeric debris may exceed the tissue tolerance and transport potential of the implantation site [27, 38]. This in turn can stimulate what is said to be a 'nonspecific foreign-body reaction' rather than a true inflammatory response [27, 38]. Thus, a large implant made of a fast-degrading polymer is likely to produce a more pronounced inflammation than a small implant composed of a slow-degrading polymer. PGA polymers have been associated with a higher rate of tissue reaction, even including the formation of fibrous capsules, sterile cysts and sinuses. On the other hand, pure polylactic acid (PLA) polymers have a low or nonexistent rate of tissue reaction, while once again, copolymers are intermediate [27, 38, 44].

Histological evaluation of these inflammatory sites has shown typical nonspecific foreign-body reactions. Similar foreign-body reactions were found on histological examination of implant sites of patients without clinical evidence of an inflammatory response [40]. These specimens were obtained upon reoperation for fixation failure. No explanation is available for why some patients have clinical signs of the foreign body reaction while others do not. Most studies have shown the inflammatory response, when clinically present, to occur several months after implantation. Bostman [40] postulates that this time to occurrence of the reaction is reflective of the estimated degradation time of PGA and PLLA/PGA implants which is 90–120 days. Patients who have had plates and screws made solely of PLLA, implanted for fixation of zygomatic fractures, have shown inflammatory reactions from 3.3 to 5.7 years after surgery [35]. These findings seem to correlate with degradation rates of PLLA, stated in some studies to be from 2 to over 4 years [39].

PLA polymers and PLA-PGA copolymers are biocompatible with the dura [45–47]. PLA biocompatibility has also been specifically tested in reference to neural tissue, including brain and spinal cord tissue as well as peripheral nerves. No effect on neuronal cells, nonneuronal cells or axonal growth has been noted [45, 48]. No significant toxicity, carcinogenicity, teratogenicity or mutagenesis has been associated with either PLA or PGA [27, 38].

LactoSorb plates and screws became commercially available for craniofacial applications in 1996. Most of the interest in bioresorbable plates for cranial reconstruction has been in the pediatric patient population because of complications with metallic implants related to bone growth. LactoSorb plates have been used in neurosurgery for fixation of craniotomy flaps, repair of depressed skull fractures and for repair of craniosynostosis [33, 49–53]. Encouragingly, it has been found that the dissolution and gradual loss of tensile strength of the devices minimize growth restrictions as well as the potential for transcranial migration [54]. In addition, good results have been obtained in both the pediatric and adult population when LactoSorb plates and screws were used for cranial fixation and reconstruction.

LactoSorb plates are designed to withstand similar external forces and approximate the strength of traditional titanium plates. In order for a bioresorbable plate to perform similarly to a titanium implant, it must retain similar strength characteristics long enough for osteosynthesis to occur. Because PGA, PLLA, and copolymers are all significantly less rigid than titanium, the design of plate-like implants must be adjusted somewhat. In general, resorbable plate designs incorporate a thicker plate, in order to recapitulate the mechanical properties of a standard titanium implant. Flexural strength is significantly improved in the LactoSorb plate, for example, due to its 'I-beam'-like construction (raised rails along the side of the plate). In vitro studies of flexural strength show the LactoSorb plate has an initial strength comparable to Lorenz titanium plates and retains 70% of this strength for 6–8 weeks [55, 56]. The improved strength does, however, create a much higher profile implant than the traditional metallic plate.

The most common reported clinical difficulties with the LactoSorb products are related to implantation technique. LactoSorb screws are not self-tapping which increases the time necessary to place the screws. Second, unlike metal plates, which can be shaped by hand or with instruments at room temperature, polymer plates must be heated before they can be shaped. Heating is achieved by use of a bag of calcium chloride which, when injected with sterile water, will liberate heat for approximately 20 min. By placing the bag around the LactoSorb plate, the implant can be made malleable. Some authors have stated that the 20-min window may be too small, making a second calcium chloride bag necessary, which involves adding time and expenses. Despite these initial technical difficulties, most authors agree that the LactoSorb system is a safe, effective system for cranial fixation and reconstruction, which, after minimal experience with the system, adds very little time to the operation compared to the traditional titanium plating systems.

Six studies of the use of bioresorbable plates for cranial fixation, either alone or in conjunction with facial reconstruction and orthosis, have been published with a combined total of 115 patients [33, 49–53]. No patients were noted to have significant complications from inflammatory reactions, seizures or failure of the fixation. In fact, clinical studies of patients who have had LactoSorb plates implanted and have been followed for greater than 9 months show no evidence of inflammatory reactions [49, 57]. It is believed that the intermediate rate of degradation for this predominately PLLA copolymer allows for efficient removal of its byproducts without overwhelming the body's mechanisms of clearance [50, 58].

Because of its relatively high profile, LactoSorb can produce a palpable and sometimes visible implant. Studies have noted this factor to occur occasionally; however, the authors state that in all cases the external evidence of the

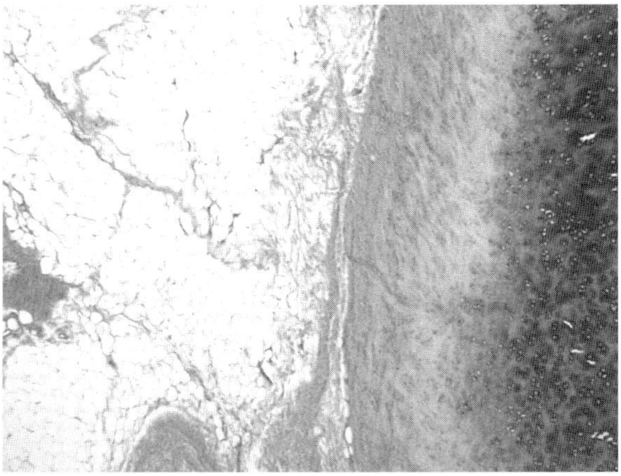

Fig. 4. Explanted LactoSorb plate. Histological examination of explanted LactoSorb plate demonstates complete resorption of implant material 1 year following surgery (bone on right, normal soft tissues on left) without evidence of persistent inflammatory reaction.

Table 1. Strength of MacroPore implant during degradation

Time after implantation	%
Implantation	100
6 months	90
9 months	70
12 months	50
18 months	0

implant disappears within 3–6 months [33, 51, 59]. Most studies of LactoSorb plates show the entire implant to be 95% resorbed by 9 months and completely resorbed by 1 year (fig. 4) [60].

MacroPore is characterized by a degradation time of 18–36 months. The loss of strength during degradation has been well characterized, and is predictable [61] (table1). As noted above, however, the strength and degradation characteristics of any specific MacroPore implant will be influenced by the manufacturing processes, implant size and geometry, and characteristics of the implantation site, among other factors. MacroPore can be formed into a wide variety of shapes, and it can be stored and sterilized utilizing conventional techniques. In appropriate shapes, MacroPore can be heated and shaped for conformation to the actual site of implantation, and it will hold the desired shape once cooled without loss of structural integrity [MacroPore: pers. commun.].

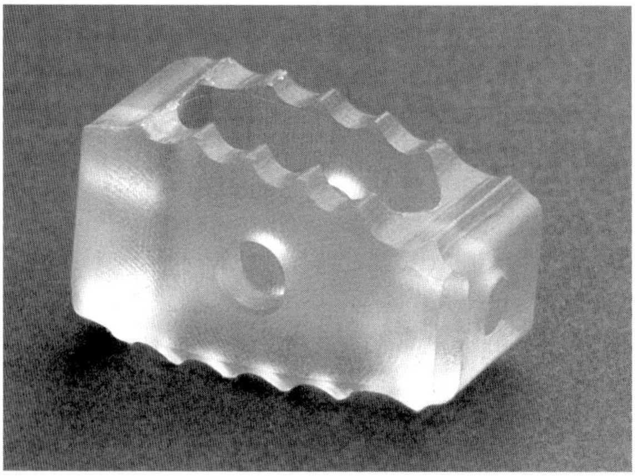

Fig. 5. Absorbable 'spacer'. This resorbable spacer represents one possible avenue of exploration for resorbable technology for spine surgery.

MacroPore devices cannot be readily visualized on routine radiographic studies, although they can be seen distinctly on CT scans prior to significant degradation [Branch: pers. commun; 62]. PLA implants do not degrade MRI images, and MRI scanning has been utilized to evaluate the tissue response of PLA implants [30, 63–65]. PLA implants are visible on MRI images as areas of homogeneous low-signal intensity, which can be distinguished from the high signal intensity of the adjacent bone [63].

MacroPore sheets have been utilized to reconstruct iliac crest donor site defects [66]. Iliac crest reconstruction may diminish pain, prevent bowel herniation through large defects [67], improve cosmesis, and optimize donor site regeneration [66]. The benefits of a protected healing space have been recognized in promoting optimal bone healing [47, 68]. Specifically, if soft tissue is prevented from prolapsing into a bone defect, the regrowth of bone may be better than with graft materials alone. In terms of the iliac crest, once the bone is harvested, the donor site is backfilled with allograft or bone matrix material if desired. A MacroPore sheet is then heated to 70°C, contoured to the defect site and allowed to cool. It is then secured with screws or tacks [66]. This is an example of the potential use of MacroPore as a barrier type of implant.

MacroPore implants are being utilized in pilot studies as load-sharing implants in spine fusion constructs [62]. The versatile nature of this material allows it to be formed into 'cages', 'dowels' and 'interbody spacer' shapes (fig. 5). This, coupled with the desirable strength and degradation characteristics, lack of artifact on imaging, low potential for foreign body reaction and the biocompatibility with the dura and nervous tissue, makes it a very promising material.

One such study examines the use of MacroPore devices in instrumented posterior lumbar interbody fusion constructs [62]. The devices are placed following complete discectomy, along with morsellized autograft bone, and maintain the disc space height during the early phase of bone healing. Preliminary results show equivalent clinical outcomes to those obtained with the use of allograft bone spacers. The devices produce no artifact on postoperative imaging, allowing better visualization of the maturing bone fusion [62].

Other products are being developed worldwide in order to expand the applications of bioabsorbable products. Bostman et al. [40] used a biodegradable rod for internal fixation of extremity fractures and osteotomies. The composition of the rods was either polyglycolide or a lactide-glycolide copolymer (polyglactin). A small percentage of the 516 patients treated required reoperation for fixation failure (1.2%). The incidence of bacterial wound infections was low (1.7%). The most significant complication was a foreign-body reaction in 7.9% of the patients. The reaction caused a painful, reddened, fluctuant swelling at the operative site 2–4 months after surgery. Godard et al. [69] have investigated a bioresorbable implant for spinal arthrodesis, which is reported to undergo ossification. Brunon et al. [70] have used a bioresorbable plate developed from PLLA for anterior cervical interbody stabilization in 5 patients. The development of bioabsorbable plates, screws, and rods for use in the spine is an area of intense activity at the present time.

Conclusion

Absorbable bone substitutes and fixation devices are being developed for spinal surgery. Advances in material technology may allow for the avoidance of autograft harvest morbidity and allograft preparation costs and toxicities. Resorbable implants may result in decreased morbidity and better radiographic evaluation of spinal fusion procedures. The pace of new development in this field is remarkable. As new products are brought to market, thorough and rigorous testing in well-designed clinical trials will be required to establish their ultimate worth.

References

1 Delecrin J, Takahashi S, Gouin F, Passuti N: A synthetic porous ceramic as a bone graft substitute in the surgical management of scoliosis: A prospective, randomized study. Spine 2000;25: 563–569.

2 Khan S, Sandhu H, Parvataneni H, Girardi F, Cammisa F: Bone graft substitutes in spine surgery. Bull Hosp Jt Dis 2000;59:5–10.

3 Bostman M, Yang X, Kennan M, Sandhu H, Dicarlo E, Lane J: An unexpected outcome during testing of commercially available demineralized bone graft materials. Spine 2001;36:1425–1428.
4 Wang J, Kanim L, Nagakawa I, Yamane B, Vinters H, Dawson E: Dose-dependent toxicity of a commercially available demineralized bone matrix material. Spine 2001;26:1429–1436.
5 Boden S: Bone repair and enhancement clinical trial design. Clin Orthop 1998;355S:S336–S346.
6 Shors EC: Coralline bone graft substitutes. Orthop Clin North Am 1999;30:599–613.
7 Kelly CM, Wilkins RM, Gitelis S, Hartjen C, Watson JT, Kim PT: The use of a surgical grade calcium sulfate as a bone graft substitute: Results of a multicenter trial. Clin Orthop 2001;382:42–50.
8 Dreesman H: Über Knochenplombierung. Beitr Klin Chir 1892;9:804–810.
9 Peltier L, Jones R: Treatment of unicameral bone cysts by curettage and packing with plaster of Paris pellets. J Bone Joint Surg Am 1978;60:820–822.
10 Coetzee A: Regeneration of bone in the presence of calcium sulfate. Arch Otolaryngol 1980;106: 405–409.
11 Hadjipavlou A, Simmons J, Yang J, Nicodemus C, Esch O, Simmons D: Plaster of Paris as an osteoconductive material for interbody vertebral fusion in mature sheep. Spine 2000;25:10–15.
12 White E, Shors E: Biomaterial aspects of interpore-200 porous hydroxyapatite. Dent Clin North Am 1986;30:49–67.
13 Yukna RA, Yukna CN: A 5-year follow-up of 16 patients treated with coralline calcium carbonate (BIOCORAL) bone replacement grafts in infrabony defects. J Clin Periodontol 1998;25: 1036–1040.
14 Zdeblick T, Cooke M, Kunz D, Wilson D, McCabe R: Anterior cervical discectomy and fusion using a porous hydroxyapatite bone graft substitute. Spine 1994;19:2348–2357.
15 Boden S, Martin G, Morone M, Ugbo J, Titus L, Hutton W: The use of coralline hydroxyapatite with bone marrow, autogenous bone graft, or osteoinductive bone protein extract for posterolateral lumbar spine fusion. Spine 1999;24:320–327.
16 Bozic K, Glazer P, Zurakowski D, Simon B, Lipson S, Hayes W: In vivo evaluation of coralline hydroxyapatite and direct current electrical stimulation in lumbar spinal fusion. Spine 1999;24: 2127–2133.
17 Baramki H, Steffen T, Lander P, Chang M, Marchesi D: The efficacy of interconnected porous hydroxyapatite in achieving posterolateral fusion in sheep. Spine 2000;25:1053–1060.
18 Thalgott J, Fritts K, Giuffre J, Timlin M: Anterior interbody fusion of the cervical spine with coralline hydroxyapatite. Spine 1999;24:1295–1300.
19 Iseda T, Nakano S, Suzuki Y, et al: Radiographic and scintigraphic courses of union in cervical interbody fusion: Hydroxyapatite grafts versus iliac crest bone autografts. J Nucl Med 2000;41: 1642–1645.
20 Emery S, Fuller D, Stevenson S: Ceramic anterior spinal fusion: Biologic and biomechanical comparison in a canine model. Spine 1996;23:2713–2719.
21 Toth J, An H, Lim T, et al: Evaluation of porous biphasic calcium phosphate ceramics for anterior cervical interbody fusion in a caprine model. Spine 1995;20:2203–2210.
22 Gunzburg R, Szpalski M: A highly porous beta tri-calcium phosphate/bone marrow graft promotes osteoinductivity in rat subcutaneous model. EuroSpine, Gothenburg, 2001.
23 Madawi A, Powell M, Crockard H: Biocompatible osteoinductive polymer versus iliac graft: A prospective comparative study for the evaluation of fusion pattern after anterior cervical discectomy. Spine 1996;21:2123–2129.
24 Schulte M, Schultheiss M, Hartig E, et al: Vertebral body replacement with a bioglass-polyurethane composite in spine metastases – Clinical, radiological, and biomechanical results. Eur Spine J 2000;9:437–444.
25 Roessler M, Wilke A, Griss P, Kienapfel H: Missing osteoconductive effect of a resorbable PEO/PBT copolymer in human bone defects: A clinically relevant pilot study with contrary results to previous animal studies. J Biomed Mater Res 2000;53:167–173.
26 Delecrin J, Aguado E, Nguyen J, Pyre D, Royer J, Passuti N: Influence of local microenvironment on incorporation of ceramic for lumbar fusion: Comparison of laminar and intertransverse sites in a canine model. Spine 1997;22:1683–1689.
27 Bostman O, Pihlajamaki H: Clinical biocompatibility of biodegradable orthopaedic implants for internal fixation: A review. Biomaterials 2000;21:2615–2621.

28 Gogolewski S: Bioresorbable polymers in trauma and bone surgery. Injury 2000;4:28–32.
29 An YH, Woolf SK, Friedman RJ: Pre-clinical in vivo evaluation of orthopaedic bioabsorbable devices. Biomaterials 2000;21:2635–2652.
30 Viljanen J, Kinnunen J, Bondestam S, Majola A, Rokkanen P, Tormala P: Bone changes after experimental osteotomies fixed with absorbable self-reinforced poly-*L*-lactide screws or metallic screws studied by plain radiographs, quantitative computed tomography, and magnetic resonance imaging. Biomaterials 1995;16:1353–1358.
31 Cutright D, Hunsuck E: The repair of fractures of the orbital floor using biodegradable polylactic acid. Oral Surg 1972;33:28.
32 Getter L, Cutright D, Bhaskar S, Augsburg J: A biodegradable intraosseus appliance in the treatment of mandibular fractures. J Oral Surg 1972;30:344.
33 Montag ME, Morales L Jr, Daane S: Bioabsorbables: Their use in pediatric craniofacial surgery. J Craniofac Surg 1997;8:100–102.
34 Bergsma E, Rozema F, Bos R, de Bruijn W: Foreign body reactions to resorbable poly(*L*-lactide) bone plates and screws used for the fixation of unstable zygomatic fractures. J Oral Maxillofac Surg 1993;51:666–670.
35 Bergsma J, de Bruijn W, Rozema F, Bos R, Boering G: Late degradation tissue response to poly(*L*-lactide) bone plates and screws. Biomaterials 1995;16:25–31.
36 Barrows T: Degradable implant materials: A review of synthetic absorbable polymers and their applications. Clin Mater 1986;1:233.
37 Pietrzak W, Sarver D, Verstynen M: Bioabsorbable polymer science for the practicing surgeon. J Craniofac Surg 1997;8:87–91.
38 Rokkanen PU, Bostman O, Hirvensalo E, et al: Bioabsorbable fixation in orthopaedic surgery and traumatology. Biomaterials 2000;21:2607–2613.
39 Vainionpaa S: Surgical applications of biodegradable polymers in human tissue. Prog Polym Sci 1989;14:679–716.
40 Bostman O, Hirvensalo E, Makinen J, Rokkanen P: Foreign body reactions to fracture fixation implants of biodegradable synthetic polymers. J Bone Joint Surg Br 1990;72:592–596.
41 Bostman O: Osteolytic changes accompanying degradation of absorbable fracture implants. J Bone Joint Surg Br 1991;73:679–682.
42 Bostman O, Parito E, Hirvensalo E, Rokkanen P: Foreign body reactions to polyglycolide screws: Observations in 24/26 malleolar fracture cases. Acta Orthop Scand 1992;63:173–176.
43 Svensson P, Janarv P, Hirsch G: Internal fixation with biodegradable rods in pediatric fractures: One year follow-up of fifty patients. J Pediatr Orthop 1994;14:220–221.
44 Van der Elst M, Klein C, Bliek-Hogervorst J, Patka P: Bone tissue response to biodegradable polymers used for intramedullary fracture fixation: A long-term in vivo study in sheep. Biomaterials 1999;20:121–128.
45 Gautier S, Oudega M, Fraguso M, et al: Poly(alpha-hydroxyacids) for application in the spinal cord: Resorbability and biocompatibility with adult rat Schwann cells and spinal cord. J Biomed Mater Res 1998;42:642–654.
46 Levy F, Hollinger J, Szachowicz E: Effect of a bioresorbable film on regeneration of cranial bone. Plast Reconstr Surg 1994;93:307–311.
47 Lundgren D, Nyman S, Mathisen T, Isaksson S, Klinge B: Guided bone regeneration of cranial defects using biodegradable barriers: An experimental pilot study in the rabbit. J Craniomaxillofac Surg 1992;20:257–260.
48 Medinaceli L, Khoury R, Merle M: Large amounts of polylactic acid in contact with divided nerve sheaths have no adverse effects on regeneration. J Reconstr Microsurg 1995;11:43–49.
49 Eppley B, Sadove A: Surgical correction of metopic suture synostosis; in Kolk C (ed): Clinics in Plastic Surgery. Philadelphia, Saunders, 1994, pp 555–562.
50 Eppley B, Sadove A: Resorbable coupling fixation in craniosynostosis surgery: Experimental and clinical applications. J Craniofac Surg 1995;6:477–482.
51 Pensler J: Role of resorbable plates and screws in craniofacial surgery. J Craniofac Surg 1997;8:129–134.
52 Kumar A, Staffenberg D, Petronio J, Wood R: Bioabsorbable plates and screws in pediatric craniofacial surgery: A review of 22 cases. J Craniofac Surg 1997;8:97–99.

53 Goldstein J, Quereshy F, Cohen A: Early experience with biodegradable fixation for congenital pediatric craniofacial surgery. J Craniofac Surg 1997;8:110–115.
54 Eppley B, Sadove A: Effects of resorbable fixation on craniofacial skeletal growth. J Craniofac Surg 1994;2:110–115.
55 Pietrzak W, Sarver D, Verstynen M: Bioresorbable impants: Practical considerations. Bone 1996;19:109S–119S.
56 Pietrzak W, Verstynen M, Sarver D: Bioabsorbable fixation device: Status for the craniomaxillofacial surgeon. J Craniofac Surg 1997;8:92–96.
57 Eppley B, Prevel C, Sadove A, Sarver D: Resorbable bone fixation: Its potential role in craniomaxillofacial trauma. J Craniomaxillofac Trauma 1996;2:56–60.
58 Eppley B, Sadove A: A comparison of resorbable and metallic fixation in healing of calvarial bone grafts. Plast Reconstr Surg 1995;96:316–322.
59 Eppley B, Prevel C: Nonmetallic fixation in traumatic midfacial fractures. J Craniofac Surg 1997;8:103–109.
60 Eppley B, Reilly M: Degradation characteristics of PLLA-PGA bone fixation devices. J Craniofac Surg 1997;8:116–120.
61 Claes L, Ignatius A, Rehm K, Scholz C: New bioresorbable pin for the reduction of bony fragments: Design, mechanical properties, and in vitro degradation. Biomaterials 1996;17:1621–1626.
62 Subach B, Branch C, Alexander J, Haid R, Rodts G: Posterior lumbar interbody fusion using an impacted bioabsorbable device. AANS/CNS Joint Section on Disorders of the Spine and Peripheral Nerves, Orlando, 2002.
63 Pihlajamaki H, Kinnunen J, Bostman O: In vivo monitoring of the degradation process of bioresorbable polymeric implant using magnetic resonance imaging. Biomaterials 1997;18:1311–1315.
64 Stroman P, Dorvil J, Marois Y, Poddevin N, Guidoin R: In vivo time course studies of the tissue responses to resorbable polylactic acid implants by means of MRI. Magn Reson Med 1999;42: 210–214.
65 Warden W, Friedman R, Teresi L, Jackson D: Magnetic resonance imaging of bioabsorbable polylactic acid screws during the first two years after anterior cruciate ligament reconstruction. Arthroscopy 1999;15:474–480.
66 Taylor W, Ames C, Cataletto M: MacroPore resorbable sheeting: Early experience in immediate iliac crest contour reconstruction. Personal communication.
67 Cowley S, Anderson L: Hernias through donor sites for iliac bone grafts. J Bone Joint Surg Am 1983;65:1023–1025.
68 Holmes R, Lemperle S, Calhoun C: Protected bone regeneration. Unpubl. data.
69 Godard J, Jacquet G, Farhat O, Steimle R: Implant intervertébral au biocopoymère (BOP) pour arthrodèse: étude de 45 cas. Chirugie 1991;117:398–404.
70 Brunon J, Duthel R, Fotso M, Tudor C: Anterior osteosynthesis of the cervical spine by phusiline bioresorbable screws and plates: Initial results apropos of 5 cases. Neurochirurgie 1994;40: 196–202.

Daniel K. Resnick, MD MS
Assistant Professor, Department of Neurological Surgery
University of Wisconsin, K4/834 Clinical Science Center
600 Highland Ave, Madison, WI 53792 (USA)
Tel. +1 608 263 9651, Fax +1 608 263 1728, E-Mail resnick@neurosurg.wisc.edu

Haid RW Jr, Subach BR, Rodts GE Jr (eds): Advances in Spinal Stabilization.
Prog Neurol Surg. Basel, Karger, 2003, vol 16, pp 55–70

Lumbar Interbody Fusion Using Bone Morphogenetic Protein: Results and Fusion Assessment

J. Kenneth Burkus[a], *Kevin T. Foley*[b], *Regis W. Haid, Jr.*[c]

[a]The Hughston Clinic, PC, Columbus, Ga., [b]Semmes-murphy Clinic, Memphis, Tenn., and [c]Department of Neurosurgery, Emory University, Atlanta, Ga., USA

No uniform criteria for determining fusion have been used in the reports of radiographic outcomes of anterior lumbar interbody fusion (ALIF) surgery [1, 2]. The most commonly reported standard for establishing the presence of a successful lumbar interbody fusion is evidence of trabecular bone formation linking the adjacent vertebral bodies. A wide range of fusion rates for the ALIF procedure has been reported [3–7]. The variability in fusion rates is, in part, determined by the surgical technique, the type and quantity of bone graft used, and the presence of an interbody fusion device. With these variables, the determination of a successful arthrodesis is largely determined by the investigator's definition of fusion.

The use of metallic interbody fusion devices creates new challenges in establishing fusion criteria. These devices obscure vertebral landmarks used in the assessment of fusion and create artifacts that degrade some imaging techniques [8–10]. The intradiscal radiographic patterns of fusion after surgery with interbody fusion cages are determined by the extent of the discectomy, the end plate preparation, the reaming techniques, the interface between the cage and the host bone, and the characteristics of the bone graft materials used. Direct surgical exploration is not a viable option for determining the status of an interbody fusion [11–13]. Indirect assessment at surgery of an anterior fusion through the manipulation of the posterior spinous processes is subjective and can identify only gross patterns of instability and cannot reliably identify micromotion across an interspace.

Other than by histologic biopsy, interbody fusion can only be assessed objectively by various radiographic imaging techniques. Although the presence of a pseudarthrosis can be determined by a single finding on an isolated radiographic study, the presence of a solid fusion cannot be determined by a single radiographic finding. Failure of fusion is established by the absence of bridging trabecular bone and the presence of a radiolucent area that extends through the entire fusion mass. Pseudarthrosis can also be identified by marginal radiolucency around the implant, progressive subsidence of implants, and angular changes in the spinal motion segment.

At present, no single study or technique is definitive for establishing the presence of a fusion after anterior interbody surgery [14]. A successful arthrodesis within a spinal motion segment can be determined by using radiographic evaluation to assess a stable spinal alignment on sequential examinations, a reduction in angular and translational changes on dynamic motion studies, an absence of fibrous tissue reaction at the device-host interface, and the presence of new bone formation and bone remodeling [15].

The most comprehensive and accurate means of radiographically assessing fusion of the lumbar spine after ALIF with intradiscal implants are plain radiographs, dynamic motion radiographs, and thin-cut computerized tomography (CT) scans. Technetium bone scans and MR imaging are not effective in assessing interbody fusion [9, 16]. Plain radiographs are effective for determining changes in spinal alignment over time. Dynamic plain radiographs can accurately assess changes in implant-host bone interface and instability patterns within the spinal motion segment. CT imaging can identify new bone formation and bone remodeling within and around the spinal implants [8, 17]. By using all three imaging technologies, the physician can accurately determine a successful and clinically relevant interbody fusion [15].

Lumbar Spine Imaging Studies

Plain Radiographs

The plain radiographic studies that are used most often to assess fusion include the following: (1) standing or weight-bearing radiographs, (2) supine radiographs, (3) dynamic flexion-extension radiographs, and (4) dynamic side-bending radiographs. Standing or weight-bearing films are more valuable than supine films in assessing sagittal plane balance and alignment; a weight-bearing radiographic technique stresses the interbody fusion can help identify instability patterns. Supine anteroposterior radiographs show lucencies around metallic implants (fig. 1).

Metallic implants create artifacts that make interpretation of plain radiographs alone inaccurate in the assessment of fusion [8, 10]. Bone growth within the implants cannot be assessed on plain radiographs. The thread patterns of

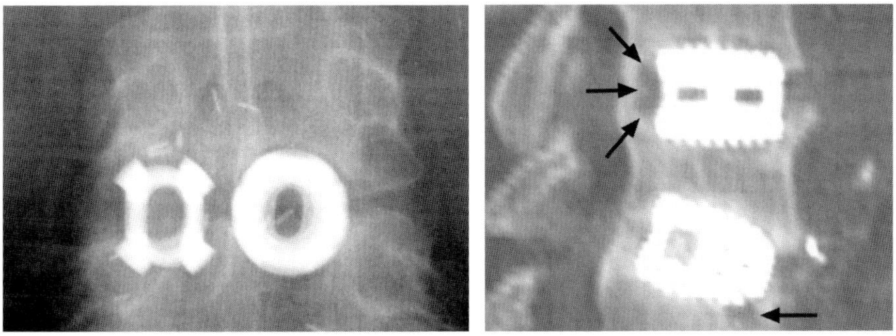

a b

Fig. 1. ***a*** Supine anteroposterior radiograph shows lucencies around both implants. ***b*** Thin-cut CT scan sagittal reconstruction confirms the lucencies surrounding the cages.

interbody fusion cages create varying amounts of artifact at the implant-host bone interface. Radiographic lucencies in this area can be misinterpreted. The following findings on plain radiographs help to identify a fusion: (1) incorporation of grafts to vertebral end plates, (2) bridging trabecular bone across the interspace, (3) absence of lucencies at the graft-host interface, (4) absence of subsidence, and (5) absence of graft or implant migration. The absence of subsidence and implant migration can only be established by a review of serial radiographs.

Dynamic Plain Radiographs

Dynamic motion studies of the lumbar spine are done to identify subtle changes within the spinal motion segment after ALIF surgery. Intra- and interobserver measurement error is always a factor in the assessment of lumbar intervertebral segmental angulation and translation on serial radiographs. In their clinical studies, examiners have considered spinal motion segments to be fused despite measured differences in both angular and sagittal translation [1, 5]. Reports of measurement error range from 1 to 5°. Brantigan [18] proposed that only 1° of motion was consistent with a fusion. Zdeblick [19] proposed 2°, and Ray [7] proposed 3° of motion as support for the presence of a solid fusion. These studies contrast with the findings of Kuslich et al. [5] who reported that angular measurements of less than 5° are not accurate. Commonly, the presence of 3–5° of motion within an instrumented spinal segment and 5 mm of translation is considered fused. These differences on dynamic studies are accepted because of measurement errors. Clinicians often find these results difficult to interpret because motion should not occur within a fused spinal segment.

Amplifying the problem of intra- and interobserver measurement error on dynamic radiographs is the fact that no standard method for obtaining flexion-extension radiographs has been established. Biplanar studies are among the most reliable plain radiographic methods. Dynamic radiographs taken with the patient in the standing position are not reliable because of variable patient compliance and the technical difficulty of properly centering the x-ray beam parallel to the appropriate interspace. With standing lateral dynamic studies, the pelvis is not locked and motion may be occurring at the hip joints rather than within the lumbar spine. Supine lateral dynamic studies obtained in the lateral decubitus position are also unreliable for the same reasons – the pelvis is not locked or properly supported. Lateral radiographic images are frequently rotated unless the lumbar spine has been supported. It is technically difficult to maintain the x-ray beam parallel to the spinal motion segment during these dynamic studies.

Flexion-extension radiographs should be obtained with the pelvis fixed so that motion occurs within the lumbar spine. Dynamic studies with the patient in the seated position restrict pelvic and hip motion and enable the technician to consistently obtain radiographs centered at the appropriate disc space with minimal rotational distortion at the interspace. Restricting motion to the lumbar spine by eliminating hip and pelvic motion and consistently obtaining radiographs that are parallel to the end plate of the instrumented spinal segment sufficiently improves the accuracy of dynamic radiographic studies and demonstrates subtle changes within the spinal motion segment (fig. 1). Biplanar radiographic techniques have been introduced to reduce measurement error [20].

Thin-Cut 1-mm CT Scans

Axial CT has also been used to establish fusion [8, 13, 21–23]. This cross-sectional imaging technique eliminates overlapping and rotational errors present on plain radiographs and allows direct visualization of the fusion mass. Thin-cut CT scans with sagittal and coronal reconstructions have a greater ability to detect radiolucent areas within a developing fusion mass. Using thin-cut CT scans, clinicians have identified and classified complex forms of spinal pseudarthrosis into distinct morphologic categories [1, 20]. In animal studies, thin-cut CT scans using 1-mm-thick axial sections through interbody fusion cages have been used to reliably identify new bone formation within metallic fusion cages and to identify pseudarthroses after interbody surgery [12, 24, 25]. These findings were correlated with histologic confirmation to establish the presence or absence of a fusion. In these animal studies, CT scans were used to show trabecular bone formation patterns within the disc space and identify bridging bone formation that crossed the interspace. CT scanning was also used to identify lucencies at the implant-bone interface. In our clinical experience, thin-cut CT scanning has been the most precise and accurate method of evaluating interbody fusion [26, 27].

A single CT scan may not be able to distinguish between unincorporated or necrotic bone grafts from bridging trabecular bone within a metallic fusion cage. Cunningham et al. [28] analyzed fusion through a histomorphometric assessment. They could not differentiate between residual autograft and new bone formation. However, serial CT scans can be used to identify maturation of corticocancellous grafts within fusion cages and can demonstrate incorporation of these grafts through the openings in the second-generation fusion cages [26]. CT scans can be used to accurately identify new bone formation within the disc space but outside of the interbody fusion devices [17, 26, 27].

Interbody Fusion Assessment

The assessment of fusion in a patient who has an interbody fusion device includes four key elements: (1) spinal alignment, (2) segmental spinal stabilization, (3) device-host bone interface, and (4) new bone formation and bone remodeling. Spinal alignment must be maintained over time. Similarly, with an intact fusion, no significant angular or translational change should occur on dynamic motion studies. The contact points between the device and the host cortical bone and cancellous bone must also be assessed. For an intervertebral body fusion to be considered intact and complete, there should be no radiolucent areas surrounding the devices at the interface with the host bone. Identification of new trabecular bone formation within the disc space and remodeling of the grafts within and around the interbody devices must also be assessed and is the most important aspect of the fusion criteria [17, 29], but the sentinel sign [30, 31] of the progressive anterior bone formation alone is not helpful in determining fusion.

Spinal Alignment

ALIF using stand-alone implants often improve the frontal and sagittal plain contours of the lumbar spine. Immediate postoperative improvements in frontal and sagittal plane contours are not maintained over time in all patients [32–34]. Stand-alone implants are susceptible to subsidence into the vertebral end plates. Subsidence of the implants, which occurs over the course of several years after surgery, often leads to segmental spinal instability, loss of lordosis, angular frontal plain deformities, and sagittal plain translation. It is evidence of a delayed fusion or frank pseudarthrosis (fig. 2). The ability of an implant to resist subsidence is, in part, related to its design [35]. Subsidence, loss of disc space height, and angular deformity are also related to the position of the implants within the disc space [17, 31].

Interbody fusion can only be determined to be complete if there is no change in the alignment of the spine at the instrumented fusion site for a minimum of

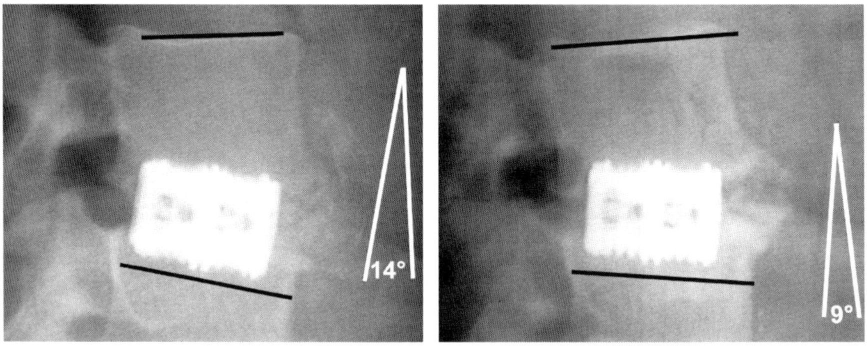

a b

Fig. 2. ***a*** Standing lateral radiograph at 6 weeks after surgery. Segmental lordosis at L4–L5 measures 14° and the implant rests on the cortical margin of the adjacent vertebral end plate. ***b*** At 18 months after surgery, the segmental lordosis is reduced to 9° and the implant has subsided through the vertebral end plate. Anterior radial osteophytes have formed.

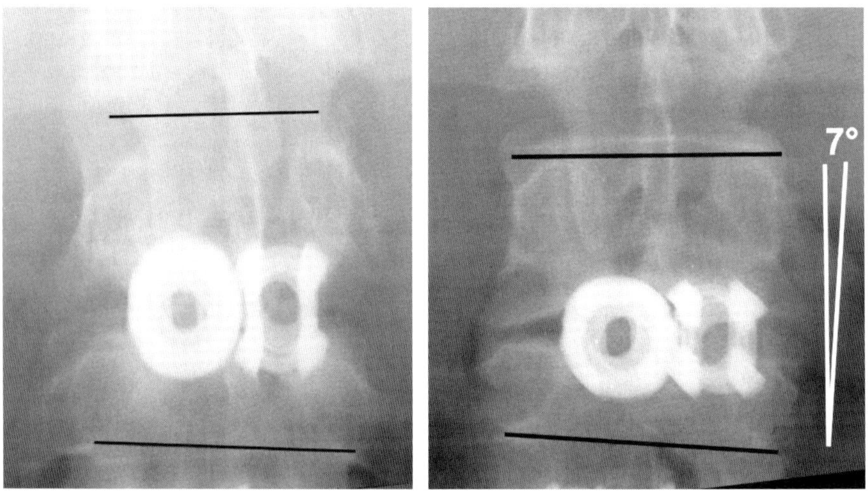

a b

Fig. 3. ***a*** Standing anteroposterior radiographs at 3 months after surgery show no significant frontal plane deformity. ***b*** Standing anteroposterior radiograph at 1 year after surgery shows a 7° angular deformity across the instrumented interspace.

6 months. Standing anteroposterior and lateral radiographic views must show no significant change in segmental lordosis (≤3°), sagittal translation (≤5 mm), or frontal plane angulation (≤3°) on sequential radiographs taken at least 6 months apart. Interbody fusion cannot be considered intact if there are progressive changes in any frontal or sagittal plane angular or translational measurements (fig. 3).

Segmental Spinal Stabilization

Subtle changes in the lumbar contours can be identified on dynamic lateral radiographs; changes in segmental lordosis and sagittal plane translation can be identified on these studies. Incorporating known measurement error, criteria for fusion on dynamic radiographic studies include angular motion of 3° or less and reduction in sagittal plane or frontal plane translation of 5 mm or less. The documentation of persistent motion across a fused motion segment has led some clinicians and researchers to conclude that the error in measuring dynamic plane radiographs often precludes an accurate determination of fusion.

Device-Bone Interface

The host bone reaction to an interbody fusion device helps to ascertain fusion. Although the composition and shape of the implant influence the region around the device, the host bone reaction to the implant remains an important aspect of determining fusion. The presence of sclerosis or cystic radiolucencies on the margins of the implant within the subchondral bone can result from bony reabsorption and fibrosis tissue reaction secondary micromotion in the presence of a pseudarthrosis. Radiolucency surrounding the implants represents the interposition of fibrous tissue at the host bone-implant interface. It is commonly agreed that this is also a sign of micromotion and instability. End plate sclerosis that extends through the subchondral bone and alters the trabecular pattern of the vertebral body is also consistent with micromotion and pseudarthrosis. Plain radiographs, dynamic extension radiographs, and thin-cut CT scans are helpful in assessing the device-bone interface. These changes can be seen on plain radiographs but are best detailed on thin-cut CT scans.

Progressive collapse of the interspace and migration of implants are gross radiographic signs of instability, delayed union, and pseudarthrosis. Plain radiographs can also identify migration and subsidence of the implants within the disc space. Dynamic lateral extension radiographs help to identify subtle patterns of motion at the disc space and can help to identify interface lucencies. If a fusion is not present, hyperextension lateral radiographs can increase the gap between the implant and host bone. This gap appears as increased radiolucency surrounding the implant or may appear as a gap in the anterior fusion mass.

Thin-cut CT scans are best at detailing cystic changes within the vertebral end plates, sclerosis, and interface lucency. Heithoff et al. [10] found CT scans of little value in assessing fusion for the first-generation BAK cages. It is difficult to assess for fusion in patients with the thick-walled and square-threaded BAK cage because of the radiographic scatter inherently associated with its

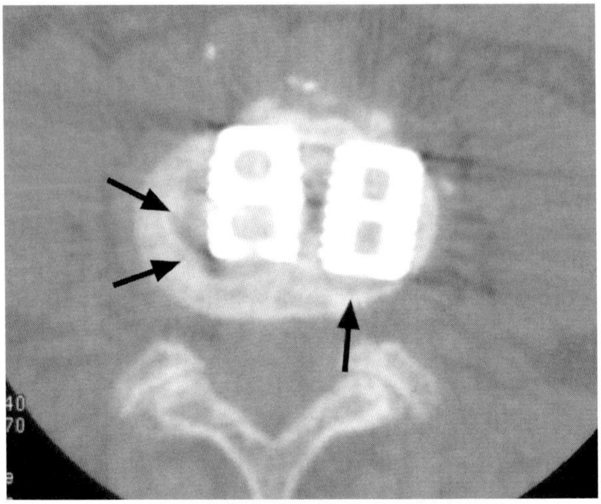

Fig. 4. Axial CT scan at the device-bone interface shows lucent lines surrounding the contact points of the implant and the host bone.

design. However, end plate sclerosis and the presence of cyst formation within the end plate adjacent to the implants can be readily determined even on these first-generation implants (fig. 4). The interface between the host bone and titanium implants can be more easily assessed with second-generation cages such as the INTER FIX™ (Medtronic Sofamor Danek, Memphis, Tenn., USA) and LT-Cage™ (Medtronic Sofamor Danek). The thread patterns on these cages are self-tapping and thinner than on earlier devices. The radiographic scatter and artifact are reduced. With the second-generation cages, it is possible to assess the interface between the implant and the host bone for the development of fibrous lucency.

The assessment of interbody fusion with cortical allografts must include incorporation of the graft materials in addition to the morcellized autogenous grafts. Complete fusion of an allograft-autograft montage must include incorporation of the allograft into both vertebral end plates and trabecular bone formation across the interspace [22, 36]. With threaded cylindrical bone dowels and femoral rings, it is possible to determine incorporation of the allograft to end plates of the host vertebra. On plain radiographs and CT scans, it is common to find early trabecular bone formation crossing the interspace. In the presence of spanning trabecular bone formation around the implant, there is often incorporation of the allograft to only one vertebral end plate. The lucencies surrounding the contact points of the allograft to one end plate often resolve over time [34, 37, 38]. They are commonly present at 1 year after surgery and do not

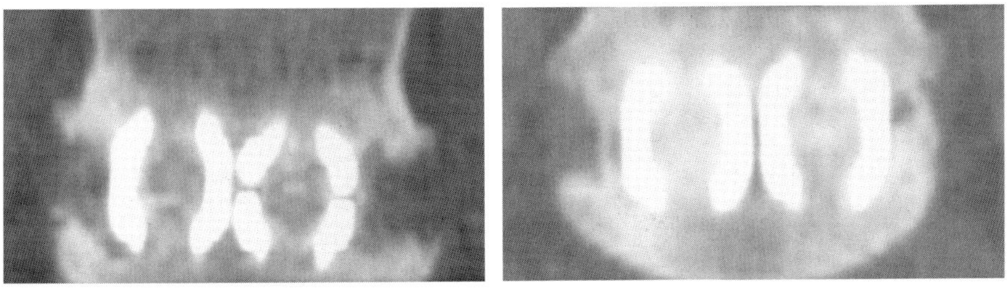

a b

Fig. 5. ***a*** Coronal CT scan reconstruction immediately after interbody surgery with LT-Cage devices and autogenous grafts shows the cages are well seated within the L5–S1 disc space. There are autogenous bone grafts within the cages; no grafts were placed lateral to the cages. ***b*** Coronal CT scan reconstruction at 1 year after surgery shows maturation of grafts with the cages and new bone formation outside of the cages and within the confines of the disc space in the lateral fusion zones.

resolve until 2–3 years after surgery. These unilateral lucencies on dynamic plain radiographs are not associated with poor clinical outcomes, subsidence, or instability. However, they do represent incomplete incorporation and fusion of the allograft.

New Bone Formation and Bone Remodeling

New bone formation and bone remodeling in and around interbody fusion cages can be assessed radiographically. Carbon fiber implants and cortical allografts are readily assessed radiographically. The ability to assess bone formation around titanium implants depends, in part, on the size of the implant, the configuration of the implant, and the porosity of the implant. The first-generation BAK implant is thick-walled and square-threaded. It also has two small openings that are bordered by an internal strut for driving the implant. The configuration of this thick-walled titanium implant is not conducive to radiographic visualization of bone graft within or immediately adjacent to the cage. Second generation titanium implants produce significantly less scatter and artifact on plain radiographs and CT scans. The LT-Cage, INTER FIX and Ray TFC™ (Surgical Dynamics, Norwalk, Conn., USA) fusion cages [10] are hollow, fenestrated cylinders with no internal driving device. These cages are significantly more porous and their thread patterns are also not square and do not produce as much scatter (fig. 5).

The appearance of bone within an interbody fusion cage is not always indicative of a fusion after surgery using autograft. CT scanning cannot be used to distinguish between unincorporated necrotic bone present in the cage and new trabecular bone formation. Identification of new bone formation outside

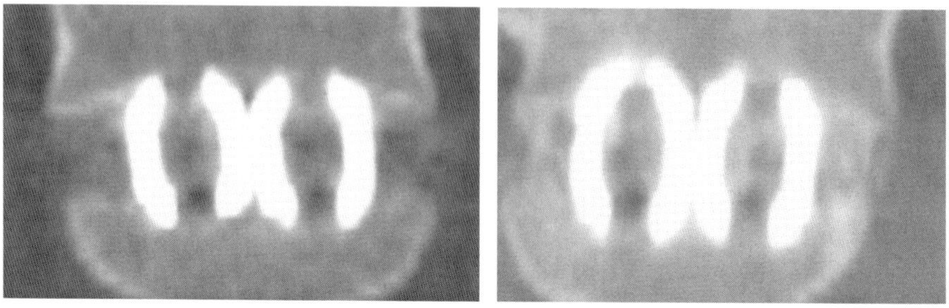

a b

Fig. 6. ***a*** Coronal CT scan reconstruction shows two LT-Cage devices centrally placed in the L5–S1 disc space 48 h after surgery. The cages were filled with InFUSE bone graft substitute (rhBMP-2 and an absorbable collagen sponge). No autogenous grafts were placed within the disc space or cage. ***b*** At 1 year after surgery, there is new formation within both cages. There is also new bone formation outside the cages in the lateral fusion zones. All new bone formation remains confined to the disc space.

the cages in an area where no bone graft was placed is the most important radiographic sign indicating fusion. Similarly, identification of annular ossification and bridging osteophytes crossing a disc space are secondary signs of new bone formation after a successful interbody fusion.

Recombinant Human Bone Morphogenetic Protein-2

Assessing new bone formation after interbody surgery with InFUSE™ Bone Graft (Medtronic Sofamor Danek) substitute does not have the inherent limitations of differentiating between de novo new bone formation and residual necrotic bone. InFUSE is recombinant human bone morphogenetic protein (rhBMP-2) applied to an absorbable collagen sponge. Its use replaces the need for autogenous bone grafts and eliminates the complications associated with iliac crest graft harvesting. In animal experimental models and in all human studies, InFUSE has been used without any autogenous or autologous grafts [24–27, 39].

In a prospective human study, osteoinduction after lumbar interbody surgery was shown to occur with the use of InFUSE [25, 26]. These early findings were confirmed in a larger study involving 143 treated with InFUSE [27]. New bone formation occurred in all patients treated with the LT-Cage and InFUSE (rhBMP-2). The overall fusion rate at 24 months was greater than 94% in these patients. In a smaller sample of these rhBMP-2-treated patients, bone formation, as evidenced by progressive density on thin-cut CT scans, almost doubled within 6 months of surgery and increased almost 2.5 times by 24 months [26] (fig. 6). Similar to the bone formation within the cages, new

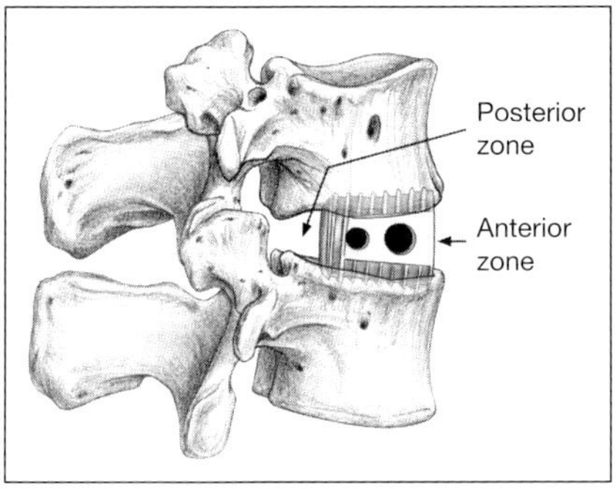

Fig. 7. Anterior and posterior fusion zones.

bone formation had occurred outside of the cages in the rhBMP-2 group by 6 months after surgery, and it occurred in all patients by 24 months [26, 27]. New bone formation within the cages occurred most markedly during the first 6–12 months after surgery; rates of new bone formation exceeded those of the autograft control group. All new bone formation outside of the cages occurred within the confines of the disc space. All CT scan slices and all reconstructed images were studied to evaluate new bone formation. No new bone formation extended outside of the annulus fibrosus; no bone growth was observed extending posteriorly into the spinal canal or posterolaterally into the neuroforamina.

Fusion Zones

New bone formation in a region or zone of the interspace that is free of autogenous graft or growth factors represents osteoinduction within the soft tissue elements of the spinal motion segment. Identifying osteoinduction within the disc space is the most accurate means of determining fusion after an ALIF procedure. New bone formation only occurs in a spinal motion segment that is adequately stabilized and, therefore, represents a fused motion segment. Five fusion zones have been established for interbody fusion devices. The zones of fusion can be assessed on plain radiographs and CT scans.

The anterior zone is an area of bone formation in front of the cages along the anterior margins of the disc space (fig. 7). Bone formation in this zone is the least reliable indication of interbody fusion. The formation of radial osteophytes, which is indicative of instability, often masquerades as an early 'sentinel sign'. On the basis of anterior bone formation alone, it is impossible to tell if it is a good sign or a bad sign. For a fusion to be present, trabecular bone

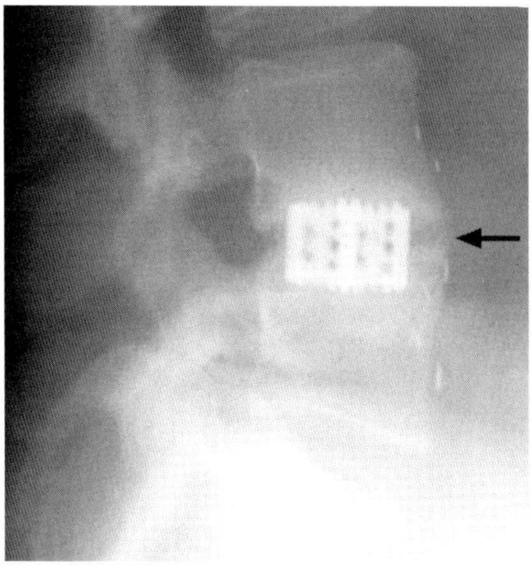

Fig. 8. Lateral plain radiograph shows bone anterior to the cage within the L4–L5 disc space. There has been significant subsidence of the device through the L5 end plate. This sentinel sign does not represent a fusion.

formation in the anterior zone must be complete from end plate to end plate. Bone formation that extends past the confines of the disc space can be an early indication of a developing pseudarthrosis (fig. 8). Frequently the sentinel sign represents radial bone spur formation, not interbody fusion. The isolated sentinel sign may indicate progressive instability instead of progressive fusion.

The posterior zone is the posterior margin of the interspace (see fig. 7). Trabecular bone formation in this zone is most likely the best radiographic indication of interbody fusion. Bone formation in the posterior zone is the most reliable indication of fusion.

The lateral zone or the lateral margins of the disc space are divided into left and right regions (fig. 9). Bone formation between the lateral borders of the implants and the annulus is difficult to visualize on plain radiographs. On anteroposterior and Ferguson views at the L4–5 and L5–S1 interspace, the posterior facet joints overlie the lateral fusion zones and early bone formation in the lateral zone on these plain radiographs. CT scans are essential in visualizing early trabecular bone formation in the lateral zones (fig. 10). Only the final stages of ossification of the annulus fibrosus are apparent on plain anteroposterior radiographs. Bone formation in these zones is also a very good predictor of fusion and typically occurs here before it does in the posterior zone. Bone formation with the two lateral zones is often asymmetric; this may be related to asymmetric cage placement.

The between zone is the area of bone formation between the implants (fig. 9, 11). Bone formation in this zone is best visualized with thin-cut CT scans and in those patients where the implants have been adequately spaced away from each other.

9 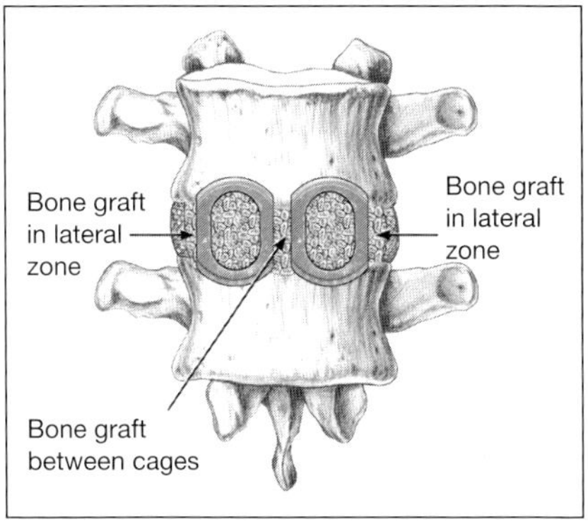

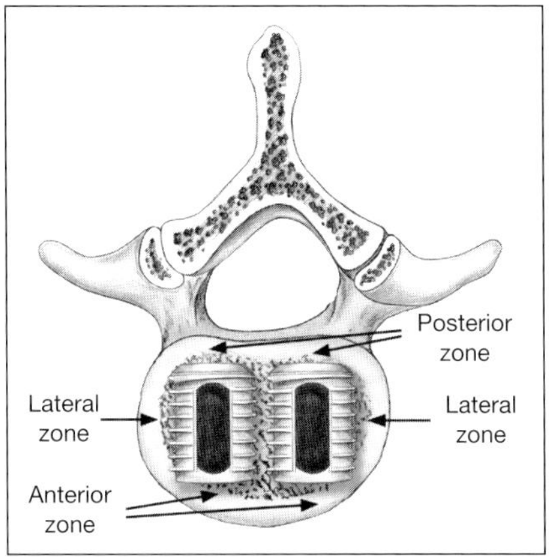 10

Fig. 9. Anteroposterior view of the lateral zones and the between zone. The interbody fusion cages are placed equidistant from the midline of the disc space. However, there is space between the cage walls and the annulus fibrosus that compromises new bone formation in the lateral zone.

Fig. 10. Drawing of an axial CT scan shows the position of the anterior, posterior, and lateral zones.

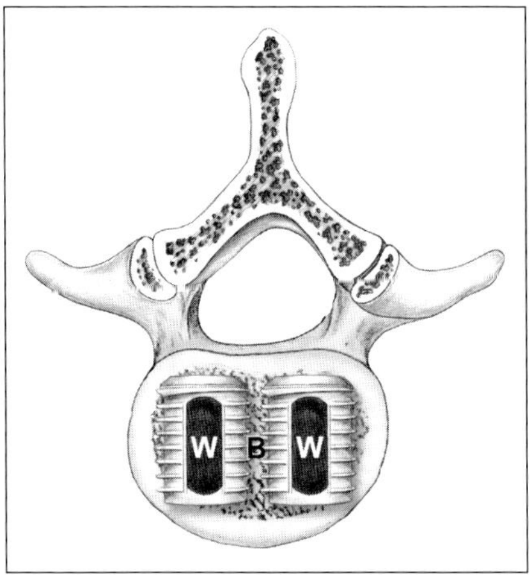

Fig. 11. Drawing of an axial CT scan highlights the within (W) and between (B) zones.

The within zone is the area of bone formation within the interbody fusion device (fig. 9, 11). It is very difficult to differentiate between living and dead bone within the cages. The size, configuration, and material of the cages also significantly influence the ability to accurately assess bone formation in this zone. Assessment of bone formation is not practical with a single CT scan. It is best assessed over time with serial CT scans.

Conclusion

Radiographic criteria have been established to reliably assess fusion after ALIF with threaded and impacted implants and for titanium, carbon fiber, and allograft devices. Determination of fusion involves the radiographic evaluation of spinal alignment, stabilization of the spinal motion segment dynamic studies, assessment of the device-host interface, and identification of new bone formation and bone remodeling. Each of the fusion criteria must be met to ensure that an arthrodesis is complete.

Changes in the sagittal or frontal plane contours over time indicate a delayed fusion. Progressive subsidence or any change in sagittal or frontal plane contours also represents a failed fusion. A fusion can be considered intact if there is no change in spinal alignment within the spinal motion segment over a 6-month period.

Dynamic radiographic studies must be obtained in a manner that applies stress to the instrumented spinal motion segment and in a manner that can be successfully replicated on serial radiographs. The pelvis must be stabilized and radiographs must be taken parallel to the vertebral end plates. A fusion is considered intact only if there is no significant motion on dynamic studies.

Changes in or the appearance of lucencies at the implant-end plate interface are indicative of a failed fusion. Second-generation cages permit a closer evaluation of the device-bone interface. The development of cystic or sclerotic changes within the subchondral bone of the vertebral end plates is suggestive of a fusion failure. If a pseudarthrosis is present, hyperextension lateral radiographs frequently highlight radiolucencies at the device-bone interface and can identify a gap within an anterior 'sentinel fusion'.

The formation of new bone adjacent to or within the intradiscal implants is the most reliable finding for establishing fusion. New bone formation occurs outside the intradiscal implants when fusion has occurred. New bone formation within the lateral and posterior zone is the most reliable radiographic indication of a fusion. Remodeling of autogenous grafts or allografts is also consistent with an intact fusion.

References

1 Frymoyer JW, Hanley EN Jr, Howe J, Kuhlmann D, Matteri RE: A comparison of radiographic findings in fusion and nonfusion patients ten or more years following lumbar disc surgery. Spine 1979;4:435–440.

2 Weiner BK, Fraser RD: Spine update: Lumbar interbody cages. Spine 1998;23:634–640.

3 Crock HV: Anterior lumbar interbody fusion: Indications for its use and notes on surgical technique. Clin Orthop 1982;165:157–163.

4 Harmon PH: Anterior excision and vertebral body fusion operation for intervertebral disc syndromes of the lower lumbar spine. Clin Orthop 1963;26:107–127.
5 Kuslich SD, Ulstrom CL, Griffith SL, Ahern JW, Dowdle JD: The Bagby and Kuslich method of lumbar interbody fusion. History, techniques, and 2-year follow-up results of a United States prospective, multicenter trial. Spine 1998;23:1267–1278.
6 Lane JD, Moore ES: Transperitoneal approach to the intervertebral disc in the lumbar area. Ann Surg 1948;127:537–551.
7 Ray CD: Threaded titanium cages for lumbar interbody fusions. Spine 1997;22:667–679.
8 Cizek GR, Boyd LM: Imaging pitfalls of interbody spinal implants. Spine 2000;25:2633–2636.
9 Djukic S, Lang P, Hoaglund F, Genant HK: The postoperative spine. Magnetic resonance imaging. Orthop Clin North Am 1990;21:603–624.
10 Heithoff KB, Mullin JW, Holte D, Renfrew DL, Gilbert TJ: Failure of radiographic detection of pseudarthrosis in patients with titanium lumbar interbody fusion cages. Proceedings of the 14th Annual Meeting North American Spine Society, Chicago, 1999, pp 14–17.
11 Kant AP, Daum WJ, Dean SM, Uchida T: Evaluation of lumbar spine fusion. Plain radiographs versus direct surgical exploration and observation. Spine 1995;20:2313–2317.
12 Sandhu HS, Toth JM, Diwan AD, Seim HB 3rd, Kanim LE, Kabo JM, Turner AS: Histologic evaluation of efficacy of rhBMP-2 compared with autograft bone in sheep spinal anterior interbody fusion. Spine 2002;27:567–575.
13 Steinmann JC, Herkowitz HN: Pseudarthrosis of the spine. Clin Orthop 1992;284:80–90.
14 Watkins R: Anterior lumbar interbody fusion surgical complications. Clin Orthop 1992;284:47–53.
15 Burkus JK, Foley K, Haid R, LeHuec JC: Radiographic assessment of interbody fusion devices: Fusion criteria for anterior lumbar interbody surgery. Surgical Interbody Research Group. Neurosurg Focus 2001;10/4:1–9.
16 Hannon KM, Wetta WJ: Failure of technetium bone scanning to detect pseudarthroses in spinal fusion for scoliosis. Clin Orthop 1977;123:42–44.
17 Gilbert TJ, Heithoff KB, Mullin WJ: Radiographic assessment of cage-assisted interbody fusions in the lumbar spine. Semin Spine Surg 2001;13/4:311–315.
18 Brantigan JW: Carbon fiber interbody fusion cages: Indications, results and radiographic interpretation of fusion. Spine State Art Rev 1997;11:287–306.
19 Zdeblick TA: A prospective randomized study of lumbar fusion. Preliminary results. Spine 1993; 18:983–991.
20 Pearcy M, Burrough S: Assessment of bony union after interbody fusion of the lumbar spine using a biplanar radiographic technique. J Bone Joint Surg Br 1982;64:228–232.
21 Heggeness MH, Esses SI: Classification of pseudarthroses of the lumbar spine. Spine 1991; 16(suppl):S449–S454.
22 Rothman SL, Glenn WV Jr: CT evaluation of interbody fusion. Clin Orthop 1985;193:47–56.
23 Siambanes D, Mather S: Comparison of plain radiographs and CT scans in instrumented posterior lumbar interbody fusion. Orthopedics 1998;21:165–167.
24 Boden SD, Martin GJ Jr, Horton WC, Truss TL, Sandhu HS: Laproscopic anterior spinal arthrodesis with rhBMP-2 in titanium interbody threaded cage. J Spinal Disord 1998;11:95–101.
25 Boden SD, Zdeblick TA, Sandhu HS, Heim SE: The use of rhBMP-2 in interbody fusion cages. Definitive evidence of osteoinduction in humans: A preliminary report. Spine 2000;25:376–381.
26 Burkus JK, Dorchak JD, Sanders DL: Prospective randomized study of radiographic assessment of interbody fusion using rhBMP-2. Proceedings of the 16th Annual Meeting North American Spine Society, Seattle, 2001, p 98.
27 Gornet M, Burkus JK, Dickman C, Zdeblick TA: RhBMP-2 with tapered cages: A prospective, randomized lumbar fusion study. Proceedings of the 16th Annual Meeting North American Spine Society, Seattle, 2001, pp 21–22.
28 Cunningham BW, Kanayama M, Parker LM, Weis JC, Sefter JC, Fedder IL, McAfee PC: Osteogenic protein versus autologous interbody arthrodesis in the sheep thoracic spine: A comparative endoscopic study using the Bagby and Kuslich interbody fusion device. Spine 1999;24:509–518.
29 McAfee PC: Interbody fusion cages in reconstructive operations on the spine. J Bone Joint Surg Am 1999;81:859–880.

30 McAfee PC, Boden SD, Brantigan JW, Fraser RD, Kuslich SD, Oxland TR, Panjabi MM, Ray CD, Zdeblick TA: Symposium: A critical discrepancy: A criteria of successful arthrodesis following interbody fusions. Spine 2001;26:320–334.
31 McAfee PC, Cunningham, Lee GA, Orbegoso CM, Haggerty CJ, Fedder IL, Griffith SL: Revision strategies for salvaging or improving failed cylindrical cages. Spine 1999;24:2147–2153.
32 Dennis S, Watkins R, Landaker S, Dillin W, Springer D: Comparison of disc space heights after anterior lumbar interbody fusion. Spine 1989;14:876–878.
33 Dorchak JD, Burkus JK, Foor BD, Sanders DL: Dual paired proximity and combined BAK/proximity interbody fusion cages: Radiographic results. Proceedings of the 15th Annual Meeting North American Spine Society, New Orleans, 2000, pp 83–85.
34 Kumar A, Kozak JA, Doherty BJ, Dickson JH: Interspace distraction and graft subsidence after anterior lumbar fusion with femoral strut allograft. Spine 1993;18:2393–2400.
35 Burkus JK, Dorchak JD, Estes BT, et al: Subsidence evaluation of reduced lateral profile threaded constructs. 7th International Meeting on Advanced Spine Techniques, Barcelona, 2000.
36 Wimmer C, Krismer M, Gluch H, Ogon M, Stockl B: Autogenic versus allogenic bone grafts in anterior lumbar interbody fusion. Clin Orthop 1999;360:122–126.
37 Flynn JC, Hoque MA: Anterior fusion of the lumbar spine. End-result study with long-term follow-up. J Bone Joint Surg Am 1979;61:1143–1150.
38 Sacks S: Anterior interbody fusion of the lumbar spine. Indications and results in 200 cases. Clin Orthop 1966;44:163–170.
39 Zdeblick TA Ghanayem AJ, Rapoff AJ, Swain C, Bassett T, Cooke ME, Markel M: Cervical interbody fusion cages: An animal model with and without bone morphogenetic protein. Spine 1998; 23:758–765.

J. K. Burkus, MD
The Hughston Clinic
PC, 6262 Veterans Parkway, Columbus, GA 31909 (USA)
Tel. +1 706 576 3239, Fax +1 706 571 2502, E-Mail jkb66@knology.net

Haid RW Jr, Subach BR, Rodts GE Jr (eds): Advances in Spinal Stabilization.
Prog Neurol Surg. Basel, Karger, 2003, vol 16, pp 71–83

Overview of Spinal Navigation

Mark R. McLaughlin, Juan Bartolomei

Neuro-Group, PA, Lawrenceville, N.J., USA

An important advance in spinal surgery has been the development and application of image-guided techniques for spinal navigation and fixation. Image-guided technology includes both spinal stereotaxis as well as fluoroscopy-based image guidance systems. Both of these techniques offer significant advantages over commonly used plain radiography and fluoroscopy for complex spine procedures. Image-guided spine surgery has been utilized for cervical, thoracic, and lumbar fixation [1, 3–5, 7, 9–11, 13, 15–17, 19–22, 24, 28, 31, 34, 35]. This chapter will highlight the newest techniques in image-guided spine surgery and discuss their advantages and nuances compared to standard open techniques.

Unreliability of Intraoperative Radiography

Traditionally, intraoperative image guidance in spine surgery was directed primarily by plain radiography and fluoroscopy. Although these conventional imaging techniques offer surgeons better visualization compared with simple open exposure and recognition of the anatomy, they still have a limited accuracy [6, 7, 14, 23, 27, 29, 35]. Intraoperative plain films and fluoroscopy lack a three-dimensional (3-D) perspective of the anatomy. In addition, imaging in the thoracic region with these two techniques is problematic related to the rib cage and difficulty in localizing the appropriate level. Berlemann et al. [2] found that only 41% of 119 thoracolumbar pedicle screws were accurately placed with plain radiography at the time of surgery. Weinstein et al. [33] found a 21% failure rate in pedicle screw placement in a cadaver study. He found that success was independent of experience or approach and that 92% of the failures were cortical perforations within the spinal canal. Odgers et al. [23] reviewed a series of 72 patients undergoing placement of pedicle screws utilizing plain radiography for image guidance. Out of a total of 238 pedicle screw placements, 24 penetrated the pedicle wall and 2 resulted in neurological injury. Other studies have also documented a significant incidence of pedicle violation with standard techniques [6, 18, 29]. Anatomical variations have been described within the cervical spine that suggest image guidance may improve accuracy of screw placement [13, 17, 18, 26, 30, 34].

Numerous techniques have been described attempting to increase the accuracy of pedicle screw placement. These include open laminar techniques, evoked and spontaneous EMG potentials to record pedicle wall breakthrough, and intrapedicular or epidural endoscopy [8, 12]. Each of these techniques has significant limitations. Although intuitively open laminar techniques seem to the safest method of placing pedicle screws, there are various anatomical anomalies that sometimes can mislead a surgeon. In addition, optimal screw trajectory is difficult to predict based solely on anatomy. Evoked and spontaneous EMG potentials have been utilized to determine pedicle wall breakthrough; however, this technique presents information to the surgeon after potential neurological injury has occurred. Intrapedicular or epidural endoscopy is problematic primarily in the thoracic spine region given the small epidural space and presence of thoracic spine cord.

Image-Guided Technology

There are multiple advantages of image guidance in complex spine surgery. This technology can determine preoperatively the feasibility of performing certain difficult spinal instrumentation procedures and can assist the surgeon in navigating surgical instruments intraoperatively in real time. This technology can improve accuracy in the placement of spinal instrumentation minimizing the risk of neurological and vascular injury. In addition to reducing potential complications, there is an added advantage of achieving optimal bone purchase at each instrumented level. Once the surgeon and operating room team are familiar with the use of image-guided techniques, operating time can be reduced compared with other conventional technologies. Lastly, intraoperative exposure of patient and surgeon to ionizing radiation can be reduced or eliminated depending on the technique used [25].

Spinal Stereotaxis

The steps involved in utilizing spinal stereotaxis include both preoperative data acquisition and correlation of this data with the intraoperative field. First, a preoperative CT or MRI scan is obtained with 1-mm slices at a single

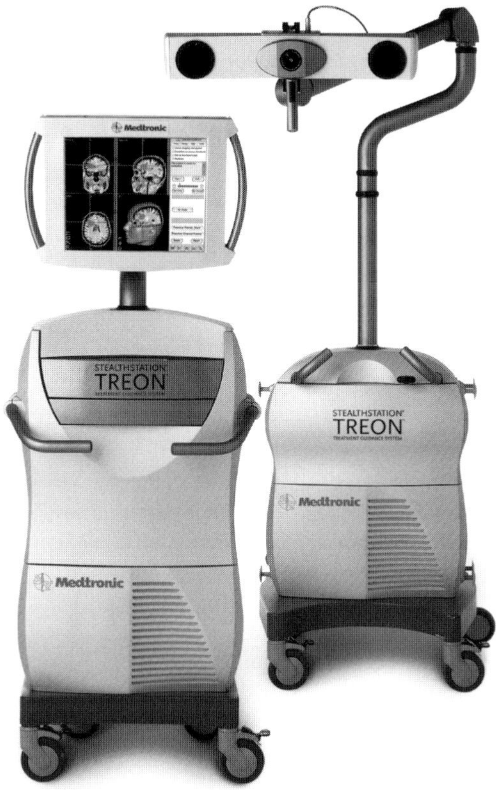

Fig. 1. The Stealthstation (Medtronic Sofamor Danek) includes a high-powered computer and high-resolution monitor. The display generates triplanar images and a 3-D model of the patient's spine. After registration, the digitized instruments are passed through the operative field and are displayed on the monitor.

gantry angle. Although the patient is in a prone position during surgery, a preoperative data set is obtained while the patient is in the supine position. Although there are slight differences in position, these are not quantifiably significant with the exception of cases of severe instability. Respiratory variation during scanning or surgery is not relevant to the navigation accuracy either [10, 11, 26]. Once the data set has been acquired, a 3-D model is built on the computer (fig. 1).

The patient is positioned in a standard fashion for surgery, adequate exposure is obtained and the reference arc is then firmly attached to a spinous

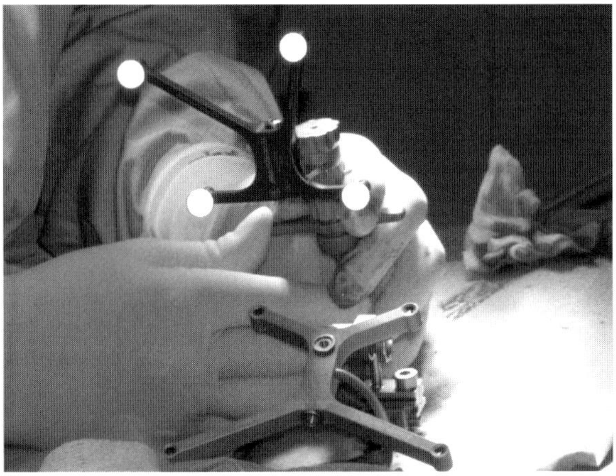

Fig. 2. The reference arc is attached firmly to one of the spinous processes exposed in the operative field. Theoretically the arc should be attached at each vertebral level being registered and instrumented. We have found for short segment fixation that only one level registration yields clinically relevant accuracy.

process (fig. 2). It has been our experience that the spinous process is the most secure and reliable landmark for anchoring the reference arch. The arc should be placed at each vertebral level being registered and instrumented. At L5, S1 it is useful to place the reference arc on the sacral spinous process with the angled arch toward the feet. This allows for free movement of the surgeon's hands and instruments without interference of the arc. For upper lumbar and thoracic instrumentation, the arc should be placed pointing cephalad.

Once the reference arc has been secured, it must be visible to the optical camera (fig. 3). The surgeon can then register analogous anatomical points on the computer and on the patient's spine. For registration in the lumbar and thoracic regions specific landmarks include the middle posterior lateral aspect of the transverse process tips bilaterally, the inferior and superior aspect of the spinous process tips, the mamillary tubercles as the base of the transverse processes (when present) (fig. 4).

These points are easily identifiable both on the computer model as well as the patient's spine. Once the reference arc is placed and registration is complete the computer will then verify the location of the patient's spinal anatomy in relation to the operating room with submillimetric precision. Accuracy is confirmed by correlating the patient's anatomy with the computer model. Digitized instruments then can be moved within the operative field and using both passive and active light-admitting diodes (LED). Frameless navigation can be performed. Standard lumbar instrumentation equipment is available and digitized

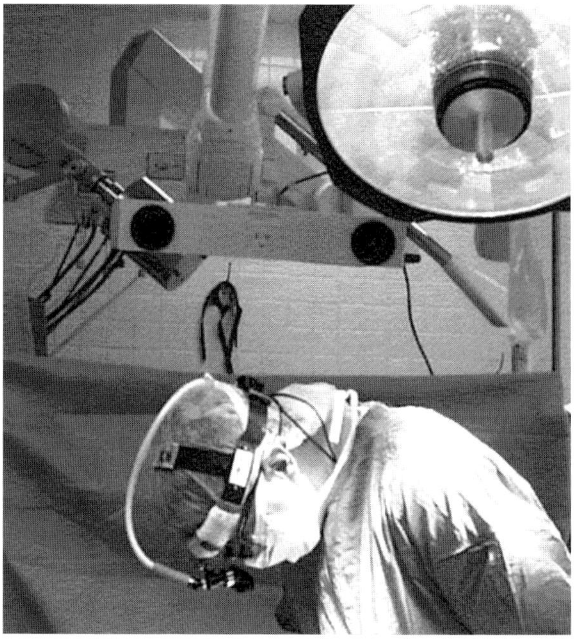

Fig. 3. The optical camera must be positioned approximately 6 ft away from the reference arc. It must have unobstructed views of the LEDs on the reference arc and the digitized instruments.

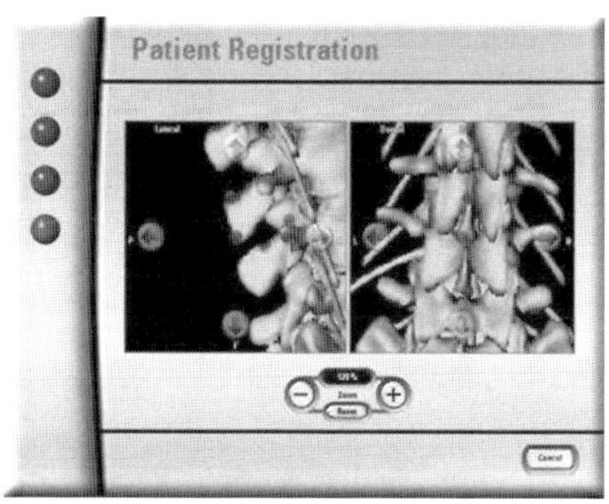

Fig. 4. Registration is carried out by locating homologous points of anatomy between the exposed osseous anatomy and the model generated on the computer workstation. Typically the spinous processes, transverse processes, and pars intra-articularis can be identified and correlated with the computer-generated model.

including a probe-all drill guide and tap that can contact the spine. With each movement, the surgeon can look on the computer screen and visualize the instruments in relation to the patient's spine. Images are available in the axial, sagittal and coronal planes as well as a 3-D image. This allows the surgeon to see the anatomy in any of the three necessary planes. As an instrument is passed through the surgical field, its position is projected onto the computer screen with this triplanar view.

The advantages of frameless stereotaxis were discussed previously. Instrumentation can be placed more accurately decreasing the risk of vascular and neurological injury. Operating time can be decreased as a result of increased speed of hardware placement. The exposure of surgeon and patient to ionizing radiation is also decreased because there is less need for reliance on traditional imaging techniques such as fluoroscopy or plain films.

Limitations of frameless spinal stereotaxis include the additional cost of obtaining a preoperative CT or MRI scan. Also any significant unexpected movement related to instability at the time of positioning or surgery renders this type of spinal navigation inaccurate. This is because the anatomical relationships will differ from the preoperative data set. If the patient has had prior surgery, potential anatomical landmarks used for registration may not be available. Lastly, any disruption of the reference arc will require re-registration. Complicated multilevel fusions can pose a difficult problem in avoiding any unintended manipulation of the reference arc.

Virtual Fluoroscopy

The introduction of virtual fluoroscopy has offered surgeons several advantages over frameless spinal stereotaxis. Virtual fluoroscopy combines the optical tracking technology of spinal stereotaxis with fluoroscopic images. This technique does not require any preoperative data set acquisition and allows for instantaneous registration of the patient's anatomy. Virtual instruments are then superimposed on standard fluoroscopic images and data sets can be updated instantaneously by simply obtaining a new fluoroscopic image. Imaging studies utilized as anatomic data are obtained from lateral or AP fluoroscopic intraoperative views. Only one or two images are required to obtain a complete data set. The C-arm can then be removed from the field. The FluoroNav system (Medtronic Sofamor Danek, Memphis, Tenn., USA) allows for four images to be displayed simultaneously in navigated computer-generated representations of the digitized instruments (fig. 5). The advantages of utilizing virtual fluoroscopy include minimizing the surgeon's exposure to radiation and eliminating the need for protective aprons. Also, there is an ergonomic benefit being able to stand flush against the table when placing instrumentation rather than uncomfortably leaning against the C-arm. Equipment needed for virtual fluoroscopy includes a C-arm with LED attachments and fiducial array, a computer work station compatible with most stereotactic systems, an optical camera, a reference arc, and digitized instruments (fig. 6).

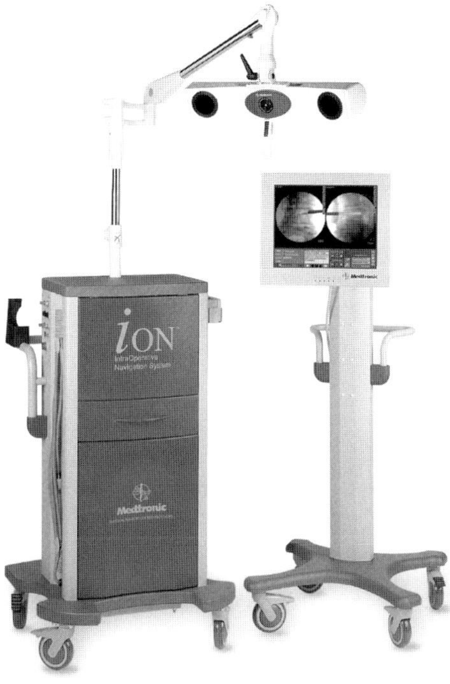

5

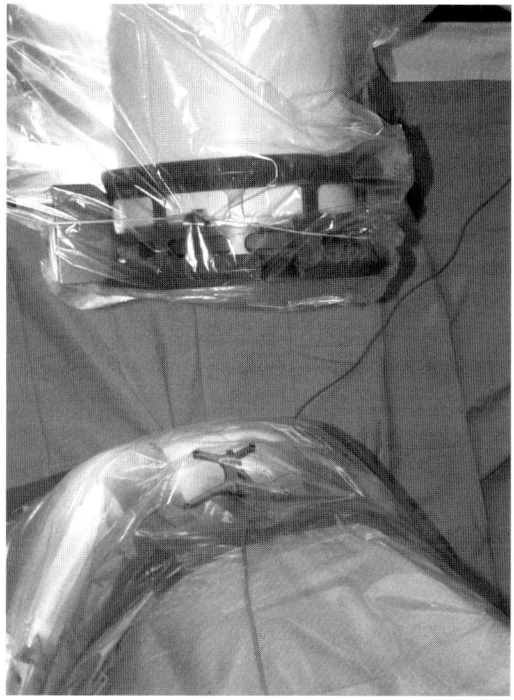

6

Fig. 5. The Fluoronav system (Medtronic Sofamor Danek) includes a workstation with a high-powered computer and a high-resolution monitor, an optical camera, and an attachment with LEDs and fiducial display for the C-arm.

Fig. 6. The C-arm is modified slightly in that a fiducial display is attached to the receiver. This metallic attachment contains LEDs that the optical camera sees to begin the registration process.

Similar to the use of frameless stereotaxis, the patient is positioned in a standard fashion and the relevant anatomy is exposed. Again, the reference arc is attached to the spine, and lateral, AT or oblique fluoroscopic images can be obtained depending on the surgeon's preference. The initial image is demonstrated with an overlaid array of spherical fiducials, which are called the calibration target. The anatomy is then instantaneously registered and the computer combines the known geometry of the calibration target with the fluoroscopic image. Signals are sent from LEDs on the reference arc, instruments, and C-arm to the optical camera, which then transmits this data to the computer. The computer calculates the anatomy of the spine relative to the C-arm. No point for point registration is required.

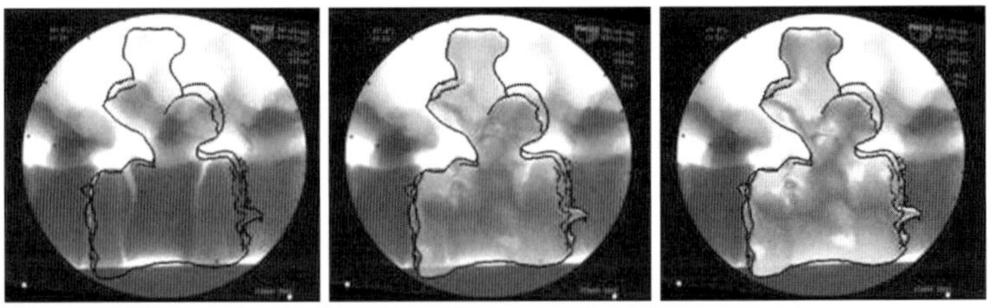

Fig. 7. Fluoro to CT registration. Through computer deformation algorithms, the software merges the selected vertebral body with the fluoroscopic images. This minimizes extensive tissue dissection and it becomes convenient when there are no bony anatomical landmarks (i.e. postlaminectomy) for registration.

The surgeon can choose any instrument needed for pedicle screw placement and a single universal instrument handle is attached. The software system projects to the computer screen a virtual instrument in relation to fluoroscopic image of the spine.

Various instruments can be projected onto the screen. As the instruments move in real time with surgeon manipulation, the changes are replicated instantaneously on the computer screen. The surgeon is thus aware of the depth and specific location of the instrument at all times. Distances such as pedicle length can be calculated and screw angulation for optimal screw trajectory can be determined with simple movements of the hand.

Because virtual fluoroscopy relies on fluoroscopic images, it is most useful in navigating bony anatomy. Tumor resections and soft tissue abnormalities are not suited to virtual fluoroscopy but are best suited for standard frameless stereotaxis. Patients with 3-D or coronal deformities are also unsuitable candidates for virtual fluoroscopy and would be better suited for frameless stereotactic techniques as well.

Another spinal navigational system has recently gained popularity with the advancement in fluoro to CT registration technology in which the two fluoroscopic images are used to noninvasively merge into the preoperative CT image data set (Vector Vision, Brainlab, Germany) (fig. 7). A preoperative CT scan with the standard image-guided protocol is necessary prior to using the fluoro to CT registration technology. This protocol consists of 1-mm axial cuts incorporating one or two levels above and below the area of interest or the surgical field where instrumentation is going to be placed. The images are then transported via ether net or zip drive into the working station where a 3-D image is created. With the 3-D image operative planning can be performed such as identification of entry and target points for pedicle, transarticular, and lateral mass screw insertion or biopsies.

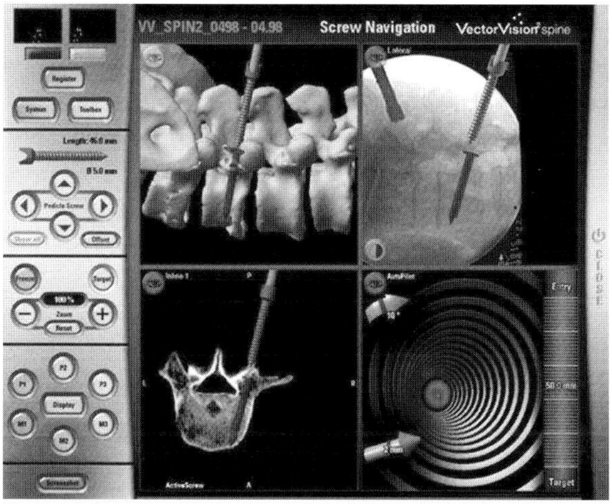

Fig. 8. Computer screen displaying (clockwise) 3-D image, lateral fluoro image, axial CT, and Auto Pilot view while inserting a pedicle screw.

Once the images are transformed into a 3-D rendition, surgical exposure is obtained in a standard fashion and the reference array is clamped to the spinous process. A new device is also available that allows the reference array to be placed anteriorly into the vertebral body if an anterior surgical approach is desired. This has been described previously with other systems [32]. By adjusting the flexible joints, the reference clamp can be positioned without obstructing the surgical field. Once the array is secured AP and lateral fluoroscopic images over the area to be instrumented are obtained. There are three methods for registration. Like other systems there is the paired point registration in which anatomical landmarks are identified and registered on both the spine and on the CT images, and there is the surface matching algorithm in which ten or more points are rapidly collected on the surface of the spine and registered to the CT images. As mentioned above, unique to the Brain Lab system is the fluoro to CT registration.

Fluoro to CT registration is performed by matching on the computer screen the vertebral body of interest in a spine model to the AP and lateral films obtained. Once the vertebral bodies are identified and matched, it takes approximately 5 min for the software to register and have a navigational 3-D image. Once registered, the software allows the surgeon to navigate in 3-D, CT, and fluoro images or a combination of all by adjusting the computer screen (fig. 8).

When targeting a specific end point such as a lesion biopsy or placement of a pedicle screw, the Brain Lab provides a software called Auto Pilot view that

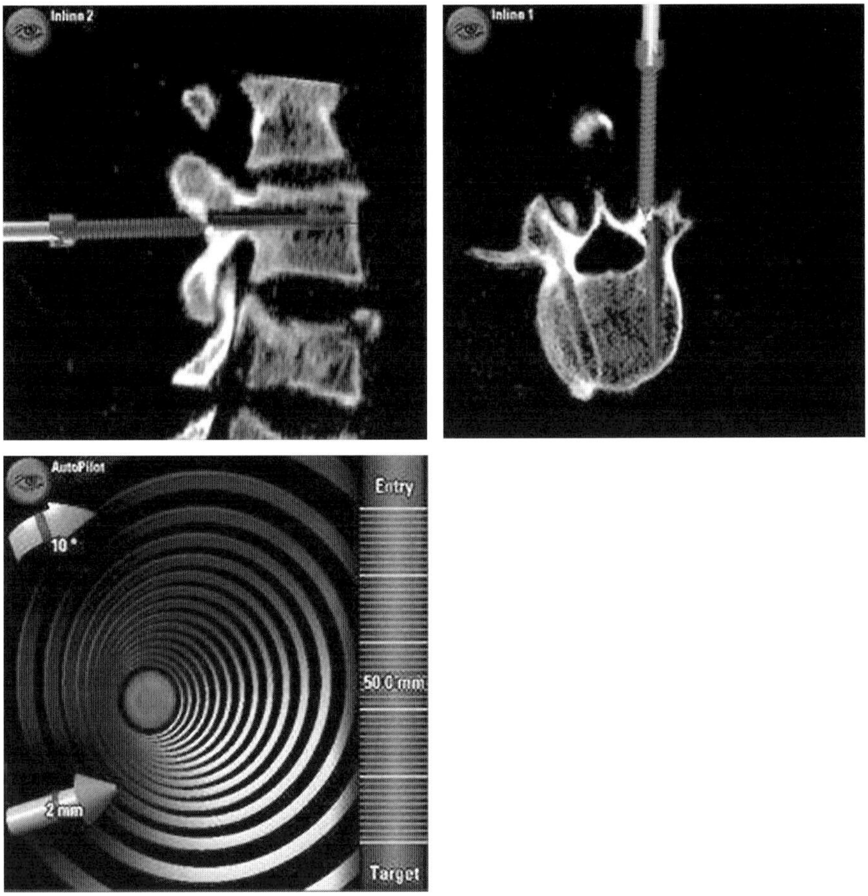

Fig. 9. Auto Pilot view. Concentric circles form a tunnel which provides immediate directional feedback for pedicle screw insertion or biopsy guidance.

enables safe navigation and instant feedback. The tool consists of a series of aligned concentric circles forming a tunnel on a direct path to the target. The first concentric circle is the entry point and the target point is the smallest black circle at the end of the tunnel. If during navigation there are any deviations from the trajectory, the tunnel will curve as the last and first circle become noncongruent. The software provides immediate feedback providing distance to end point or any compensatory changes in direction (i.e. angle) necessary to safely reach the desired target. This tool can be used on difficult cases were the anatomy might be distorted such as in scoliotic patients or when performing percutaneous pedicle screw insertion where visible landmarks are not available (fig. 9).

The Brain Lab system allows the surgeon to adapt any desired instrument into the image-guided field. This is performed by clamping a passive marker array to any instrument (i.e. penfield, pedicle finder, tap, or awl) and inserting the tip of the instrument into the calibration matrix box. This allows any instrument to be utilized during the surgery.

Conclusions

Image-guided spine surgery enhances a surgeon's ability to navigate instruments and spinal instrumentation throughout the entire spine. These techniques not only minimize morbidity related to instrumentation, but also optimize screw purchase, decrease operating time, and minimize patient and surgeon exposure to ionizing radiation. Frameless stereotactic techniques offer certain advantages in the 3-D navigation of the spine. This technology is particularly helpful in the placement of C1,2 transarticular screw fixation and in patients with tumors infiltrating the spinal column. Virtual fluoroscopy, which is a combination of computer-assisted stereotaxis with C-arm fluoroscopic guidance, allows a surgeon to manipulate instruments within a surgical field while viewing a virtual image of the instrument in real time on a computer screen. Both of these techniques represent significant advances in spinal stabilization and will most definitely advance future minimally invasive percutaneous techniques. One remaining challenge in spinal navigation is improving registration accuracy when the spinal alignment is deformed during surgery. Also, severe spinal deformities tend to pose significant obstacles when trying to register the images using fluoroscopy. Innovative advances using fluoro to CT merge registration technology and the 3-D fluoroscopy units appear to provide new horizons for the improvement of real time registration and safe navigation.

References

1 Abdel-Malek K, et al: Bone registration method for robot assisted surgery: Pedicle screw insertion. Proc Inst Mech Eng 1997;211/3:221–233.

2 Berlemann U, et al: Reliability of pedicle screw assessment utilizing plain radiographs versus CT reconstruction. Eur Spine J 1997;6:406–410.

3 Bolger C, Wigfield C: Image-guided surgery: Applications to the cervical and thoracic spine and a review of the first 120 procedures. J Neurosurg 2000;92:175–180.

4 Brodwater BK, Roberts DW, Nakajima T, Friets EM, Strohbehn JW: Extracranial application of the frameless stereotactic operating microscope: Experience with lumbar spine. Neurosurgery 1993;32/2:209–213.

5 Carl AL, et al: In vitro simulation. Early results of stereotaxy for pedicle screw placement. Spine 1997;22:1160–1164.

6 Castro WH, Halm H, Jerosch J, Malms J, Steinbeck J, Blasius S: Accuracy of pedicle screw placement in lumbar vertebrae. Spine 1996;21:1320–1324.

7 Cinotti G, et al: Pedicle instrumentation in the thoracic spine. A morphometric and cadaveric study for placement of screws. Spine 1999;24/2:114–119.

8 Clements DH, et al: Evoked and spontaneous electromyography to evaluate lumbosacral pedicle screw placement. Spine 1996;21:600–604.

9 Foley KT, Rampersaud YR: Stereotactic image guidance of cervical spine lateral mass fixation. Tech Neurosurg 1999;5/2:95–100.

10 Foley KT, Smith KR, Bucholz RD: Stereotactic applications in spine surgery. Contemporary Update on Disorders of the Spine, Snowbird, 1994.

11 Foley KT, Smith MM: Image-guided spine surgery. Neursurg Clin N Am 1996;7/2:171–186.

12 Frank EH, Chamberland DL: An endoscopic pedicle probe: Preliminary development. Neurol Res 1997;6:657–661.

13 Glossop ND, Hu RW, Randle JA: Computer-aided pedicle screw placement using frameless stereotaxis. Spine 1996;21:2026–2034.

14 Heller JG, Carlson GD, Abitol JJ, Garfin SR: Anatomic comparison of the Roy-Camille and Magerl techniques for screw placement in the lower cervical spine. Spine 1991;16: S552–S557.

15 Kalfas J, Kormos D, Murphy M, et al: Application of frameless stereotaxy to pedicle screw fixation of the spine. J Neurosurg 1995;83:641–647.

16 Kim KD, et al: Universal calibration of surgical instruments for spinal stereotaxy. Neurosurgery 1999;44:173–177.

17 Laine T, et al: Improved accuracy of pedicle screw insertion with computer-assisted surgery. A prospective clinical trial of 30 patients. Spine 1997;22:1254–1258.

18 Laine T, Lund T, Ylikoski M, Lohikoski J, Schlenzka D: Accuracy of pedicle screw insertion with and without computer assistance: A randomized controlled clinical study in 100 consecutive patients. Eur Spine J 2000;9:235–240.

19 Ludwig SC, et al: Transpedicle screw fixation of the cervical spine. Clin Orthop 1999;359: 77–88.

20 Merloz P, Tonetti J, Pillet L: Pedicle screw placement using image-guided techniques. Clin Orthop 1998;354:39–48.

21 Nolte L, et al: Image-guided computer-assisted spine surgery: A pilot study on pedicle screw fixation. Stereotact Funct Neurosurg 1996;66/1–2:108–117.

22 Nolte LP, Zamorano LJ, Jiang Z, Wang Q, Langlotz F, Berlemann U: Image-guided insertion of transpedicular screws: A laboratory set-up. Spine 1995;20:497–500.

23 Odgers CJ, et al: Accuracy of pedicle screw placement with the assistance of lateral plain radiography. J Spinal Disord 1996;9:334–338.

24 Patel N, et al: Interactive image-guided surgery of the spine: Use of the ISG/Elekta Viewing Wand to aid intraoperative localization. Br J Neurosurg 1997;11/1:60–64.

25 Rampersaud YR, Foley KT, Shen AC: Radiation exposure to the spine surgeon during fluoroscopically assisted pedicle screw insertion. Spine 2000;25:2637–2645.

26 Rampersaud YR, Simon DA, Foley KT: Accuracy requirements for image-guided spinal pedicle screw placement. Spine 2001;26:352–359.

27 Robertson PA, et al: Reliability of axial landmarks for pedicle screw placement in the lower lumbar spine. Spine 1998;23/1:60–66.

28 Roessler K, Ungersboeck K, Dietrich W, Aichholzer M: Frameless stereotactic guided neurosurgery: Clinical experience with an infrared based pointer device navigation system. Acta Neurochir 1997;139:551–559.

29 Schulze CJ, Munzinger E, Weber U: Clinical relevance of accuracy of pedicle screw placement: A computed tomographic-supported analysis. Spine 1998;23:2215–2220.

30 Schwarzenbach O, Berlemann U, Jost B, et al: Accuracy of computer-assisted pedicle screw placement: An in vivo computed tomography analysis. Spine 1997;22:452–458.

31 Tessman C: Exploring frameless stereotactic image guided surgery. AORN J 1999;69:498–512.

32 Vinas FC, Holdener H, Zamorano L, et al: Use of interactive-intraoperative guidance during vertebrectomy and anterior spinal fusion with instrumental fixation. Minim Invasive Neurosurg 1998;41:166–171.

33 Weinstein JN, Spratt KF, Spengler D, et al: Spinal pedicle fixation: reliability and validity of roentgenogram-based assessment and surgical factors on successful screw placement. Spine 1988;13:1012–1018.
34 Welch WC, Subach BR, Pollack IF, Jacobs GB: Frameless stereotactic guidance for surgery of the upper cervical spine. Neurosurgery 1997;40:958–963.
35 Xu R, et al: Anatomic considerations of pedicle screw placement in the thoracic spine. Roy-Camille technique versus open-lamina technique. Spine 1998;23:1065–1068.

Mark R. McLaughlin, MD
Neuro-Group, PA, 123 Franklin Corner Road
Lawrenceville, NJ 08648 (USA)
Tel. +1 609 895 8898, Fax +1 609 895 8330, E-Mail mclaughlin@spineuniverse.com

Haid RW Jr, Subach BR, Rodts GE Jr (eds): Advances in Spinal Stabilization.
Prog Neurol Surg. Basel, Karger, 2003, vol 16, pp 84–95

Virtual Fluoroscopy: Overview and Future Implications

Y. Raja Rampersaud[a], *Kevin T. Foley*[b, c]

[a] Divisions of Orthopaedic and Neurosurgery, University of Toronto, Toronto, Canada;
[b] Division of Neurosurgery, University of Tennessee and
[c] Image-Guided Surgery Center, Memphis, Tenn., USA

The utilization of neuronavigation in spinal surgery continues to grow. Numerous advances in this field have facilitated more practical clinical applications and have led to greater acceptance of this technology. The successful combination of neuronavigational technology with a practical intraoperative imaging modality (i.e. fluoroscopy) has significantly increased the clinical utility of computer-assisted surgery. Consequently, the introduction of computer-assisted fluoroscopy ('virtual fluoroscopy') has had a significant impact across multiple surgical specialties.

The complex anatomy of the spine necessitates reliable preoperative and intraoperative imaging. In spinal surgery, a significant number of surgical complications are a direct result of poor intraoperative anatomical localization. However, due to technical limitations and cost considerations, detailed intraoperative imaging modalities such as computed tomography (CT) or magnetic resonance imaging (MRI) are not readily available. Consequently, the need to improve intraoperative visualization has led to the development of image-guided navigational systems for spinal surgery. The first such system was three-dimensional (3D) and relied on preoperative imaging (CT based) [1, 2]. Although conventional 3D image guidance technology has gained significant recognition and acceptance, it is by no means widely utilized by spine surgeons. This technology is still considered to be early in its evolution and is not without limitations. From a clinical perspective, the greatest limitation of current 3D systems is the time-consuming and often frustrating process of registration. Another limitation is the current inability to update the preoperative imaging to reflect the intraoperative position of the spine. At present, intersegmental changes in the position of the spine either due to a change in the patients' overall position compared to their preoperative position or following a reduction maneuver cannot be updated without the presence of an intraoperative CT or MRI. This limitation mandates that each segment be individually registered to provide maximal navigational accuracy at that respective segment. As previously stated, this can often be a rate-limiting step to the novice user of a conventional 3D image guidance system. Furthermore, the accuracy provided by these systems is often felt to be unnecessary for the majority of spinal procedures. These limitations continue to drive the need to develop more user-friendly and practical computer-assisted techniques, such as virtual fluoroscopy.

C-arm fluoroscopy is an intraoperative imaging technique that is familiar to all spine surgeons. It is routinely employed for real-time intraoperative localization of patient anatomy and surgical instruments in a variety of spinal procedures. Fluoroscopic localization facilitates improved accuracy and in many instances reduces surgical exposure in a variety of spinal procedures such as pedicle screw insertion, interbody cage placement, odontoid screw insertion, and atlantoaxial transarticular screw fixation. This imaging technology has also enabled the development of percutaneous spinal procedures, such as vertebroplasty. Despite the advantages of intraoperative fluoroscopy, there are several limitations. Without a second fluoroscope, only a single projection can be visualized at one time. This limitation makes it necessary to reposition the C-arm during procedures that require multiple planes of visualization. Frequent repositioning of the C-arm is tedious, time-consuming, and frustrating. In addition, maintaining ideal sterility is a challenge. Furthermore, the position(s) of the C-arm is often ergonomically challenging to the surgeon. Finally, the potential deleterious effect of repeated radiation exposure to the surgeons' hands is always an important consideration [3].

Combining neuronavigational technology with a standard C-arm fluoroscope has enabled the optimization of this versatile intraoperative imaging modality. A computer-assisted image-guided fluoroscopy (virtual fluoroscopy) system provides the user with real-time multiplanar anatomical localization of a tracked surgical instrument in relation to patient-specific fluoroscopic-based images [4–8]. These systems eliminate the need for special preoperative imaging studies, manual image to patient registration (see above), C-arm repositioning, or the associated ergonomic challenges of using a C-arm fluoroscope. Furthermore, patient and occupational radiation exposure is significantly reduced, as is the need for wearing lead protection. Virtual fluoroscopy is currently being used for a wide variety of spinal applications. It is also being used for assistance in osseous cranial navigation (e.g. transsphenoidal access to the parasellar region) [9]. In addition, these systems are being extensively used for a variety of orthopedic trauma procedures and more recently total joint replacement. A novel variant of this technology is also being utilized in interventional radiology.

System Overview

A typical virtual fluoroscopy system consists of a surgical navigational computer system, a commercially available digital C-arm fluoroscope, a calibration target that attaches to the C-arm, and a variety of modified surgical instruments that are capable of being tracked by the image guidance system. The process of virtual fluoroscopy can be divided into four basic steps: (1) acquisition of one or more fluoroscopic images, (2) capturing the position of the patient and C-arm at the time of image acquisition, (3) mathematically recreating the fluoroscopic image formation process of the C-arm for each image acquired, and (4) superimposing the relative position of a tracked surgical instrument onto the virtual fluoroscopic image(s) [6, 8]. In step 1, conventional fluoroscopic images acquired in any plane are automatically transferred to the computer for image processing. In step 2, information about the relative position of the patient and the C-arm at the time of image acquisition (i.e. generation of the fluoroscopic image) is captured by a position-sensing camera array. The most commonly used tracking device is an electro-optical camera that detects the position of light-emitting diodes or passive reflectors attached to the object(s) of interest. Other means of position sensing (e.g. electromagnetic) can also be used. The patient position is defined by attachment of a dynamic reference array (DRA), which rigidly attaches to the portion of the patient's anatomy that is to be imaged. The C-arm position is defined by position markers or signal emitters built into the calibration target that is affixed to the image intensifier. In step 3, utilizing a mathematical algorithm, the computer recreates the fluoroscopic image formation process of the C-arm (i.e. virtual fluoroscopy). The algorithm calibrates the acquired fluoroscopic image by taking into account the positional data acquired in the second step. The calibration process compensates for factors such as gravity-dependent changes in the C-arm image center, the effect of external electromagnetic fields generated by electrical equipment in the operating room, and the effect of changes in the C-arm's position with respect to the earth's magnetic field. These factors are unique to every C-arm position; therefore, it is necessary that every acquired image be independently calibrated. Essentially the computer creates multiple live virtual fluoroscopic beams that are maintained in their original spatial orientation relative to the patient. In step 4, the computer determines the position of one or more trackable surgical instruments using a position-measuring camera and then superimposes an image of the instrument(s) in the virtual fluoroscopic display. Dedicated image-guided instruments such as awls, probes, taps, and screwdrivers are commercially available. Alternatively, any rigid surgical instrument may be customized with a tracking device or tracked with the assistance of a universal tool array. The system can display the position of the surgical instrument(s)

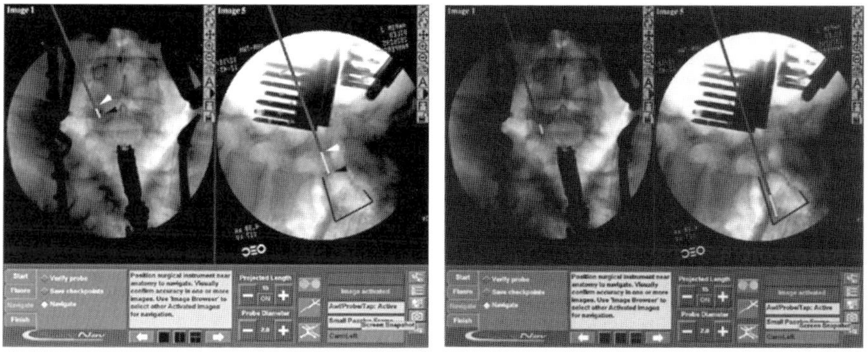

a b

Fig. 1. AP and lateral virtual fluoroscopic views of the lumbar spine. Note the high-grade spondylolisthesis. ***a*** The pedicle probe (dark line) has been positioned at the pedicle entry point (white arrowhead). Its trajectory (light line) has been virtually extended 15 mm to the base of the pedicle (black arrow). ***b*** Pedicle probe advancement is displayed in both the AP and lateral images simultaneously.

in any of the previously acquired fluoroscopic images, in multiple planes, simultaneously. The system also allows the actual projection of a surgical instrument (in one color) and the simultaneous projection of the linear extension of that instrument's proposed trajectory (in a second color) (fig. 1).

Accuracy Validation

Bench top testing of these systems has shown excellent (submillimetric) correlation of the live fluoroscopic position of a probe and its virtual fluoroscopic projection. In a simulated operating room setting, Foley et al. [4] investigated the in vitro accuracy of the FluoroNav (Medtronic Surgical Navigation Systems, Louisville, Colo., USA) system. In this study, the difference in positioning of an implanted pedicle probe (tip and trajectory angle) was measured comparing live and virtual fluoroscopic images. The mean error in probe tip localization was 0.97 ± 0.40 mm (99% confidence interval = 2.2 mm, maximum probe tip error = 3 mm). The mean trajectory angle difference between the virtual and actual probe images was $2.7 \pm 0.6°$ (99% confidence interval = 4.6°, maximum trajectory angle difference = 5°).

Clinical Spinal Applications

As this form of 2D neuronavigation is based on fluoroscopy, the use of a good fluoroscopic technique is necessary. Specifically, the anatomic region of interest should be placed in the center of the fluoroscopic image to minimize parallax. Furthermore, a true image should always be obtained if possible (e.g. in a true anterior-posterior (AP) view, the spinous process should bisect the pedicle). Prior to clinical use, it must be clearly understood that virtual fluoroscopy systems typically cannot improve the image quality generated by a given C-arm and it cannot compensate for a surgeon's misinterpretation of fluoroscopic (2D) osseous anatomic data. Therefore, a sound knowledge of fluoroscopic spinal anatomy is essential for the successful use of a virtual fluoroscopy system.

Virtual fluoroscopy is presently being used for the following spinal procedures: open pedicle screw placement (C7–S1), percutaneous pedicle screw placement (T10–S1), lumbar interbody cage insertion, C1–C2 transarticular screw placement, lateral mass screw placement, odontoid screw fixation and transoral decompression.

Posterior Spinal Procedures

For posterior spinal procedures, patient setup and surgical exposure are identical to the surgeon's normal technique. The DRA is rigidly affixed to the spinous process of the vertebra. For a typical degenerative case (without gross instability), the end vertebrae can be utilized for this purpose (e.g., attach the DRA to L4 for screw placement at L4, L5, and S1). The fluoroscopic views preferred by the surgeon are then acquired. These may include lateral views, AP views, or oblique (owl's eye) views down the length of the pedicle. Once processed (see System Overview), the desired images are simultaneously displayed and anatomical correlation of the tracked instrument compared to its virtual position is carried out. Utilizing virtual multiplanar fluoroscopic information, the starting point and trajectory for a given task are chosen. Clinical judgment and tactile feedback are used to refine the trajectory as necessary. These systems can provide the virtual projection of any desired length and diameter onto the chosen trajectory. The use of tracked awls, probes, and taps permits continuous visualization of the instruments along their course (fig. 2).

Percutaneous Pedicle Screws

Virtual fluoroscopy systems do not require direct exposure of the spine for registration, thus percutaneous navigation may be performed as follows. Through a small incision, the DRA is rigidly affixed to the desired spinous process. The appropriate fluoroscopic projections (AP, lateral, and oblique) are obtained and calibrated. From the skin surface, the trajectory of the tracked probe is virtually extended through the pedicle to visualize the anticipated course of the pedicle screw. Preoperative CT and MRI are used to decide the optimal entry point and trajectory for the pedicle screw. Using a cannulated

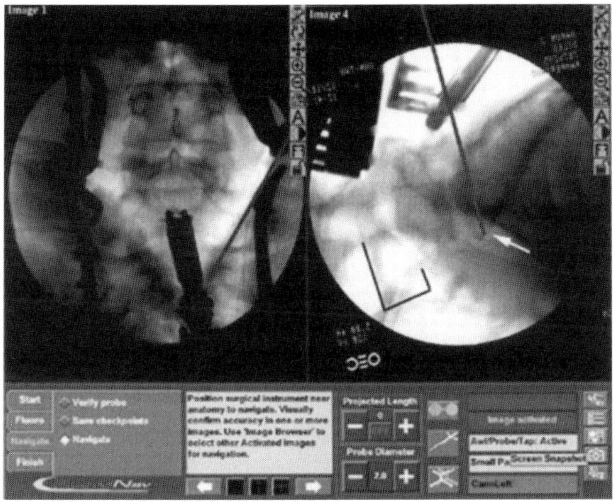

Fig. 2. AP and lateral virtual fluoroscopic views of the lumbar spine (same patient as in fig. 1). The ability to follow the course of the pedicle probe simultaneously in the AP and lateral planes enables reliable placement of the probe along an intended trajectory. Advancement of image-guided pedicle probe trough the S1 pedicle to the sacral promontory (white arrow) is demonstrated.

screw system the pedicle is probed and tapped under virtual fluoroscopic assistance (fig. 3) [10].

Anterior-Cervical Spine

The surface anatomy of the anterior cervical spine is typically prohibitive to anatomical registration using conventional 3D neuronavigation. Furthermore, the anatomy of the anterior cervical spine and the nature of anterior cervical spinal procedures typically do not allow the practical or safe attachment of a DRA directly to the spine. At the craniocervical junction, the anatomical relationship of the occiput-C1-C2 can often be maintained by the use of a Mayfield apparatus. As a result of the rigid relationship between the Mayfield apparatus and the occiput, a DRA directly attached to the Mayfield combined with automatic registration enables virtual fluoroscopic navigation during procedures at the craniocervical junction (e.g. odontoid screw insertion or transoral decompression). For anterior procedures of the subaxial cervical spine, the DRA can be directly attached to one or more vertebral bodies using threaded distraction pins. As noted for posterior procedures, the multiplanar position and trajectory of tracked surgical tools are provided in real time. Specific to anterior cervical procedures, information with respect to the anatomical midline and depth is also utilized.

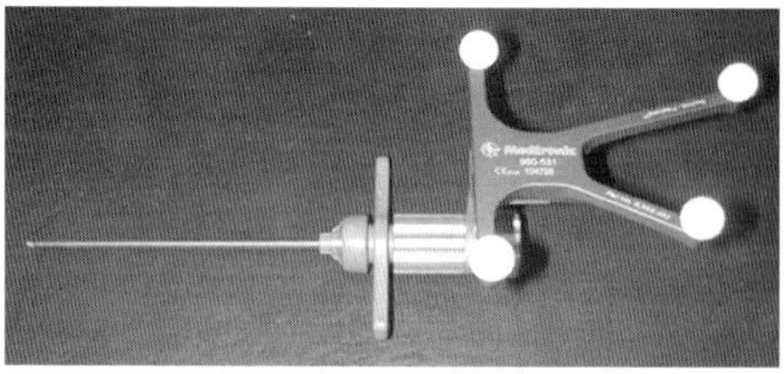

3a

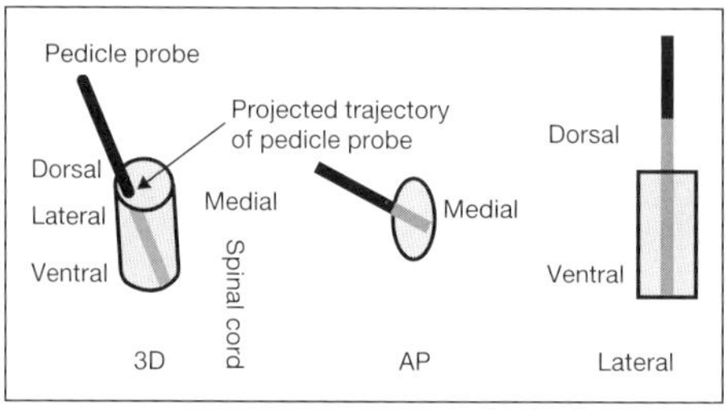

3b

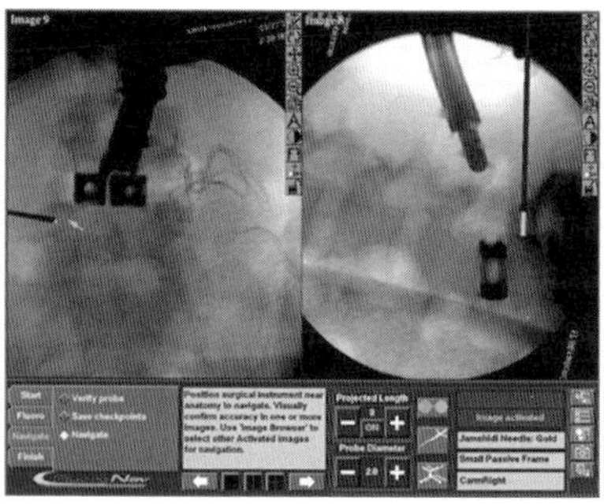

3c

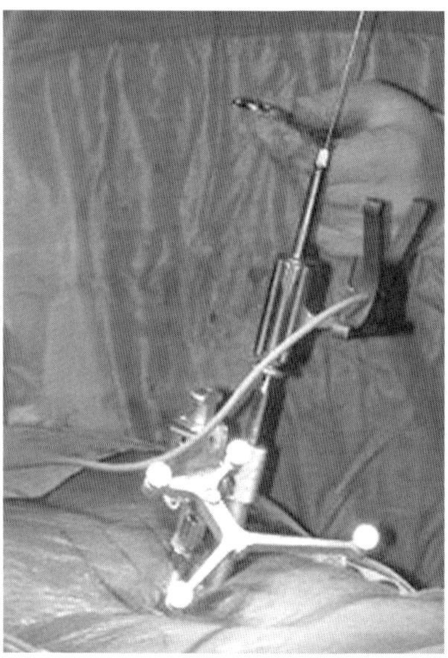

3d

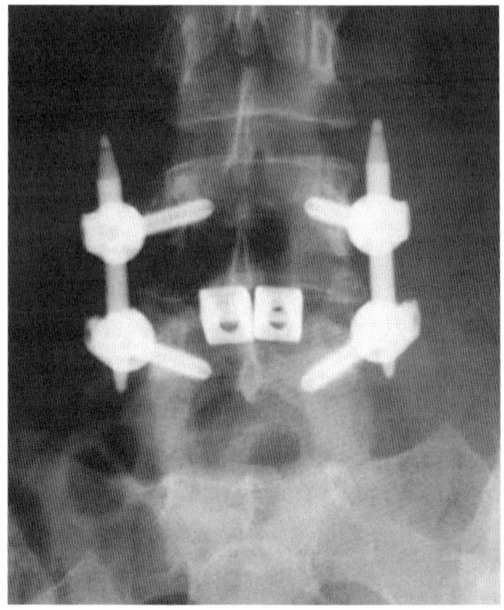

3e

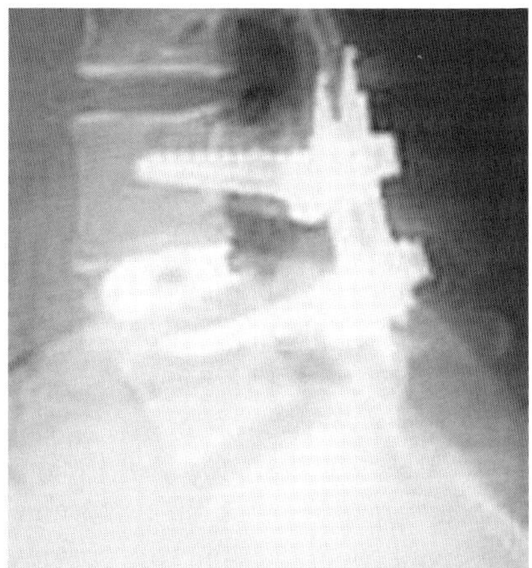

3f

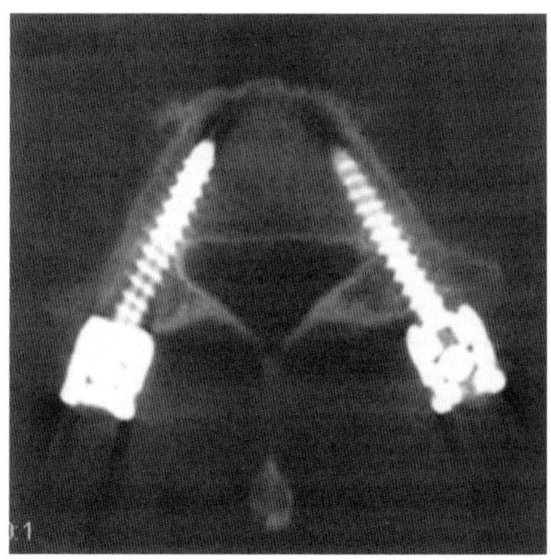

3g

Clinical Outcomes

The authors have significant clinical experience utilizing the FluoroNav™ system (Medtronic Surgical Navigation Technologies, Louisville, Colo., USA). In a current prospective study the clinical accuracy of virtual fluoroscopy for the placement of thoracic and lumbosacral pedicle screws is being evaluated (unpubl. data). In this study, postoperative CT of 360 pedicle screws [45 patients; lumbosacral (L1–S1) = 279; thoracic T (T3–T12) = 81] were independently reviewed by a spinal fellow and neuroradiologist. All screws were placed at an academic teaching center using the FluoroNav system. Residents and fellows placed over 50% of the screws. The relative position of the screw to the pedicle was assessed and graded as follows: A = completely in; B = <2 mm; C = 2–4 mm; D = >4–6 mm. Any borderline position was automatically downgraded. If an osseous breach occurred, the direction of the breach was further classified. To date, 49 out of 360 screws (13.6%) breached the pedicle wall (fig. 4). Overall pedicle breaches were grade B in 11.9%, grade C in 1.4% and grade D in 0.3% of screws. The majority (87.5%) of breaches were minor (grade B). Overall medial and lateral breaches occurred equally. Due to anatomic constraints, breaches were 3 times more likely to occur in the thoracic spine. Thirty-five percent of breaches were secondary to a pedicle screw that was larger than the size of the pedicle. There were no clinically significant screw misplacements and no screws required revision. In this series, the potential for any neurological injury (medial pedicle breach, greater than 2 mm) was 0.6%. This study represents a worse case scenario assessment (CT analysis). The overall misplacement rate in this ongoing study is less than or comparable to reported misplacement rates using other techniques [11–13].

Fig. 3. ***a*** Percutaneous pedicle screw insertion can be accomplished utilizing multiplanar virtual fluoroscopy and an image-guided pedicle probe such as a bone biopsy needle. ***b*** As depicted, the pedicle can be pictured as a cylinder. ***c*** A percutaneously placed pedicle probe is positioned at the pedicle entry point (the 'top' of the pedicle cylinder on the lateral view and the lateral edge of the pedicle cylinder on the AP view). Its trajectory is then virtually extended to the 'bottom' of the pedicle cylinder (the junction of the pedicle and the vertebral body). By maintaining a probe trajectory that is lateral to the medial edge of the pedicle (arrow – AP view) at the 'bottom' of the pedicle, the pedicle can be percutaneously probed with minimal risk of a medial pedicle breach. When using this technique, it is imperative that true AP and lateral views are utilized. ***d*** After the pedicle is probed, a guide wire is introduced and a cannulated pedicle screw can be placed. Postoperative AP (***e***) and lateral x-ray (***f***) following a minimally invasive posterior lumbar interbody fusion augmented with the Sextant™ percutaneous pedicle screw system (Medtronic – Sofamor Danek, Memphis, Tenn., USA). ***g*** Postoperative CT image (see ***e***, ***f***) demonstrating ideal placement of percutaneously placed L5 pedicle screws utilizing virtual fluoroscopic assistance.

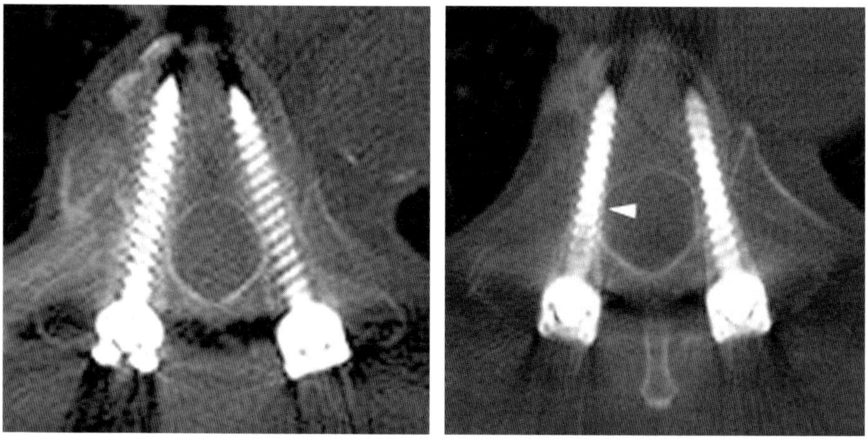

a *b*

Fig. 4. Postoperative CT images demonstrating pedicle screw placement using virtual fluoroscopic assistance. ***a*** At T6 both screws (5.5 mm) are in excellent position within the pedicles. ***b*** At T4, the left screw is in good position and the right screw demonstrates a minor breach (<2 mm) of the medial pedicle wall (arrowhead). In this case the screw diameter (5.5 mm) was greater than that of the pedicle.

Using a novel instrumentation technique, Foley et al. [10] placed percutaneous lumbar pedicle screws utilizing the FluoroNav system. Twelve patients were successfully treated using this technique. The versatility of the imaging system allowed registration of unexposed spine elements for the percutaneous procedure. Screw placement was without complication in all cases.

Although the authors only have clinical experience using the FluoroNav system, other commercially available virtual fluoroscopy systems seem to have similar accuracy and likely will demonstrate similar clinical results. In an in vitro study comparing a virtual fluoroscopy system to a conventional 3D image-guided technique, Choi et al. [7] demonstrated comparable accuracy. The overall screw misplacement rate (17.9%) demonstrated in this in vitro study is comparable to the clinical findings of Rampersaud et al. (see above, unpubl. data). Based on extensive in vitro data and in vivo experience the authors have concluded that FluoroNav appears to be a safe adjunct for the placement of thoracic and lumbosacral pedicle screws.

Disadvantages

Although virtual fluoroscopy has many advantages over conventional fluoroscopy, its primary limitation is 2D image generation. Also, the quality of the fluoroscopically generated images and the surgeon's ability to meaningfully interpret these views are unchanged compared to conventional fluoroscopy.

For all current image guidance systems, the navigational accuracy is greatest at the spinal segment to which the DRA is attached. The rigid relationship between the DRA and the spinal segment to which it is attached allows for accurate tracking and compensation for any motion occurring at that specific spinal segment. As a result of intersegmental motion and other technical reasons, overall navigational accuracy decreases as one moves further away from the DRA. Consequently, to maintain maximal navigational accuracy, the DRA should be moved to each spinal segment of interest with new fluoroscopic images acquired at each segment. This, however, is clinically impractical for multilevel cases. Unless gross segmental spinal instability is present, acceptable clinical accuracy is typically maintained for 2–5 spinal segments for one DRA position (1 segment: above, 1: at and 1–3: below). However, clinical judgment must be used to determine whether the system is adequately correlating to the segment of interest before navigation is carried out. For spinal procedures such as C1–2 transarticular screws where a low margin of error exists the DRA must be attached to the vertebrae of interest. Furthermore, by obtaining a live image to confirm the position of a tracked instrument the fluoroscope can serve as its own internal validation system.

Although virtual fluoroscopy provides the advantages of intraoperative imaging, it is still limited by the inability to easily track multiple spinal segments. Therefore, it is still necessary (for the reasons mentioned above) to move the DRA and acquire new fluoroscopic images several times during long segment procedures. The overall number of C-arm positional changes and images required, however, is still much less when compared to conventional C-arm fluoroscopy.

Under ideal circumstances surgical navigational systems can be very accurate. However, there are numerous potential sources of error that can significantly affect the clinical accuracy of any image guidance system. These include errors related to imaging, tracking, registration algorithm(s), and the tracked surgical tools. These errors, although typically submillimetric, are cumulative and can result in a clinically significant overall navigational error. One of the potentially largest, but often understated sources of errors is the surgeon. Like any other tool, a virtual fluoroscopic navigational system is only as good as its user. Sound knowledge of the limitations associated with these systems is paramount for their optimal use.

Future Implications

The future of virtual fluoroscopy is one of versatility. The practical implementation of an easy to use intraoperative imaging modality combined with surgical navigational technology has enabled a robust platform from which only improvement is possible. Virtual fluoroscopy has the potential to bring practical 3D intraoperative image guidance to the operating room. This is currently evolving in two pathways. The first is a direct method utilizing a novel isocentric C-arm (Siemens). This C-arm is capable of generating a 3D image data set, therefore allowing 3D neuronavigation without the hassles of 3D registration. Furthermore, because it is an intraoperative imaging device certain limitations such as positional (patient) intersegmental motion and intraoperative image update of conventional 3D neuronavigation are eliminated. The second pathway involves technology that allows automated registration of intraoperative 2D fluoroscopic images to a preacquired 3D image data set [14]. The goal of both techniques is to eliminate the time-consuming step of tactile anatomic registration, while providing unparalleled 3D anatomic information and practical intraoperative imaging capabilities. 2D to 3D image fusion also allows incorporation of multiple imaging modalities (e.g. CT, MRI, ultrasound or angiographic). The added anatomical detail of a 3D image data set without the need for tactile registration is ideally suited for the refinement and development of percutaneous or minimal access spinal surgery.

Virtual fluoroscopy is also facilitating another exciting area of research that involves practical solutions for tracking multiple segments of the spine. Combined with segmentation of an image data set this will allow the user to maintain optimal navigational accuracy over numerous segments and update the relative position of individual segments in real time. Finally, it is only logical that this technology will likely be integrated directly into the C-arm fluoroscope, thus providing a versatile intraoperative imaging-navigational system.

Conclusion

Virtual fluoroscopy is a safe and beneficial adjunct to complex spinal surgery. The use of this technology has shown improved or comparable pedicle screw misplacement rates when compared to published results utilizing anatomical landmarks with or without fluoroscopy and conventional 3D image guidance, respectively. As with all neuronavigation devices, advantages and disadvantages specific to virtual fluoroscopy exist and must be considered in the decision to utilize this technology. The real-time multiplanar information provided by these systems can be a powerful adjunct to the surgeon's ability to perform complex tasks during spinal surgery. However, it must never be forgotten that this technology is intended to serve as an adjunct to the surgeon's clinical judgment and technical skills, not a replacement.

References

1 Foley KT, Smith MM: Image-guided spine surgery. Neurosurg Clin N Am 1996;7/2:171–186.

2 Rampersaud YR, Foley KF: Image-guided spinal surgery. Operative Tech Orthopaed 2000;10/1: 64–68.

3 Rampersaud YR, Foley KT, Shen AC, Williams S, Solomito M: Radiation exposure to the spine surgeon during fluoroscopically assisted pedicle screw insertion. Spine 2000;25:2637–2645.

4 Foley KT, Rampersaud YR, Simon DA: Virtual fluoroscopy: Multi-planar x-ray guidance with minimal radiation exposure. Eur Spine J 1999;8(suppl 1):S36.

5 Nolte LP, Slomczykowski MA, Berlemann U, Strauss MJ, Hofstetter R, Schlenzka D, Laine T, Lund T: A new approach to computer-aided spine surgery: Fluoroscopy-based surgical navigation. Eur Spine J 2000;9(suppl 1):S78–S88.

6 Foley KT, Simon DA, Rampersaud YR: Virtual fluoroscopy. Operative Tech Orthopaed 2000;10/1: 77–81.

7 Choi WW, Green BA, Levi ADO: Computer-assisted fluoroscopic targeting system for pedicle screw insertion. Neurosurgery 2000;47:872–878.

8 Foley KT, Simon DA, Rampersaud YR: Virtual fluoroscopy: Computer-assisted fluoroscopic navigation. Spine 2001;26:347–351.

9 Jane JA, Thapar K, Alden TD, Laws ER Jr: Fluoroscopic frameless stereotaxy for transsphenoidal surgery. Neurosurgery 2001;48:1302–1308.

10 Foley KT, Gupta SK, Justis JR, Sherman MC: Percutaneous pedicle screw fixation of the lumbar spine. Neurosurg Focus 2001;10/4:1–8.

11 Merloz P, Tonetti J, Pittet L, Coulomb M, Lavallee S, Sautot P: Pedicle screw placement using image guided techniques. Clin Orthop 1998;354:39–48.

12 Laine T, Lund T, Ylikoski M, Lohikoski J, Schlenzka D: Accuracy of pedicle screw insertion with and without computer assistance: A randomised controlled clinical study in 100 consecutive patients. Eur Spine J 2000;9:235–240.

13 Youkilis AS, Quint DJ, McGillicuddy JE, Papadopoulos SM: Stereotactic navigation for placement of pedicle screws in the thoracic spine. Neurosurgery 2001;48:771–778.

14 Theodore N, Sonntag VKH: Spinal surgery: The past century and the next. Neurosurgery 2000;46: 767–776.

Y. Raja Rampersaud MD, FRCSC
Toronto Western Hospital, University Health Network
Edith Cavell Wing, 1-039, 399 Bathurst St., Toronto, ON M5T 2S8 (Canada)
Tel. +1 416 603 5399, Fax +1 416 603 3437, E-Mail raja.rampersaud@uhn.on.ca

Haid RW Jr, Subach BR, Rodts GE Jr (eds): Advances in Spinal Stabilization.
Prog Neurol Surg. Basel, Karger, 2003, vol 16, pp 96–106

Placement of Thoracic Pedicle Screws

David W. Polly, Jr., Timothy R. Kuklo

Department of Orthopaedic Surgery and Rehabilitation,
Walter Reed Army Medical Center, Washington, D.C., USA

Thoracic pedicle screws are experiencing a significant increase in utilization in North America, as well as in the rest of the developed world [2, 5, 20, 21, 30–34]. Consequently, there is a heightened interest in factors leading to successful use.

When placing pedicle screws in the thoracic spine, the surgeon primarily uses his or her knowledge of general thoracic pedicle anatomy along with a preoperative plan founded on sound biomechanical principles for the initial approach. Preoperative patient-specific imaging studies aid the surgeon in adapting general anatomy knowledge to patient-specific anatomy. These include a detailed study of the preoperative radiographs for pedicle position and size, in addition to possible computerized tomography (CT) and magnetic resonance (MR) imaging, which can further detail the pertinent anatomy. In concert with a thorough understanding of this anatomy, tactile feedback, however, remains the primary means of confirmation for successful screw placement.

More recent screw placement guidance tools include conventional fluoroscopy (fig. 1), two-dimensional (2-D) fluoroscopy (fig. 2), computer-aided image guidance (fig. 3), intraoperative advanced imaging (such as CT or MR), physiological monitoring guidance and emerging three-dimensional (3-D)

The opinions or assertions contained herein are the private views of the authors and are not to be construed as official or as reflecting the views of the United States Army or the Department of Defense. The authors are employees of the United States government. This work was prepared as part of their official duties and as such, there is no copyright to be transferred.

Fluoro guidance

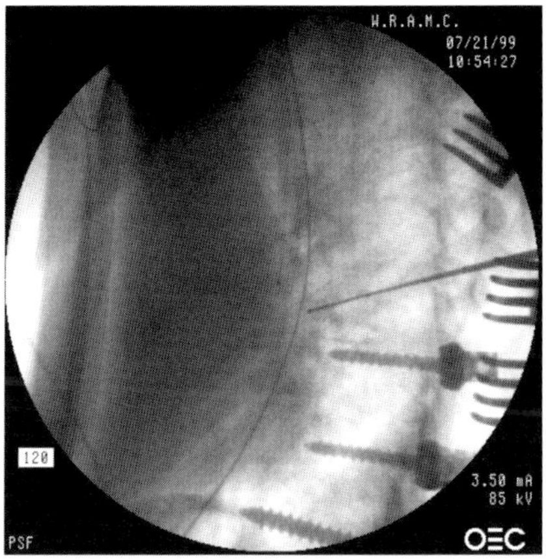

Fig. 1. This is conventional image guidance with use of intraoperative fluoroscopy. This image demonstrates the typical 22° sagittal inclination of the thoracic pedicle when utilizing the anatomic axis.

2-D guidance

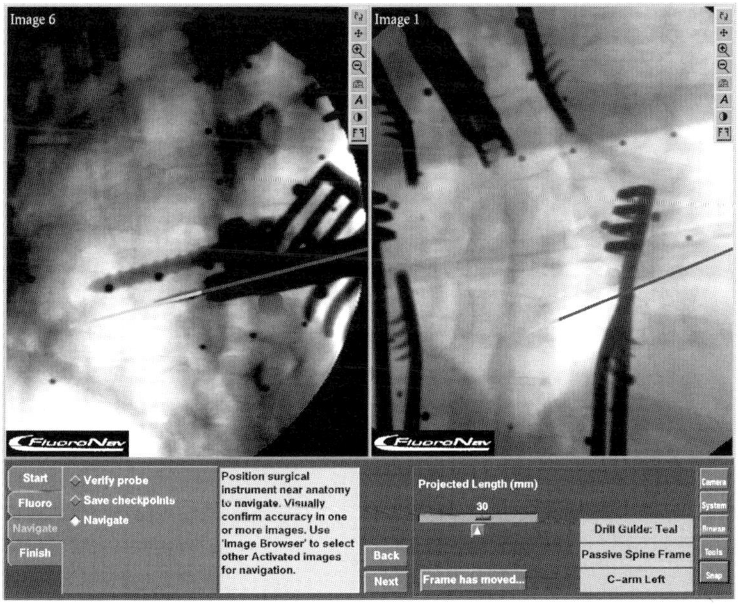

Fig. 2. This example of 2-D image guidance demonstrates two planar images allowing the surgeon to navigate simultaneously in these planes. Advantages of this include familiarity of the display (fluoroscopy) and the ability to update the images intraoperatively as needed.

3-D image guidance

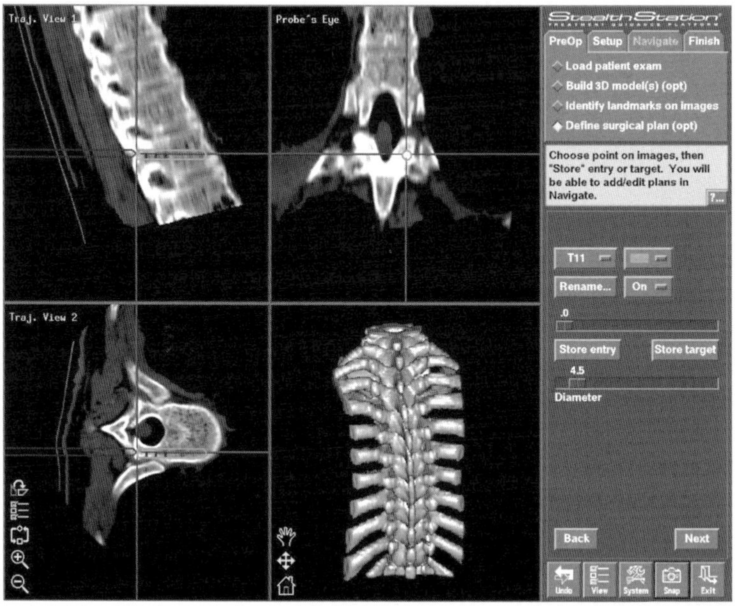

Fig. 3. This example of 3-D image guidance demonstrates the utility of multiplanar navigation. It allows for simultaneous sagittal, coronal and axial planar navigation. This allows for true optimization of pedicle screw fit, fill and trajectory.

fluoroscopic guidance. Screw tract and screw placement confirmation is ultimately achieved by palpation, imaging, physiological monitoring or a combination of all of these techniques. Successful screw placement can be defined in a number of ways [2, 11]. With successful surgical outcome as the primary goal, successful screw placement may be a necessary, but not sufficient requirement.

Pedicle Anatomy

Applied thoracic pedicle anatomy has been well studied, and normative tables and graphs have been developed [7, 8, 14, 16, 22, 24, 35–38, 40, 41]. Currently, there are primarily two accepted screw trajectories – the straight-ahead trajectory (initially popularized by Roy-Camille, then Suk and Lenke), and the anatomic trajectory (utilized by Harms and others, the term initially suggested by Polly) [31].

Advantages of the straight-ahead trajectory include permitting the use of a fixed head (monoaxial) screw, as well as offering increased insertional torque and pull-out strength when compared to the anatomic trajectory [17, 19]. The major disadvantage is that this trajectory may require the screw to traverse a narrower portion of the pedicle isthmus to remain fully contained. The anatomic trajectory (directed along the sagittal pedicle axis – a 22° inclination from dorsal rostral to ventral caudal) permits the surgeon to navigate a larger portion of the pedicle isthmus and place a longer screw within the bone. It may also provide a 'toenail' effect, which typically provides the advantage of not sustaining direct in-line pull-out forces to the screw. Any potential benefit in construct performance, as opposed to individual screw performance, is unknown.

Pedicle Screw Tract Placement

A number of techniques have been used to successfully navigate the pedicle. Initial techniques utilized tactile feedback along with knowledge of the pedicle anatomy to place screws. The 'cancellous feel', familiar to surgeons experienced in lumbar pedicle screw placement, can also be used for thoracic screw placement. Since cortical bone has a distinctly different feel, a progressive cancellous resistance to the advancing pedicle probe is highly reassuring. Likewise, a sudden change in this feel is a cause for reassessment.

The neurocentral junction, however, is a predictable point where a distinct change in the 'feel' occurs. This is because the physeal growth plate is distinctly more dense than the cancellous bone of the pedicle and the vertebral body. Breeching this physeal scar has a similar feel to violating a cortical margin and requires a certain level of experience (or anatomic confirmation) to differentiate acceptable from unacceptable pedicle tract navigation.

Surgical Pedicle Navigation Techniques

Proposed techniques for pedicle navigation include the 'freehand' technique as well described by Lenke et al. [20]. Similarly, drilling has been utilized by many surgeons while the use of a small diameter drill followed by placement of k-wires with conventional radiographic confirmation has been popularized by Suk et al. [32]. The 'funnel technique' of breeching the dorsal cortex with a burr and then navigating the pedicle with a small size curette (such as a 2-0 Cloward curette) has been popularized by Gaines [10], and espoused by others for cervical pedicle navigation (find the hole, do not make the hole). Nonetheless, each of these techniques requires tactile feedback as the primary means of confirmation.

This tactile feedback can be supplemented with a number of adjunctive technologies [1]. Conventional fluoroscopy has been widely used, with a high level of accuracy [2]. It has the advantage of being a real time evaluation in a familiar format. Disadvantages include the presence of the fluoroscopic unit at the operative field, the conventional difficulties associated with planar radiography (visualizing the upper thoracic spine, penetrating large body mass patients, surgeon impairment from lead gowns) and exposure to both the patient and the operative team. A skilled technologist is also required.

2-D image guidance (such as FluoroNav, Medtronic Sofamor Danek, Memphis, Tenn., USA) acquires intraoperative images through a tracking arc attached to the patient and displays the images on a computer screen to assist the surgeon to navigate the pedicle [27, 28] (fig. 2). The major advantage of this system is that it permits the surgeon to navigate in multiple conventional fluoroscopic planes simultaneously. This concept, the use of conventional imaging linked in multiple planes, is a comfortable concept for many surgeons due to the familiarity of the radiographic images. The disadvantages include the requirement for a sophisticated unit that requires an additional user familiar with the technical operation of the system.

3-D image guidance, or frameless stereotactic image guidance, utilizes preoperative axial imaging studies (most typically CT) with intraoperative registration to correlate segmental anatomy and display multiplanar images for navigation [4] (fig. 3). The most significant advantage of this technique is the display of axial images during the navigation process. This is perhaps the most critical anatomic information required by the surgeon during pedicle navigation. Disadvantages include the need for the sophisticated unit (and subsequent cost), obtaining the preoperative axial imaging studies (and additional cost), transferring the information to the unit and then obtaining appropriate intraoperative segmental registration of acceptable precision. There is a significant time investment necessary in the early use of the technology.

Physiological intraoperative guidance is based on stimulating a pedicle probe during screw tract navigation, thus looking for a neural response from either a nerve root or the spinal cord. This technique has been extensively researched in the lumbar spine where the nerve root level myotomes provide good discrimination. In the thoracic spine, this has proven to be more difficult. Monitoring from the rectus abdominis appears to give reasonable evoked potentials for T6–T12 [29]. To date, this technique has proven to be less reliable rostral to T6. Newer technologies may allow real time monitoring of nerve root proximity, as well as directional information.

Future technological developments may include sophisticated haptic feedback that can discriminate between bone, nerve and blood vessels. Ideally, this technology should permit differentiation between cortical and cancellous bone, thus providing an excellent adjunct in pedicle navigation. The merging of multiple modalities could further enhance the margin of safety provided for navigating these narrow access corridors.

Evaluation of the Pedicle Tract

Classically, evaluation of the pedicle tract is done by direct bony palpation. This includes 'five-wall' confirmation, or palpation of the medial, lateral, superior, inferior and anterior walls. However, the predictive value of this maneuver varies between surgeons, and is not foolproof [18]. If a breech is detected, there is a high positive predictive value; however, if no breech is detected, the negative predictive value is not as good. An 'experience' factor is also present and appears to play a significant role.

Confirmation of a bony pedicle breach requires further analysis by the surgeon to determine whether or not a screw can still be placed safely. One technique, described by Dvorak et al. [6], places a pedicle screw along a trajectory lateral to the pedicle, but within the confines of the pedicle-rib complex, and ultimately into the vertebral body. This has subsequently been termed the 'in-out-in' technique or the 'pedicle-rib' technique. O'Brien et al. [23] have demonstrated the anatomy of this corridor. So simply having a small lateral cortical breach is of no particular clinical consequence. It also appears that a small medial breach can be tolerated [2, 11]. Further, Polly et al. [26] analyzed volumetric spinal canal intrusion from medially positioned screws in a computer model and found that a screw must have over a 2-mm medial breach to have the same volumetric spinal canal intrusion as a perfectly positioned pediatric laminar hook. However, in spinal deformity, a medial breach on the concave apex would not be tolerated, and any change in neurological monitoring is always a cause for significant concern [25].

Following insertion, screw purchase is routinely evaluated. If the screw is loose (poor purchase), then it is not acceptably placed, whereas good purchase does not necessarily confirm adequate placement. Again, screw removal and direct palpation may assist the surgeon in identifying a breach. Similarly, electrophysiological monitoring can suggest a medial cortical violation, especially from T6–T12, but it is less reliable at detecting lateral or anterior breaches. Intraoperative imaging (fluoro or plain film) can also be used to assess placement, yet interpretation of the images can be challenging. Several checks have been found to be helpful. First, with multiple level fusions, one can appreciate the progressive orientation of the screws on the PA view, and a break in the progression will alert the surgeon to a potentially misplaced screw. Further, the pedicle can usually be identified, and the screw should appear to be tracking

Case example

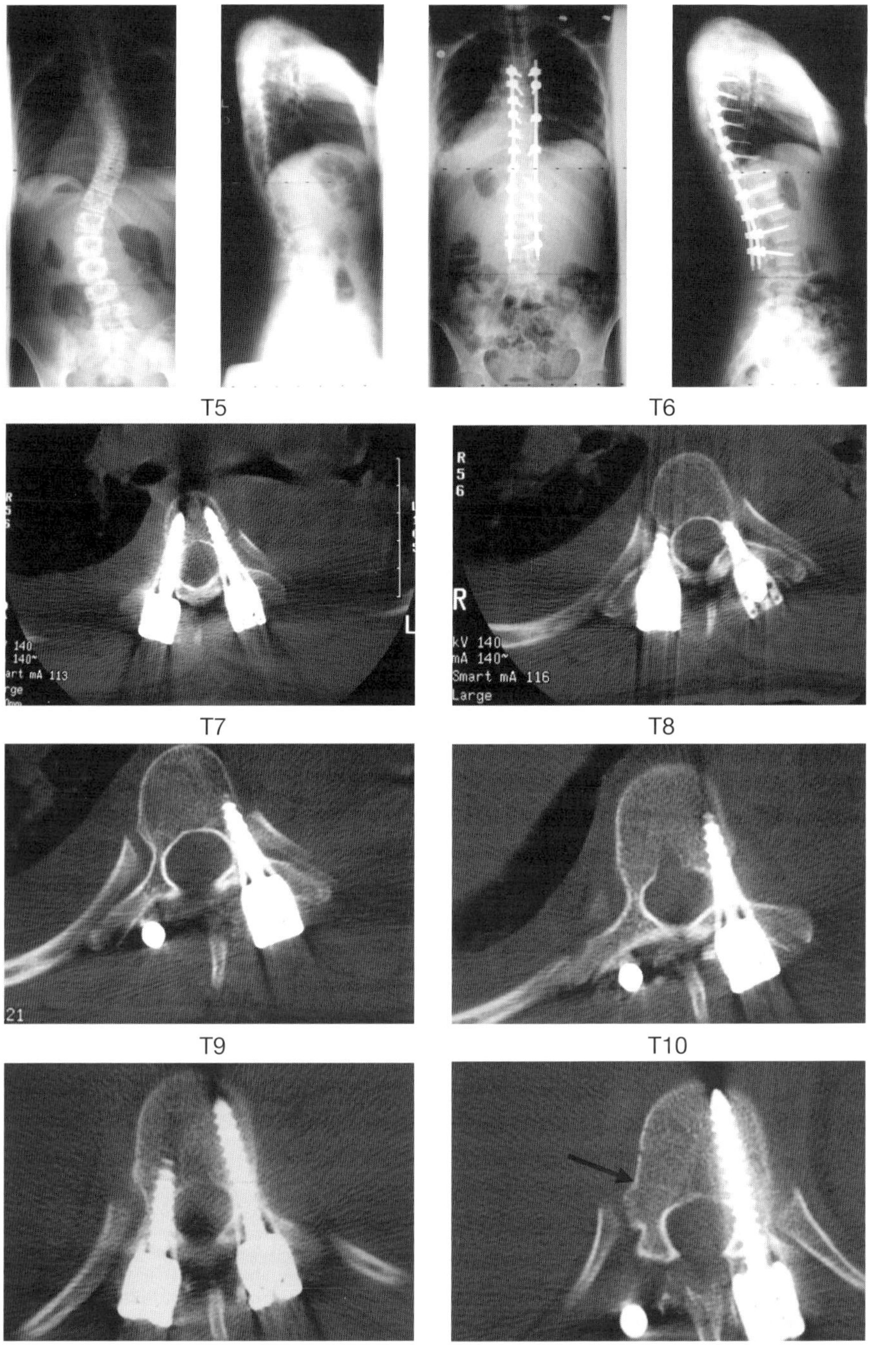

4a 4b 4c 4d 4e 4f 4g

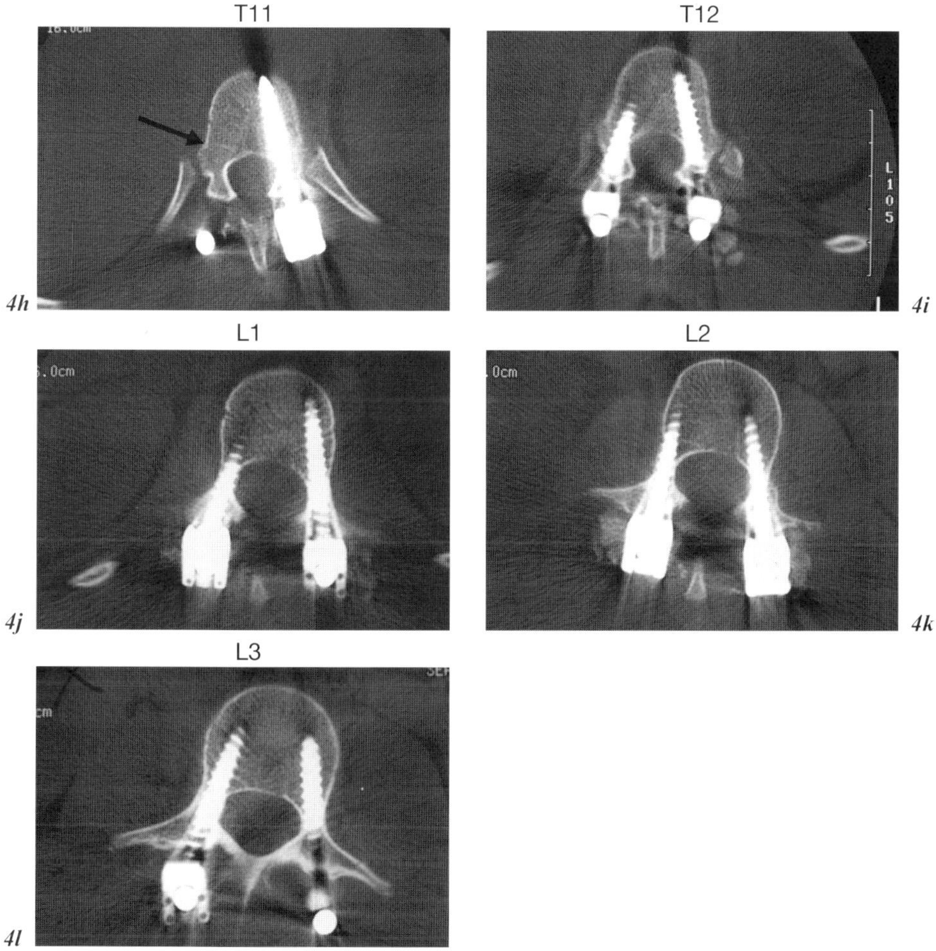

Fig. 4. a–l This is an example of a right thoracic left lumbar progressive scoliotic deformity in a skeletally immature individual (curve pattern Lenke 3CN, King curve type double major). Because of the curve magnitude (>50°), and her immaturity, she met operative indications. The lumbar modifier (Lenke C) and the thoracolumbar junctional kyphosis mandated fusion of both curves. The preoperative coronal and sagittal radiographs demonstrate the deformity, the postoperative radiographs demonstrate the excellent correction in the coronal and sagittal planes while preserving the motion of the intervertebral disks from L3 to the sacrum. The sequential CT images demonstrate the axial views of the screw position at each level T5 through L3. The physeal scar (or neurocentral growth plate) is well visualized on the right at T10 and T11.

through the pedicle projection. Multiple views, especially in spinal deformity, can be of further help. To date, the accuracy of planar radiography to determine pedicular screw placement in the thoracic spine has not been validated. Currently, CT scanning is considered the gold standard, although it is more realistically a worst case analysis since there is some magnification artifact even with titanium implants [3, 9, 12, 13, 39]. Intraoperative CT scanners have been utilized at some institutions. Obviously, this requires a significant infrastructure and operating room modifications. For particularly high-risk screw placement, one strategy might involve a planned intraoperative transport to a scanner within the institution. Again, this requires significant coordination and increased operative time. We have found that the routine use of postoperative CT scans in patients who have undergone placement of thoracic pedicle screws has added an extra margin of safety and an invaluable educational opportunity for the operating surgeons to critically assess their technique (fig. 4a–l).

Successful Screw Placement

Successful screw placement can be defined in a number of ways. The most obvious criteria would be the presence or absence of neurological or visceral compromise as a result of the screw placement [15]. By all definitions, presence of these conditions would be considered an unsuccessful screw placement. The second criterion may be screw purchase. In other words, does the screw have enough purchase to hold against the applied loads? However, even if placed with anatomic precision, placement can still be unsuccessful if there is inadequate bone stock. Third, did the screws successfully achieve the goal of instrumentation, i.e. was the deformity corrected or was the spine stabilized sufficiently to achieve the long-term biological solution of fusion?

Conclusions

Individual decisions and techniques, including the use of neuronavigational aids, are premised to successfully and safely achieve the goals of surgical treatment. Placement of thoracic pedicle screws is only one component of the surgical process. However, for the surgery to be a success, the screws must be placed safely and effectively. This can be achieved through a variety of techniques using one of several accepted strategies. The surgeon must have enough resources available to accomplish the task. Given the variety of experience, skill and patient-specific anatomy, different resources will be required.

References

1 Amiot LP, Labelle H, DeGuise JA, et al: Computer-assisted pedicle screw fixation: A feasibility study. Spine 1995;20:1208–1212.

2 Belmont PJ, Klemme WR, Dhawan A, Polly DW: In vivo accuracy of thoracic pedicle screws. Spine 2001;26:2340–2346.

3 Berlemann U, Heini P, Müller U, Stoupis C, Schwarzenbach O: Reliability of pedicle screw assessment utilizing plain radiographs versus CT reconstruction. Eur Spine J 1997;6:406–411.

4 Carl AL, Khanuja HS, Sachs BL, et al: In vitro simulation: Early results of stereotaxy for pedicle screw placement. Spine 1997;22:1160–1164.

5 Cinotti G, Gumina S, Ripani M, et al: Pedicle instrumentation in the thoracic spine. Spine 1999;24/21:114–119.

6 Dvorak M, MacDonald S, Gurr KR, Bailey SI, Haddad RG: An anatomic, radiographic, and biomechanical assessment of extrapedicular screw fixation in the thoracic spine. Spine 1993;18:1689–1694.

7 Ebraheim NA, Jabaly G, Xu R, et al: Anatomic relations of the thoracic pedicle to the adjacent neural structures. Spine 1997;22:1553–1557.

8 Ebraheim NA, Xu R, Ahmad M, et al: Projection of the thoracic pedicle and its morphometric analysis. Spine 1997;22/3:233–238.

9 Farber GI, Place HM, Mazur RA, Jones CDE, Damiano TR: Accuracy of pedicle screw placement in lumbar fusions by plain radiographs and computed tomography. Spine 1995;13:1494–1499.

10 Gaines RW: The use of pedicle screw internal fixation for the operative treatment of spinal disorders. J Bone Joint Surg Am 2000;82:1458–1476.

11 Gertzbein SD, Robbins SE: Accuracy of pedicular screw placement in vivo. Spine 1990;15:11–14.

12 Kim KD, Johnson JP, Bloch O, Masciopinto JE: Computer-assisted thoracic pedicle screw placement: An in vitro feasibility study. Spine 2001;26:360–364.

13 Klemme WR, Belmont PJ, Polly DW: Transpedicular thoracic screws: General concepts and insertion technique using fluoroscopic guidance. Semin Spine Surg 2002;14/1:43–47.

14 Kothe R, Panjabi MM, Liu W: Multidirectional instability of the thoracic spine due to iatrogenic pedicle injuries during transpedicular fixation. A biomechanical investigation. Spine 1997;22:1836–1842.

15 Kuklo TR, Lehman RA, Schroeder T: Perils and pitfalls of thoracic pedicle screw placement. Semin Spine Surg 2002;14/1:97–102.

16 Kuklo TR, Polly DW: Anatomy of the thoracic pedicle. Semin Spine Surg 2002;14/1:3–7.

17 Lehman RA, Kuklo TR: Pedicle screw salvage using anatomic trajectory. Scoliosis Research Society Annual Meeting, Seattle, 2002.

18 Lehman RA, Kuklo TR, Orchowski JR, Potter BK, Polly DW: Probing for detection of thoracic pedicle breach: Is it valid? Scoliosis Research Society Annual Meeting, Seattle, 2002.

19 Lehman RA, Polly DW, Kuklo TR, Belmont PJ, Cunningham B, Kirk KL: Advantage of straight forward versus anatomic trajectory for placement of thoracic pedicle screws: A biomechanical study. Scoliosis Research Society Annual Meeting, Seattle, 2002.

20 Lenke LG, Rinella A, Kim Y-J: Free hand thoracic pedicle screw placement. Semin Spine Surg 2002;14/1:48–57.

21 Liljenqvist UR, Halm HF, Link TM: Pedicle screw instrumentation of the thoracic spine in idiopathic scoliosis. Spine 1997;22:2239–2245.

22 McCormack BM, Benzel EC, Adams MS, et al: Anatomy of the thoracic pedicle. Neurosurgery 1995;37:303–308.

23 O'Brien MF, Lenke LG, Mardjetko S, et al: Pedicle morphology in thoracic adolescent idiopathic scoliosis: Is pedicle fixation an anatomically viable technique? Spine 2000;25:2285–2293.

24 Panjabi MM, O'Holleran JD, Crisco JJ, et al: Complexity of the thoracic spine pedicle anatomy. Eur Spine J 1997;6:19–24.

25 Polly DW, Belmont PJ, Klemme WR, Robinson M: In vivo accuracy of transpedicular thoracic screws in patients with and without coronal-plane spinal deformities. Scoliosis Research Society Annual Meeting, Cleveland, 2001.

26 Polly DW, Young JS, Johnson C, Kuklo TR: Comparison of volumetric intrusion of pedicle screws versus hooks. Scoliosis Research Society 36th Annual Meeting, Cleveland, 2001.
27 Rampersaud YR, Simon DA, Foley KT: Accuracy requirements for image-guided spinal pedicle screw placement. Spine 2001;26:352–359.
28 Rampersaud YR: Advanced image guidance for thoracic pedicle screws. Semin Spine Surg 2002;14/1:58–65.
29 Raynor BA, Lenke LG, Kim YJ, et al: Can triggered EMG thresholds predict safe thoracic pedicle screw placement? Scoliosis Research Society Annual Meeting, Cleveland, 2001.
30 Roy-Camille R, Saillant G, Mazel C: Internal fixation of the lumbar spine with pedicle screw plating. Clin Orthop 1986;203:7–17.
31 Roy-Camille R, Saillant G, Mazel C: Plating of thoracic, thoracolumbar, and lumbar injuries with pedicle screw plates. Orthop Clin North Am 1986;17:147–159.
32 Suk SI, Kim WJ, Lee SM, et al: Thoracic pedicle screw fixation in spinal deformities: Are they really safe? Spine 2001;26:2049–2057.
33 Suk SI, Lee CK, Kim WJ, et al: Segmental pedicle screw fixation in the treatment of thoracic idiopathic scoliosis. Spine 195;20:1399–1405.
34 Suk SI, Lee CK, Min HJ, et al: Comparison of Cotrel-Dubousset pedicle screws and hooks in the treatment of idiopathic scoliosis. Int Orthop 1994;18:341–346.
35 Ugur HC, Attar A, Uz A, et al: Thoracic pedicle: Surgical anatomic evaluation and relations. J Spinal Disord 2001;14/1:39–45.
36 Vaccaro AR, Rizzolo SJ, Allardyce TJ, et al: Placement of pedicle screws in the thoracic spine. I. Morphometric analysis of the thoracic vertebrae. J Bone Joint Surg Am 1995;77:1993–1999.
37 Vaccaro AR, Rizzolo SJ, Balderston RA, et al: Placement of pedicle screws in the thoracic spine. II. An anatomic and radiographic assessment. J Bone Joint Surg Am 1995;77:1200–1206.
38 Xu R, Ebraheim NA, Ou Y, Yeasting RA: Anatomic considerations of pedicle screw placement in the thoracic spine. Roy-Camille technique versus open-lamina technique. Spine 1998; 23:1065–1068.
39 Yoo JU, Ghanayem A, Petersilge C, Lewin J: Accuracy of using computed tomography to identify pedicle screw placement in cadaveric human lumbar spine. Spine 1997;22:2668–2671.
40 Zindrick MR, Knight GW, Sartori MJ, et al: Pedicle morphology of the immature thoracolumbar spine. Spine 2000;25:2726–2735.
41 Zindrick MR, Wiltse LL, Doornik A, et al: Analysis of the morphometric characteristics of the thoracic and lumbar pedicles. Spine 1987;12:160–166.

David W. Polly, Jr., MD, COL, MC, USA
Department of Orthopaedic Surgery and Rehabilitation
Walter Reed Army Medical Center, Washington, DC 20307 (USA)
Tel. +1 202 782 5851, Fax +1 202 782 4365, E-Mail david.polly@na.amedd.army.mil

Haid RW Jr, Subach BR, Rodts GE Jr (eds): Advances in Spinal Stabilization.
Prog Neurol Surg. Basel, Karger, 2003, vol 16, pp 107–127

Cervical Techniques with Image-Guided Spinal Navigation

Iain H. Kalfas

Section of Spinal Surgery, Department of Neurosurgery,
Cleveland Clinic Foundation, Cleveland, Ohio, USA

Image-guided spinal navigation is a computer-based surgical technology that was developed to improve intraoperative orientation to the unexposed anatomy during complex spinal procedures [12, 17]. It evolved from the principles of stereotaxy which have been used by neurosurgeons for several decades to help localize intracranial lesions. Stereotaxy is defined as the localization of a specific point in space using three-dimensional coordinates. The application of stereotaxy to intracranial surgery initially involved the use of an external frame attached to the patient's head. However, the evolution of computer-based technologies has eliminated the need for this frame and has allowed for the expansion of stereotactic technology into other surgical fields, in particular spinal surgery.

The management of complex spinal disorders has been greatly influenced by the increased acceptance and use of spinal instrumentation devices as well as the development of more complex operative exposures. Many of these techniques place a greater demand on the spinal surgeon by requiring a precise orientation to that part of the spinal anatomy that is not exposed in the surgical field. In particular, the various fixation techniques that require placing bone screws into the pedicles of the thoracic, lumbar and sacral spine, into the lateral masses of the cervical spine and across joint spaces in the upper cervical spine require 'visualization' of the unexposed spinal anatomy. Although conventional intraoperative imaging techniques, such as fluoroscopy, have proven useful, they are limited in that they provide only two-dimensional imaging of a complex three-dimensional structure. Consequently, the surgeon is required to extrapolate the third dimension based on an interpretation of the images and a knowledge of the pertinent anatomy. This so-called dead reckoning of the anatomy can result in varying degrees of inaccuracy when placing screws into the unexposed spinal column.

Several studies have shown the unreliability of routine radiography in assessing pedicle screw placement in the lumbosacral spine. The rate of penetration of the pedicle cortex by an inserted screw ranges from 21 to 31% in these studies [6, 9, 20]. The disadvantage of these conventional radiographic techniques in orienting the spinal surgeon to the unexposed spinal anatomy is that they display, at most, only two planar images. While the lateral view can be relatively easy to assess, the anteroposterior or oblique view can be difficult to interpret. For most screw fixation procedures, it is the position of the screw in the axial plane that is most important. This plane best demonstrates the position of the screw relative to the neural canal. Conventional intraoperative imaging cannot provide this view. To assess the potential advantage of axial imaging for screw placement, Steinmann et al. [19] used an image-based technique for pedicle screw placement that combined computed tomography (CT) axial images of cadaver spine specimens with fluoroscopy. This study demonstrated an improvement in pedicle screw insertion accuracy with an error rate of only 5.5%.

Image-guided spinal navigation minimizes much of the guesswork associated with complex spinal surgery. It allows for the intraoperative manipulation of multiplanar CT images that can be oriented to any selected point in the surgical field. Although it is not an intraoperative imaging device, it provides the spinal surgeon with superior image data compared to conventional intraoperative imaging technology (i.e. fluoroscopy). It improves the speed, accuracy and precision of complex spinal surgery while, in most cases, eliminates the need for cumbersome intraoperative fluoroscopy. This chapter will focus on its use in the cervical spine.

Principles of Image-Guided Spinal Navigation

The use of an image-guide navigational system for localizing intracranial lesions has been previously described [1, 2]. Image-guided navigation establishes a spatial relationship between a preoperative CT image data and its corresponding intraoperative anatomy. Both the CT image data and the anatomy can each be viewed as a three-dimensional coordinate system with each point in that system having a specific x, y and z Cartesian coordinate. Using defined mathematical algorithms, a specific point in the image data set can be matched to its corresponding point in the surgical field. This process is called registration and represents the critical step of image-guided navigation. A minimum of three points needs to be matched or registered, to allow for accurate navigation.

A variety of navigational systems have evolved over the past decade. The common components of most of these systems include an image-processing computer workstation interfaced with a two-camera optical localizer (fig. 1).

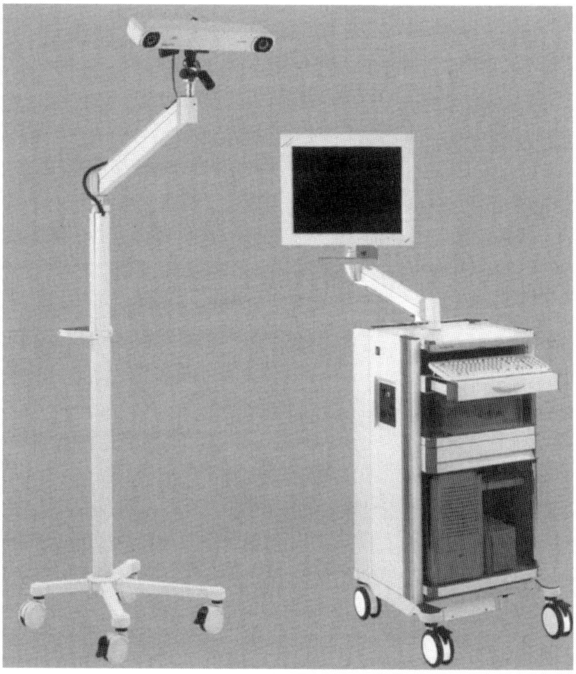

Fig. 1. Image-guided navigational workstation with infrared camera localizer system.

When positioned during surgery, the optical localizer emits infrared light towards the operative field. A hand-held navigational probe mounted with a fixed array of passive reflective spheres serves as the link between the surgeon and the computer workstation (fig. 2). Alternatively, passive reflectors may be attached to standard surgical instruments. The spacing and positioning of the passive reflectors on each navigational probe or customized trackable surgical instrument are known by the computer workstation. The infrared light that is transmitted towards the operative field is reflected back to the optical localizer by the passive reflectors. This information is relayed to the computer workstation which can then calculate the precise location of the instrument tip in the surgical field as well as the location of the anatomic point on which the instrument tip is resting.

The initial application of navigational principles to spinal surgery was not intuitive. Early navigational technology applied to intracranial surgery used an external frame mounted to the patient's head to provide a point of reference to link preoperative image data to intracranial anatomy. This was not practical for spinal surgery. The current generation of intracranial navigational technology

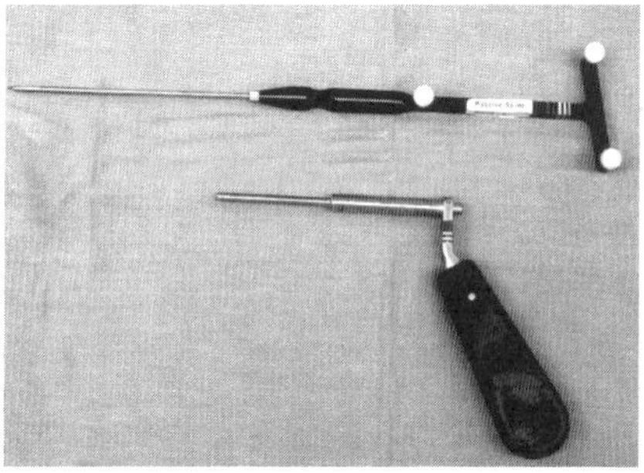

Fig. 2. Navigation probe and drill guide for spinal surgery.

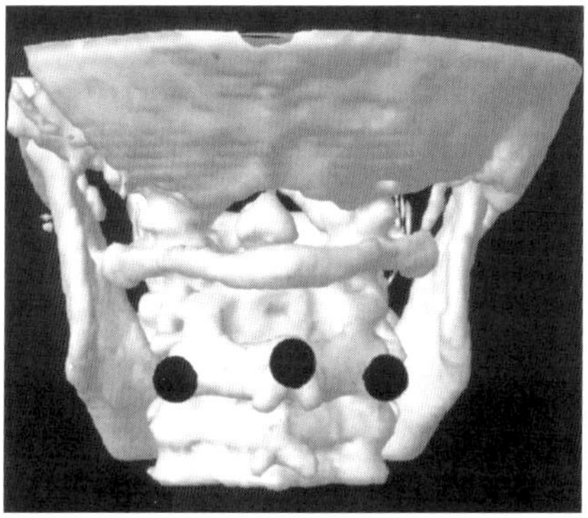

Fig. 3. Navigational workstation screen demonstrating a paired point registration plan for the insertion of C2 pedicle screws. Three discreet bony landmarks are selected at the C2 level. In this case the lateral margins of the two C2–3 facets and the spinous process tip of C2 have been selected.

uses reference markers or fiducials that are glued to the patient's scalp prior to imaging. However, the use of these surface-mounted fiducials for spinal navigation is not practical because of accuracy issues related to a greater degree of skin movement over the spinal column [4, 5]. This is less of a problem with intracranial applications because of the relatively fixed position of the overlying scalp to the attached fiducials.

The application of navigational technology to spinal surgery involves using the rigid spinal anatomy itself as a frame of reference. Bone landmarks on the exposed surface of the spinal column provide the points of reference necessary for image-guided navigation. Specifically, any anatomic landmark that can be identified intraoperatively as well as in the preoperative image data set can be used as a reference point. The tip of a spinous or transverse process, a facet joint or a prominent osteophyte can all serve as potential reference points (fig. 3). Since each vertebra is a fixed, rigid body, the spatial relationship of the selected registration points to the vertebral anatomy at a single spinal level is not affected by changes in body position.

Two different registration techniques can be used for spinal navigation, paired point registration and surface matching. Paired point registration involves selecting a series of corresponding points in a CT or magnetic resonance imaging data set and in the exposed spinal anatomy. The registration process is performed immediately after surgical exposure and prior to any planned decompressive procedure. This allows for the use of the spinous processes as registration points.

A specific registration point in the CT image data set is selected by highlighting it with the computer cursor. The tip of the probe is then placed on the corresponding point in the surgical field and the reflective spheres on the probe handle are aimed towards the camera. Infrared light from the camera is reflected back allowing the spatial position of the probe's tip to be identified. This initial step of the registration process effectively links the point selected in the image data with the point selected in the surgical field. When a minimum of three such points are registered, the probe can be placed on any other point in the surgical field and the corresponding point in the image data set will be identified on the computer workstation.

Alternatively, a second registration technique called surface matching can be used. This technique involves selecting multiple nondiscreet points only on the exposed and debrided surface of the spine in the surgical field. This technique does not require the preselection of points in the image set although several discreet points in both the image data set and in the surgical field are frequently required to improve the accuracy of surface mapping. The positional information of these points is transferred to the workstation and a topographic map of the selected anatomy is created and matched to the patient's image set [18].

Typically, paired point registration can be done more quickly than surface mapping. The average time needed for paired point registration is 10–15 s. The time needed for surface mapping is much longer with difficult cases requiring as much as 10–15 min. With the need to perform several registration processes during each surgery, this time difference can significantly impact the length of the navigational procedure and the surgery itself [16].

The purpose of the registration process is to establish a precise spatial relationship between the image space of the data with the physical space of the patient's corresponding surgical anatomy. If the patient is moved after registration, this spatial relationship is distorted making the navigational information inaccurate. This problem can be minimized by the optional use of a spinal tracking device which consists of a separate set of passive reflectors mounted on an instrument that can be attached to the exposed spinal anatomy (fig. 4). The position of the reference frame can be tracked by the camera system. Movement of the frame alerts the navigational system to any inadvertent movement of the spine. The system can then make correctional steps to keep the registration process accurate and eliminate the need to repeat the registration process. The disadvantage of using a tracking device is the added time needed

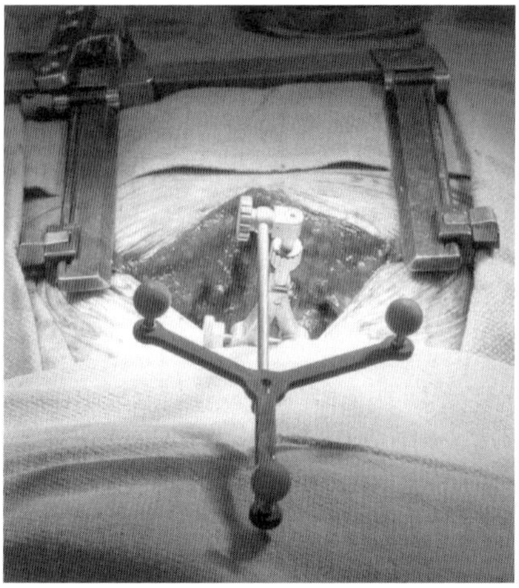

Fig. 4. Reference frame attached to a spinous process in the surgical field. The reference frame monitors inadvertent movement of the spinal anatomy that may affect navigational accuracy.

for its attachment to the spine, the need to maintain a line of sight between it and the camera and the inconvenience of having to perform the procedure with the device placed in the surgical field. It is particularly cumbersome when image-guided navigation is used during cervical procedures.

Alternatively, image-guided spinal navigation can be performed without a tracking device [12, 16]. This involves acknowledging the effect of patient movement on the accuracy of image-guided navigation and maintaining a reasonably stable patient position during the relatively short amount of time needed (i.e. 10–20 s) for the selection of each appropriate screw trajectory. Patient movement can potentially occur with respiration, from the surgical team leaning on the table or from a change of table position. Movement associated with patient respiration is negligible and does not require any tracking even in the thoracic spine. Although movement associated with leaning on the table or repositioning the table or the patient will affect registration accuracy, it can be easily avoided during the short navigational procedure. If inadvertent patient movement does occur, the registration process can be repeated. Repeating the registration process is easiest when using the shorter paired point technique as opposed to the more time-consuming surface mapping technique.

When the registration process has been completed, the probe can be positioned on any surface point in the surgical field and three separate reformatted CT images centered on the corresponding point in the image data set are immediately presented on the workstation monitor. Each reformatted image is referenced to the long axis of the probe. If the probe is placed on the spinal anatomy directly perpendicular to its long axis, the three images will be in the sagittal, coronal and axial planes. A trajectory line representing the orientation of the long axis of the probe will overlay the sagittal and axial planes. A cursor representing a cross section through the selected trajectory will overlay the coronal plane. The insertional depth of the trajectory can be adjusted to correspond to selected screw lengths. As the depth is adjusted, the specific coronal plane will also adjust accordingly with the position of the cursor demonstrating the final position of the tip of a screw placed at that depth along the selected trajectory. As the probe is moved to another point in the surgical field, the reformatted images as well as the position of the cursor and trajectory line will also change. The planar orientation of the three reformatted images will also change as the probe's angle relative to the spinal axis changes. When the probe's orientation is not perpendicular to the long axis of the spine, the images displayed will be in oblique or orthogonal planes. Regardless of the probe's orientation, the navigational workstation will provide the surgeon with a greater degree of anatomic information than can be provided by any intraoperative imaging technique.

The application of image-guided navigation to spinal surgery is directed by the complexity of the procedure and, specifically, by the need to 'visualize' the unexposed spinal anatomy. Image-guided navigation can be used with or without standard intraoperative imaging techniques (i.e. fluoroscopy). In either case, image-guided navigation provides the surgeon with an improved orientation to the pertinent spinal anatomy, which subsequently facilitates the accuracy and effectiveness of the procedure.

Clinical Applications

Prior to using image-guided navigation for spinal surgery, testing of the system was carried out in cadaver spine specimens. Image guidance was used to direct screws into the thoracic and lumbosacral pedicles of these specimens. The accuracy of screw insertion was assessed with plain film radiography and thin section CT imaging of the instrumented levels. All inserted pedicle screws were determined to be satisfactorily positioned [17].

The initial clinical application of image-guided spinal navigation was for lumbosacral pedicle fixation [8, 10, 12]. It proved to be an efficient and effective replacement for intraoperative fluoroscopy and was gradually applied to other spinal procedures such as thoracic pedicle fixation and anterior thoracolumbar decompression and screw fixation. The use of image-guided technology in the cervical spine has also evolved. It is now used for such procedures as C1–2 transarticular screw fixation, lateral mass screws at C1, pedicle screws at C2 and C7 and anterior procedures such as transoral surgery and cervical corpectomy [3, 16, 21].

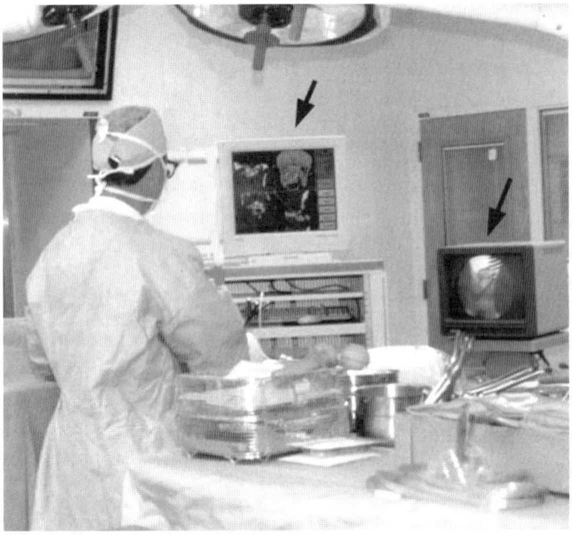

Fig. 5. Positioning of the image-guided system for a C1–2 transarticular screw fixation procedure. The camera is positioned at the head of the table in a vertical orientation. This minimizes any potential visual obstruction between the camera and the surgical field. The workstation is positioned across the table from the surgeon (left arrow). The fluoroscopic monitor sits next to the navigational workstation (right arrow).

Navigational Technique

Image-guided navigation requires the acquisition of a preoperative CT scan through the appropriate spinal segments to be instrumented. The image data is then transferred to the computer workstation via optical disc or a high-speed data link. If paired point registration is to be used, three to five reference points for each spinal segment to be instrumented are selected and stored in the image data set. For most cervical procedures, the camera can be positioned at the head of the table with the navigation workstation positioned across from the surgeon. If fluoroscopy is also used, it can be positioned next to the workstation (fig. 5).

Following a standard surgical exposure, either the paired point or surface matching registration technique is performed. When the registration process has been completed, most navigational workstations will calculate a registration error (expressed in millimeters) that is directly dependent on the surgeon's registration technique. The error presented does not represent a linear error but rather a volumetric calculation comparing the spacing of registration points in the surgical field to the spacing of the corresponding points in the image data set. This figure is, at best, a relative indicator of accuracy.

A more practical method of assuring registration accuracy is the verification step. This step is typically performed immediately after completing either registration process. The surgeon places the navigational probe on a discreet landmark in the surgical field. With the navigational system now tracking the movement and position of the probe, the trajectory line and cursor on the workstation screen will, if accurate registration has been achieved, move to the corresponding point in the image data set (fig. 6a). If registration accuracy has not been achieved, the cursor and trajectory line may rest on something other than the point selected in the surgical field (fig. 6b). If this occurs to a significant degree, the registration process needs to be repeated. This step is more of an absolute indicator of registration accuracy and is a necessary step to perform prior to proceeding with navigation.

C1–2 Transarticular Screw Fixation

This procedure involves the passage of a screw through the pars interarticularis of C2, across the facet joint and into the lateral mass of C1. The risks of screw insertion include injury to the vertebral artery if the screw is placed too laterally or ventrally, injury to the spinal cord if the screw is placed too medially, and failure to engage the lateral mass of C1 if the screw trajectory is too ventral. The insertion of a screw on either side may be contraindicated if the pars interarticularis of C2 is too narrow. The procedure is typically performed bilaterally using fluoroscopic guidance.

The selection of the appropriate screw entry site and trajectory requires a thorough understanding of the atlantoaxial anatomy. Although fluoroscopy provides real-time imaging of the relevant spinal anatomy, the views generated represent only two-dimensional images of a complex three-dimensional anatomic region. Manipulation of the fluoroscopic unit can reduce this problem but these maneuvers can be cumbersome and time-consuming. Other disadvantages include the radiation exposure and the need to wear lead aprons during the procedure. Fluoroscopy cannot provide a view of the spinal anatomy in the axial plane. It is this axial view provided by image-guided navigation that makes it superior to fluoroscopy for spinal screw fixation procedures. The application of image-guided navigation to this procedure adds a significant layer of accuracy for proper screw placement.

The technique for applying image-guided navigation to posterior C1–2 screw fixation involves acquiring a preoperative CT scan that extends from the lower occipital region to C3. The image data is transferred to the computer workstation and can be used to create a preoperative screw trajectory plan. A proposed entry point and target can be selected at the C2 and C1 levels, respectively. The image data set can then be manipulated in multiple planes between these two points to demonstrate the position of a screw placed along the selected trajectory. In addition to a sagittal image that demonstrates the same information provided by lateral fluoroscopy, two other images are

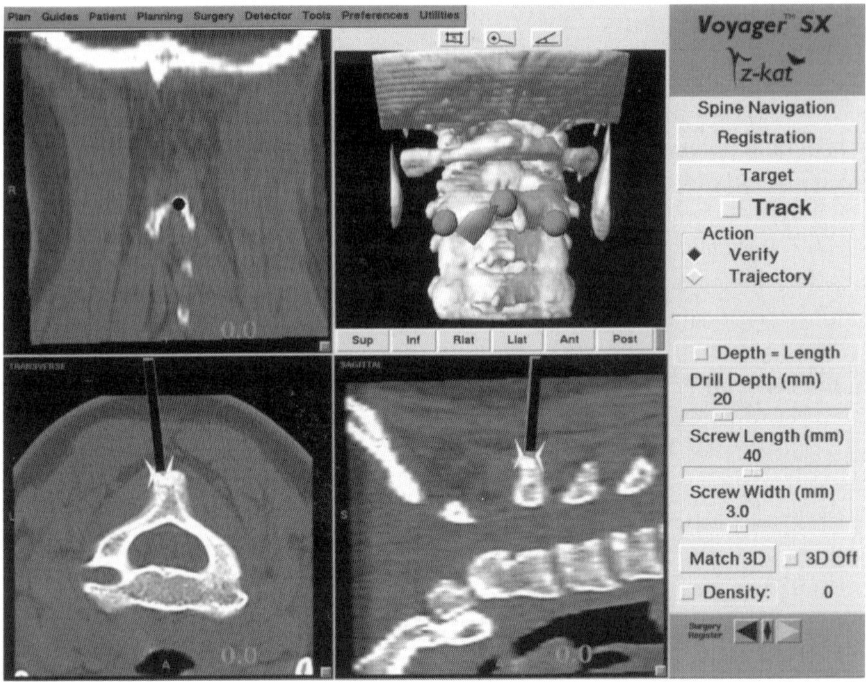
Plan Guides Patient Planning Surgery Detector Tools Preferences Utilities
Voyager™ SX
z-kat
Spine Navigation
Registration
Target
Track
Action
Verify
Trajectory
Sup Inf Rlat Llat Ant Post
Depth = Length
Drill Depth (mm)
20
Screw Length (mm)
40
Screw Width (mm)
3.0
Match 3D
3D Off
Density:
0

6a

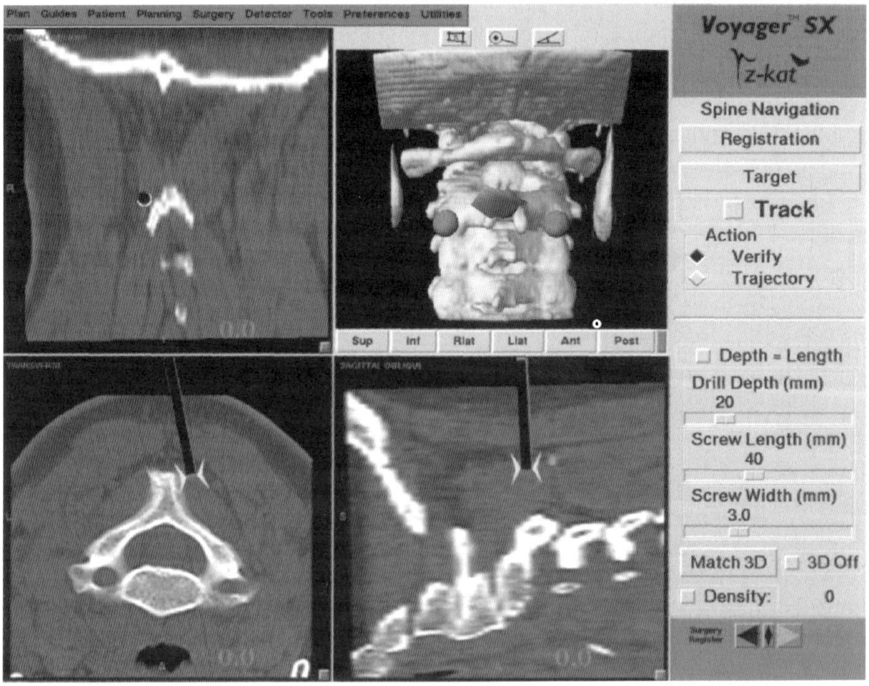
Plan Guides Patient Planning Surgery Detector Tools Preferences Utilities
Voyager™ SX
z-kat
Spine Navigation
Registration
Target
Track
Action
Verify
Trajectory
Sup Inf Rlat Llat Ant Post
Depth = Length
Drill Depth (mm)
20
Screw Length (mm)
40
Screw Width (mm)
3.0
Match 3D
3D Off
Density:
0

6b

presented. One of the images lies perpendicular to the sagittal image along the selected trajectory. It represents an orthogonal view that lies approximately midway between the coronal and axial planes through the spine. It demonstrates a second view of the selected trajectory.

An additional view demonstrates an image oriented perpendicular to the long axis of the probe and, therefore, the selected trajectory. A cursor superimposed on this image can show the position of the screw tip along the selected trajectory at millimetric increments. By scrolling through this image, the proposed position of the screw along the selected trajectory can be assessed along its entire path. While this planning technique does not assure safe screw placement intraoperatively, it can preoperatively alert the surgeon to avoid screw placement in patients with insufficient anatomy and to select an alternate approach.

Intraoperatively, the patient is positioned and the posterior C1–2 complex is exposed. A wire (cable) and bone graft stabilization procedure at the C1–2 level is performed prior to navigation and screw insertion. Performing this step first minimizes any independent motion between C1 and C2 during navigation and makes tap and screw insertion easier. If a reference frame is used, it is typically attached to the spinous process of C2.

Following placement of the graft and cable, three to five registration points are selected at the C2 level. It is not necessary to include registration points at C1. Although the spatial relationship of C1 and C2 may change between the preoperative scanned position and the intraoperative position, the ability of image-guided navigation to facilitate accurate screw placement is not significantly affected. The technical difficulty of this procedure is the accurate passage of the screw through the narrow pars interarticularis of C2. The lateral mass of C1 is a relatively large target that can be easily reached provided there is a reasonably acceptable realignment of C1 and C2 as well as an optimal positioning of the screw within the appropriate C2 anatomy. While the relative position of C1 and C2 in both the preoperative image set and in the surgical field is important, it is not critical enough to interfere with the process of image-guided navigation.

Fig. 6. ***a*** Navigational workstation screen demonstrating satisfactory verification of registration accuracy. While the navigational probe is positioned on the C2 spinous process in the surgical field, the workstation screen should show the cursor and trajectory line in a correlative position in the CT image set. ***b*** Navigational workstation screen demonstrating an unsatisfactory verification of registration accuracy. If the navigational probe is positioned on the C2 spinous process in the surgical field but the workstation screen shows the cursor and trajectory line in a noncorrelative position (i.e. not on the C2 spinous process) accurate registration has not been achieved and the registration process needs to be repeated before proceeding with navigation.

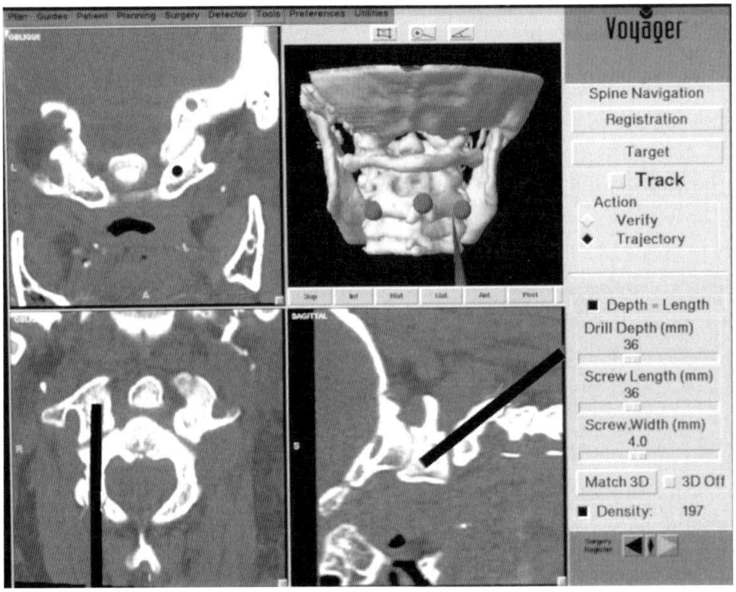

Fig. 7. Workstation screen demonstrating a trajectory for insertion of a C1–2 transarticular screw. The lower right screen shows the trajectory in the sagittal plane. The lower left screen represents an orthogonal plane lying between the axial and coronal planes. It conveys the medial-lateral trajectory. The upper left screen represents a plane that is perpendicular to the two other images. It demonstrates the location of the screw tip inserted along the selected trajectory at the indicated depth.

Two separate stab incisions are made on either side of the midline at the C7–T1 level. A drill guide is placed through one of the stab incisions, passed through the paravertebral musculature and into the operative field. A small divot is drilled at the proposed entry site in order to provide for secure placement of the drill guide. The registration process is performed at the C2 level and its accuracy confirmed using the verification step. The probe is passed through the drill guide and, as its position is adjusted in the surgical field, the images on the workstation screen will adjust accordingly to show the corresponding trajectory in two separate planes and the projected location of the screw tip in the third plane. Orientation to the correct screw position can be assessed rapidly and accurately (fig. 7). Any errors in trajectory or entry point selection can be determined and corrected by adjusting the position of the probe and the drill guide through which it passes. When the correct screw insertion parameters have been selected, the probe is removed from the drill guide and a drill inserted. A hole is drilled along the selected trajectory, tapped and the appropriate length screw inserted. The process is repeated on the opposite side.

The purpose of the drill guide is to preserve the physical trajectory and entry point information just acquired through the navigation of that pedicle. If a drill guide is not used, it may be difficult to precisely position a drill or pedicle probe on the same point and with the same trajectory previously conveyed by the navigational probe after probe removal.

While image-guided navigation does not guarantee accurate screw placement, it does provide the surgeon with a greater degree of anatomical information than fluoroscopy alone. The addition of fluoroscopy to this navigational technique provides the greatest degree of precision to the procedure. In this case however, navigational technology significantly reduces the time of intraoperative fluoroscopic usage as it is typically used only to help position the patient preoperatively and as a final check of the selected trajectory in the sagittal plane immediately following the navigational step.

Segmental C1–2 Screw Fixation

As an alternative to transarticular screw fixation, segmental fixation of C1–2 can be used for managing atlantoaxial instability [11]. The procedure involves placing a screw into each of the two lateral masses of C1 and two screws down the pedicles of C2. The polyaxial screw heads on each side are then connected with rods. Although this approach potentially reduces the risk of injury to the vertebral artery during screw insertion, it does not eliminate the risk altogether. As with the transarticular technique, precise anatomic orientation is required to avoid arterial or neural injury. Image guidance can supplement intraoperative fluoroscopy in order to provide the necessary orientation for accurate screw insertion.

As with the transarticular screw fixation technique, a preoperative CT is obtained. The posterior C1–2 spine is exposed and a wire and cable fixation procedure is carried out. Registration is first performed at C1 for placement of the C1 lateral mass screws. The three registration points typically used at C1 include the midline posterior tubercle and the bilateral points marked by the junction of the small pedicle of C1 with its lateral mass (immediately above the two exiting C2 nerve roots). Once registered, the correct trajectory into the lateral mass can be displayed on the workstation screen and the screws inserted (fig. 8).

To use image guidance for inserting C2 pedicle screws, the same registration points are used at C2 as those used for transarticular fixation (the C2 spinous process and the two lateral margins of the C2–3 facet). The entry point for the screw is more lateral and the trajectory more medially oriented than for a transarticular screw. The navigation probe is placed through a drill guide onto this entry point and the selected trajectory is displayed on the workstation screen. When the correct entry point and trajectory have been selected, the probe is removed, a drill is inserted and the pilot hole is drilled (fig. 9).

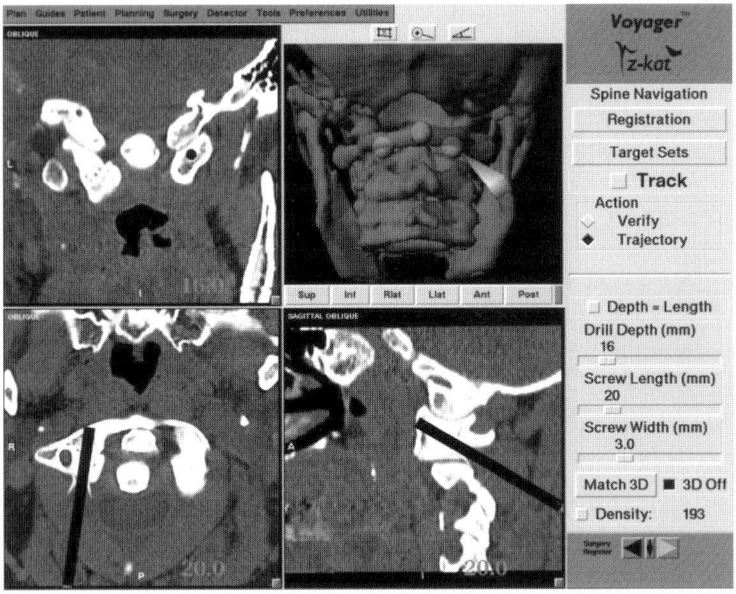

Fig. 8. Workstation screen demonstrating navigational information for placement of a screw into the lateral mass of C1.

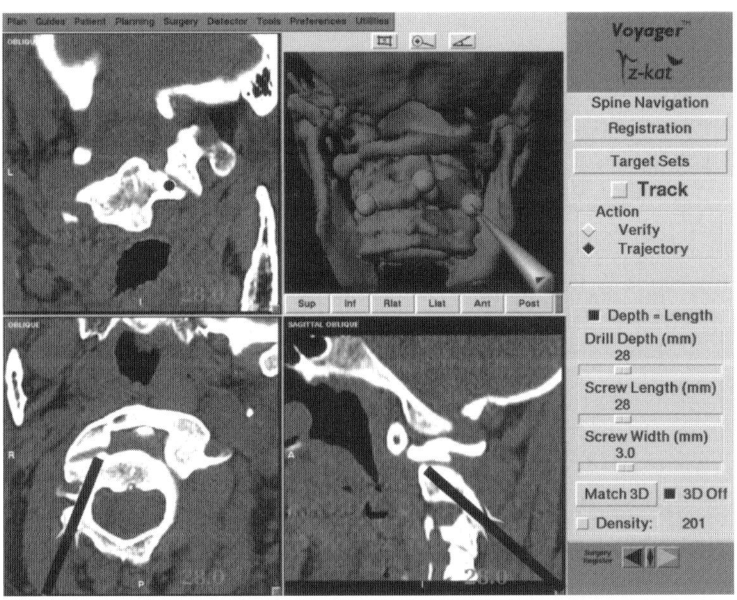

Fig. 9. Workstation screen demonstrating navigational information for placement of a screw into the pedicle of C2.

The process is repeated for the other side. The heads of the screws are then connected with two short rods.

Transoral Surgery

Transoral decompression of the upper cervical spine typically requires intraoperative fluoroscopy to help maintain proper anatomic orientation during the procedure. Although orientation in the sagittal plane is easy to obtain with fluoroscopy, depth and medial-lateral orientation are more difficult to assess. Image-guided technology can be used to orient the surgeon in multiple planes during transoral surgery [16, 21].

Unlike other spinal applications of image guidance, discreet registration points are not readily available during transoral surgery. In this setting, surface-mounted markers (fiducials) are applied to the patient prior to obtaining the preoperative CT. Typically, two fiducials are applied to the mastoid processes and two are applied to the lateral orbital margins or to both malar eminences. The nasal septum can also be used as an inherent registration point.

The patient is positioned in a three-point head holder. The registration process is performed prior to draping the patient using the surface-mounted fiducials. Because the registration points will not be accessible during the procedure, a reference frame is used for transoral navigation. This allows for changes in patient positioning during surgery without the need to re-register. The reference frame can be attached to the three-point head holder.

During the procedure, the probe can be placed into the site of the decompression. Reformatted sagittal, axial and coronal CT images are immediately generated providing the surgeon with a precise orientation to the pertinent surgical anatomy. In particular, orientation in the axial plane minimizes the risk of lateral deviation towards the vertebral artery during the decompression (fig. 10). If a posterior fixation is indicated following transoral decompression, the same CT image data set can be used for C1–2 screw placement.

Other Cervical Applications

There are several other applications for image-guided navigation in the cervical spine. Any procedure in which intraoperative imaging is required to improve a surgeon's orientation to nonexposed spinal anatomy can benefit from image guidance. The other cervical procedures to which image guidance has been applied include navigation during the removal of cervical neoplasms (fig. 11), the placement of anterior fixation screws for the management of nondisplaced odontoid fractures, lateral mass screw fixation in the subaxial

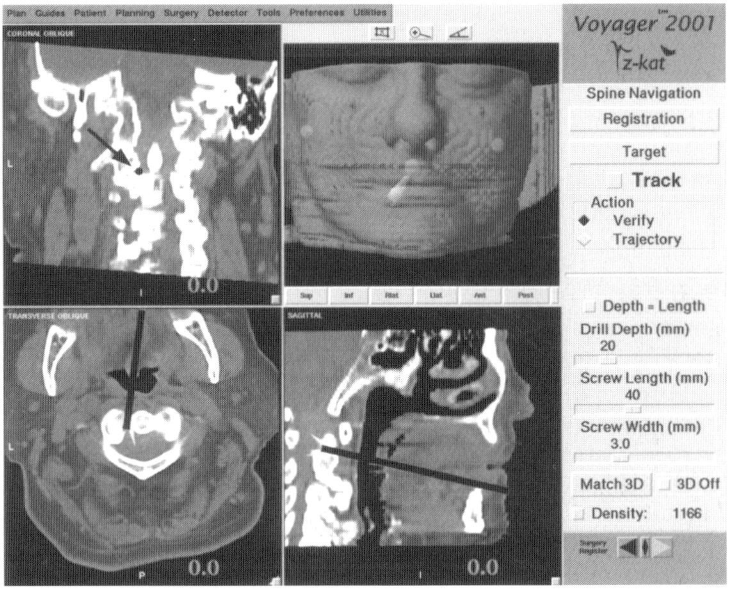

Fig. 10. Workstation screen demonstrating navigational information during transoral decompression (probe tip location and trajectory highlighted by arrows).

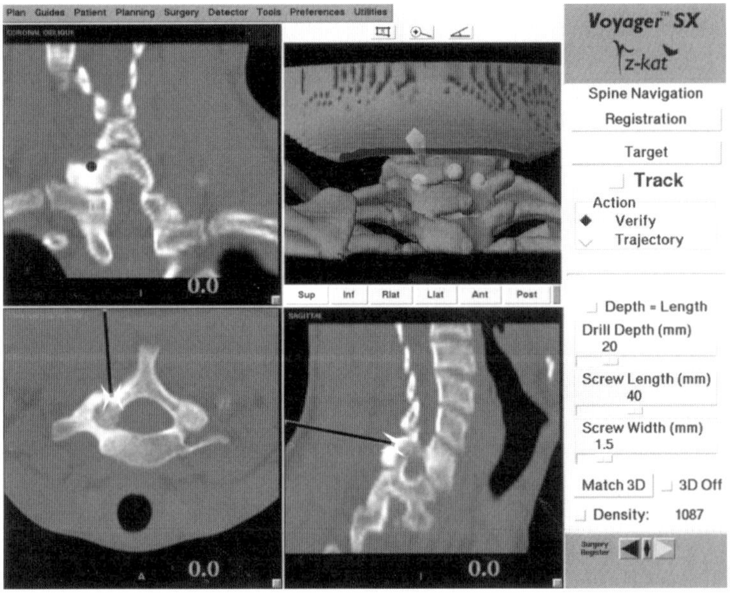

Fig. 11. Workstation screen demonstrating the use of image guidance to help localize an osteoid osteoma within the lamina and articular pillar of C7.

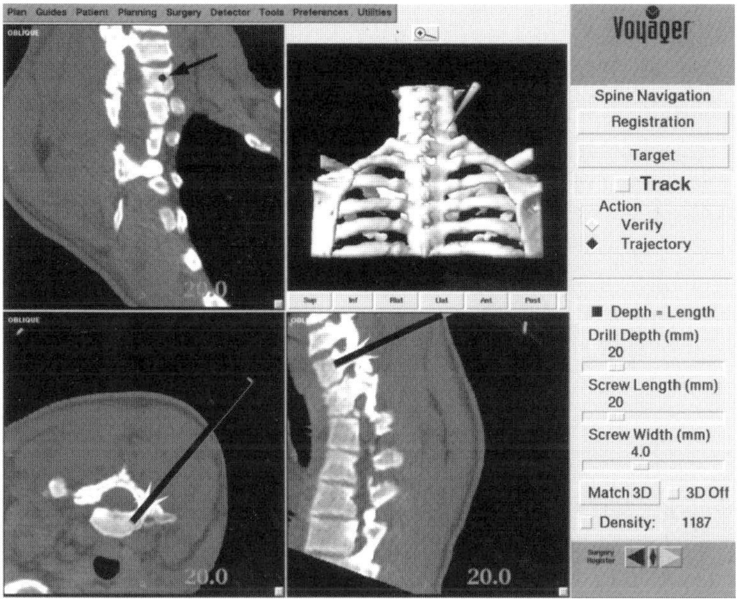

Fig. 12. Workstation screen demonstrating navigational information for the placement of a screw into the pedicle of C7.

spine, cervical corpectomy and the placement of pedicle screws into C7 (fig. 12) [3, 13–16]. While anterior cervical applications of image guidance present unique registration difficulties because of the relative lack of discreet registration points on the anterior surface of the cervical spine, sufficient navigational information can be obtained in order to improve the precision of these procedures.

Pitfalls of Image-Guided Spinal Navigation

Like any other computer-based technology, image-guided navigation is highly dependent on the quality of the information imported into the system. While obtaining the properly formatted CT images and having them correctly transferred to the navigational workstation is important, the critical step of image guidance is the registration process. If the surgeon takes too casual an approach to registration, inaccurate information will be displayed during intraoperative navigation.

Another important principle of image guidance is the need to correlate the navigational information with the surgeon's own knowledge of the surgical anatomy and the appropriate screw trajectories through that anatomy. Image-guided navigation is not a replacement for the surgeon knowing the pertinent spinal anatomy and surgical technique. It merely serves to help confirm a surgeon's estimation of the nonexposed anatomy by providing image information that typically exceeds that of intraoperative fluoroscopy.

Image-guided technology also has varying degrees of intraoperative functionality depending on the features of the navigational system used. This translates into an ease of use factor that can either simplify or complicate the overall procedure. Typically, the use of the surface mapping registration technique and a reference frame add time to the navigational procedure, frequently making it longer and more complicated than using fluoroscopy alone. The use of the paired point registration technique without a reference frame further simplifies the spinal navigation process. The option of using a reference frame is dependent on the particular navigational system used.

Fluoroscopic Navigation

Fluoroscopic navigation is the combination of standard fluoroscopy with image-guided navigational technology. It was developed to counter the user difficulties of some earlier image-guided systems that typically took much longer to use than standard fluoroscopy. Its advantage is that it allows for a reduction in fluoroscopic time during the procedure. With the patient in position prior to surgery, an anteroposterior and lateral fluoroscopic view of the pertinent spinal anatomy is obtained. This is done with a customized reference frame attached to the C-arm or to the patient. This frame serves to superimpose a specific grid on the two images obtained. The navigational workstation can then take the two images and relate the spatial position of the imaged anatomy to a navigational probe. A navigational trajectory line and cursor can be superimposed on the lateral and anteroposterior images, respectively. As the probe is moved over the exposed spinal anatomy during surgery the trajectory line and cursor will adjust their position on the stationary fluoroscopic images [7].

The disadvantage of fluoroscopic navigation is that it is still only fluoroscopy. The same difficulties experienced with standard fluoroscopy are present with fluoroscopic navigation. Specifically, only an anteroposterior and lateral images are provided. The critical plane for most spinal screw fixation procedures is the axial plane. This is the only plane that can definitively demonstrate violation of the spinal canal by a medially displaced screw. Only CT-based image-guided navigation can demonstrate this view although current developments with standard fluoroscopy will eventually allow for axial reconstructions. Furthermore, any region of the spinal column that is difficult to image with standard fluoroscopy (i.e. upper thoracic) will be difficult to image with fluoroscopic navigation.

The early goals of image-guided spinal navigation were to improve the surgeon's orientation to the intraoperative spinal anatomy in a time- and cost-efficient manner and to ultimately replace fluoroscopy. While earlier image-guided systems were difficult to use intraoperatively, several advances have made some systems much easier to use. Several years of clinical experience have helped modify and improve navigational techniques. The use of paired point registration and the optional use of a reference frame have both been found to significantly reduce the difficulties of using image-guided technology for spinal procedures. Advances in computer and localizer technology have also contributed to an improved functionality of these systems. This improved ease of use of the advanced image-guided systems coupled with superior accuracy, image manipulation and orientation capabilities provides image-guided technology with a clear advantage over any fluoroscopic-based technology.

Conclusion

Image-guided navigational technology has been successfully applied to spinal surgery. By linking digitized image data to spinal surface anatomy, image-guided spinal navigation facilitates the surgeon's orientation to unexposed spinal structures improving the precision and accuracy of the surgery. It is typically used to optimize the placement of spinal fixation screws and to monitor the extent of complex decompressive procedures. It can also be used as a preoperative planning tool.

While image-guided spinal navigation is a versatile and effective technology, it is not a replacement for the surgeon having a thorough knowledge of the pertinent spinal anatomy as well as correct surgical techniques. It merely serves as an additional source of information used by the surgeon to make selected intraoperative decisions. In this way, it is similar to more conventional intraoperative imaging techniques (i.e. fluoroscopy) except that it provides a much greater degree of information to the surgeon.

Despite the advantages of image guidance, the surgeon must ultimately assess the information provided by these systems and determine if it correlates with his or her estimation of the nonexposed anatomy and the proposed surgical plan. If good correlation exists between the two, the surgical step can be carried out. However, if sufficient correlation is not present, the surgeon needs to reassess both the spinal anatomy and the image-guided registration accuracy before proceeding.

Ideally, the clinical application of this technology to spinal surgery should facilitate a reduction in operative time, morbidity, and costs. It should be capable of minimizing or eliminating the need for conventional intraoperative imaging. It should be fast, easy to use, reliable and capable of being used briefly to provide accurate intraoperative information while minimizing any disruption to the standard routine of each surgical procedure. Ultimately, beyond each individual surgical application, image-guided navigation technology needs to be clinically versatile. It is the routine use of this technology by multiple surgical specialties that will drive its continued evolution and development as well as establishing it as a cost-effective surgical tool.

References

1 Barnett GH, Kormos DW, Steiner CP, Weisenberger J: Use of a frameless, armless stereotactic wand for brain tumor localization with two-dimensional and three-dimensional neuroimaging. Neurosurgery 1993;33:674–678.

2 Barnett GH, Kormos DW, Steiner CP, Weisenberger J: Intraoperative localization using an armless, frameless stereotactic wand. Technical note. J Neurosurg 1993;78:510–514.

3 Bolger C, Wigfield C, Melkent T, Smith K: Frameless sterotaxy and anterior cervical surgery. Comput Aided Surg 1999;4:322–327.

4 Brodwater BK, Roberts DW, Nakajima T, Friets EM, Strohbehn JW: Extracranial application of the frameless stereotactic operating microscope: Experience with lumbar spine. Neurosurgery 1993;32:209–213.

5 Bryant JT, Reid JG, Smith BL, Stevenson JM: A method for determining vertebral body positions in the sagittal plane using skin markers. Spine 1989;14:258–265.

6 George DC, Krag MH, Johnson CC, Van Hal ME, Haugh LD, Grobler LJ: Hole preparation technique for transpedicle screws: Effect on pull-out strength from human cadaveric vertebrae. Spine 1991;16:181–184.

7 Foley KT, Simon DA, Rampersaud YR: Virtual fluoroscopy: Computer-assisted fluoroscopic navigation. Spine 2001;26:347–351.

8 Foley KT, Smith MM: Image-guided spine surgery. Neurosurg Clin N Am 1996;7/2:171–186.

9 Gertzbein SD, Robbins SE: Accuracy of pedicle screw placement in vivo. Spine 1990;15: 11–14.

10 Glossop ND, Hu RW, Randle JA: Computer-aided pedicle screw placement using frameless sterotaxis. Spine 1996;21:2026–2034.

11 Harms J, Melcher R: Posterior C1–C2 fusion with polyaxial screw and rod fixation. Spine 2001; 26:2467–2471.

12 Kalfas IH, Kormos DW, Murphy MA, McKenzie RL, Barnett GH, Bell GR, Steiner CP, Trimble MB, Weisenberger JP: Application of frameless stereotaxy to pedicle screw fixation of the spine. J Neurosurg 1995;83:641–647.

13 Kalfas IH: Spinal surgery; in Barnett GH, Roberts DW, Maciunas RJ (eds): Image-Guided Neurosurgery: Clinical Applications of Surgical Navigation. St Louis, Quality Medical Publishing, 1998, pp 117–134.

14 Kalfas IH: Image-guided spinal navigation: Application to spinal metastasis; in Maciunas RJ (ed): Advanced Techniques in Central Nervous System Metastasis. Lebanon, AANS Publications, 1998, pp 245–254.

15 Kalfas IH: Frameless stereotaxy assisted spinal surgery; in Renganchary SS (ed): Neurosurgery Operative Color Atlas. Lebanon, AANS Publications, 2000, pp 123–134.

16 Kalfas IH: Image-guided spinal navigation. Clin Neurosurg 1999;46:70–88.

17 Murphy MA, McKenzie RL, Kormos DW, Kalfas IH: Frameless stereotaxis for the insertion of lumbar pedicle screws: A technical note. J Clin Neurosci 1994;1/4:257–260.

18 Pellizzari CA, Levin DN, Chen GTY, Chen CT: Image registration based on anatomic surface matching; in Maciunas RJ (ed): Interactive Image-Guided Neurosurgery. Park Ridge, American Association of Neurological Surgeons, 1993, pp 47–62.
19 Steinmann JC, Herkowitz HO, El-Kommos H, Wesolowski DP: Spinal pedicle fixation: Confirmation of an image-based technique for screw placement. Spine 1993;18:1856–1861.
20 Weinstein JN, Spratt KF, Spengler D, Brick C, Reid S: Spinal pedicle fixation: Reliability and validity of roentgenogram-based assessment and surgical factors on successful screw placement. Spine 1988;13:1012–1018.
21 Welch WC, Subach BR, Pollack IF, Jacobs GB: Frameless sterotactic guidance for surgery of the upper cervical spine. Neurosurgery 1997;40:958–964.

Iain H. Kalfas, MD, FACS
Department of Neurosurgery (S80)
Cleveland Clinic Foundation
9500 Euclid Ave., Cleveland, OH 44195 (USA)
Tel. +1 216 444 9064, Fax +1 216 445 6801

Haid RW Jr, Subach BR, Rodts GE Jr (eds): Advances in Spinal Stabilization.
Prog Neurol Surg. Basel, Karger, 2003, vol 16, pp 128–141

C1 Lateral Mass Fixation

Amory J. Fiore[a], *Barry D. Birch*[b], *Regis W. Haid, Jr.*[a]

[a] Department of Neurosurgery, The Emory Clinic, Atlanta, Ga., and
[b] Department of Neurosurgery, The Mayo Clinic, Scottsdale, Ariz., USA

A variety of techniques exist for fixation of the upper cervical spine. Recently, several authors have published case series reporting the use of C1 lateral mass screws for posterior cervical fixation [1–3]. In this chapter we describe our surgical technique for placement of C1 lateral mass screws, including indications and results from our experience.

C1 lateral mass screws may be used to provide additional fixation points in occipitocervical constructs, possibly increasing resistance to construct failure in the cervical spine without increasing the number of cervical levels fused. Additionally, C1 lateral mass screws may be used as a supplement to or substitute for other forms of atlantocervical fixation. Techniques for achieving atlantocervical fusion include posterior interspinous fusion with sublaminar cables and iliac crest bone graft [4, 5], C1-C2 transarticular screw fixation [5–7], and interlaminar clamp fixation [8]. While each of these methods has been successfully employed to achieve atlantocervical fusion, anatomic factors may exist in certain situations that preclude their use. Interspinous fusion at C1-C2 with sublaminar cables or interlaminar clamps cannot be performed if the posterior elements of C1 or C2 are absent or disrupted. C1-C2 transarticular screws cannot be placed successfully in the presence of a medially located vertebral artery, irreducible subluxation, severe cervicothoracic kyphosis, or destruction of the C2 pars interarticularis. In these cases constructs employing C1 lateral mass screws may be used to achieve fixation. We present a small case series in which C1 lateral mass screws were used to achieve atlantocervical fixation when anatomic characteristics precluded the use of traditional fixation methods. Also included in this series is one case where C1 lateral mass screws were used to provide additional fixation points for occipitocervical fusion.

Methods

Ten patients with cervicomedullary compression or atlantoaxial instability were treated surgically between February 1998 and February 2002. Preoperative diagnoses included C2 metastasis in 2 patients, irreducible odontoid fracture in 3 patients, atlantoaxial subluxation in 2 patients, and transverse ligament synovial cyst in 3 patients. Posterior atlantocervical fixation was planned in 9 patients, one of whom had a transoral resection of the odontoid prior to posterior fusion. In 1 patient with a C2 metastasis and pathologic fracture, an occipitocervical fusion was planned due to the high degree of instability of the atlantoaxial complex. Atlantoaxial screw fixation was chosen as the initial fixation procedure when preoperative imaging studies did not reveal anatomic factors precluding screw placement. All procedures were performed with intraoperative lateral fluoroscopy or CT-guided frameless stereotaxic navigation (Stealth Station, Sofamor Danek, Memphis, Tenn., USA). Autogenous iliac crest bone graft was harvested via a separate posterior iliac crest incision and used for arthrodesis.

Surgical Technique

The patient is positioned prone using a Mayfield head holder (OMI, Cincinnati, Ohio, USA). The neck is kept neutral with the head in the 'military tuck' position. The arms are tucked at the sides and the shoulders retracted caudally using tape. A midline incision is made extending from the inion to the spine of C3 if atlantoaxial fixation is planned. The incision is extended inferiorly as indicated by the planned procedure. A bilateral subperiosteal dissection of the paraspinal musculature is performed to expose the lateral margins of the facet joints at the C2-C3 level. Dissection is continued laterally over the dorsal arch of C1, exposing the vertebral artery in the vertebral groove on the C1 arch. Bipolar cautery and hemostatic agents such as gelfoam and fibrillar collagen are used to control bleeding from the perivertebral venous plexus. The C2 nerve root is identified and mobilized inferiorly. The lateral mass of C1 inferior to the C1 arch is exposed. The medial wall of the lateral mass is identified using a forward angle curette to identify the medial limit of screw placement. The medial aspect of the transverse foramen can also be identified and serves as the lateral limit for screw placement. The entry point for screw placement is identified 3–5 mm lateral to the medial wall of the lateral mass, at the junction of the lateral mass and inferior aspect of the C1 arch (fig. 1). The entry point may be varied depending on the distance between the medial wall of the lateral mass and the C1 transverse foramen. A high speed drill with a 3-mm round burr is used to remove a small portion of the inferior aspect of the C1 arch overlying the entry point, to create a recess for the screw head and plate or rod (fig. 2a). An assistant retracts the C2 nerve inferiorly and protects the vertebral artery with Penfield dissectors or similar instruments during drilling and screw placement. Using fluoroscopy or image guidance a 3-mm drill bit and guide are used to drill a hole with 10–15° of medial angulation to penetrate the anterior cortex of C1 (fig. 2b, 3). On lateral fluoroscopic imaging the drill is aimed toward the anterior tubercle of C1, so that the drill penetrates the ventral cortex of the lateral mass midway between the superior and inferior facets of C1 (fig. 2c, 4). The hole is tapped with a 3.5-mm tap. If lateral mass plates are used, an appropriate-sized plate is selected and contoured, after which a 3.5-mm screw is placed through the plate (fig. 5). Caudal fixation points are then finalized. If a polyaxial screw-rod

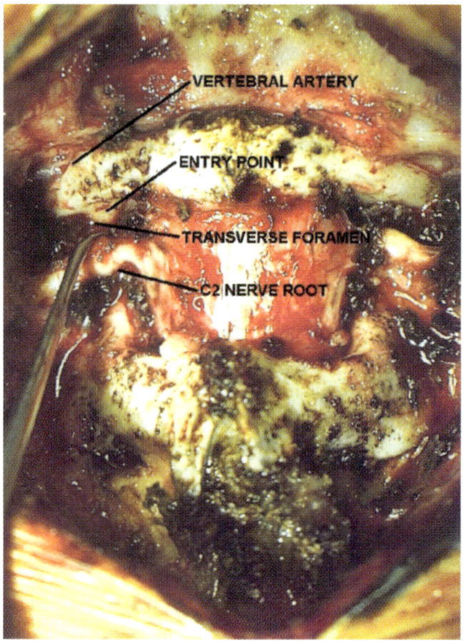

Fig. 1. Intraoperative photograph demonstrating entry point for C1 lateral mass screw, vertebral artery in vertebral groove of C1, inferior aspect of C1 transverse foramen, and C2 nerve root retracted inferiorly.

system is used, all screws are placed after which an appropriate sized and contoured rod is secured (fig. 2d). In both cases an appropriate screw length is selected to achieve bicortical fixation.

Once instrumentation placement is complete, decompression is performed if necessary. Finally, arthrodesis is performed. Posterior arthrodesis with sublaminar cable and interspinous bicortical autograft is preferred if the laminae of C1 and C2 are preserved. Otherwise, lateral arthrodesis is performed by carefully decorticating the exposed surfaces of the C1-C2 joints with a high-speed drill, and then packing cancellous iliac crest autograft over these joints. A Hemovac drain is placed prior to wound closure.

Results

Seventeen C1 lateral mass screws were placed in 8 patients (table 1). These screws were incorporated into several different constructs using lateral mass plates (Axis, Sofamor Danek) or a polyaxial screw-rod system (Vertex, Sofamor Danek) to achieve atlantocervical fixation in 9 patients and occipitocervical fixation in 1 patient. There were no intraoperative complications and no vertebral artery injuries. One patient died on postoperative day 9 from complications of aspiration pneumonia. The remaining patients were immediately mobilized postoperatively in hard cervical collars worn for 3 months. Immediate rigid fixation was achieved in all patients. Follow-up ranged from 9 days to 18 months (mean 6.6 months). Osseous fusion was documented in 2 patients on 9- and 18-month

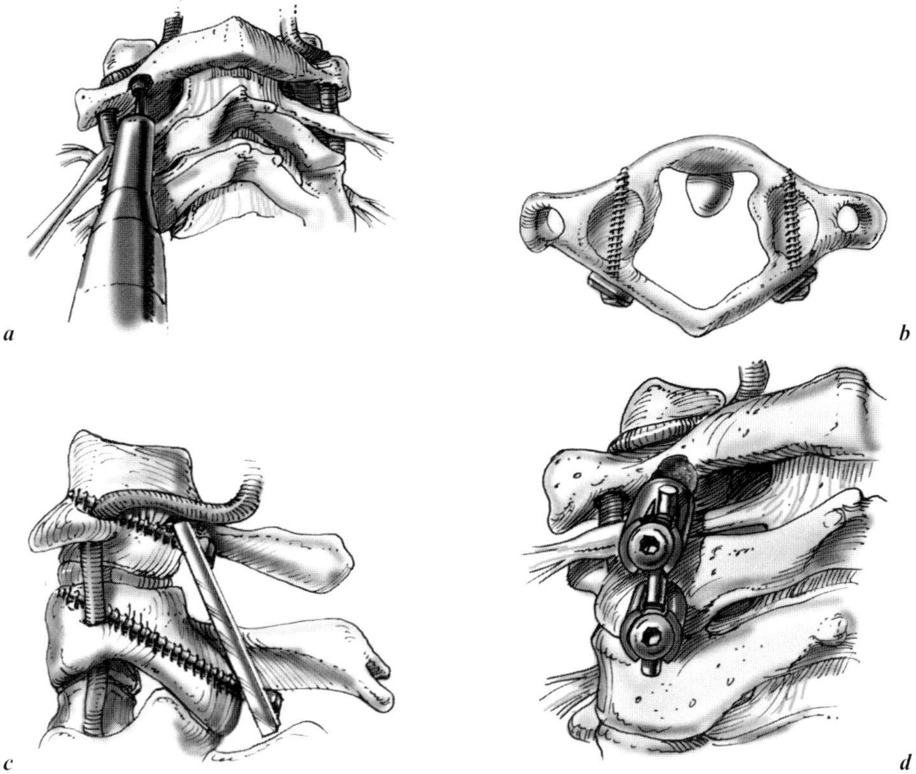

Fig. 2. ***a*** Recess for the screw head is created on the inferior aspect of the C1 arch. ***b*** Axial drawing shows medial screw angulation and relationship to transverse foramina. ***c*** Lateral view of C1-C2 construct with C1 lateral mass screw, C2 pedicle screw, and plate, demonstrating screw trajectory. ***d*** Posterior view of completed C1-C2 construct using polyaxial screw and rod system.

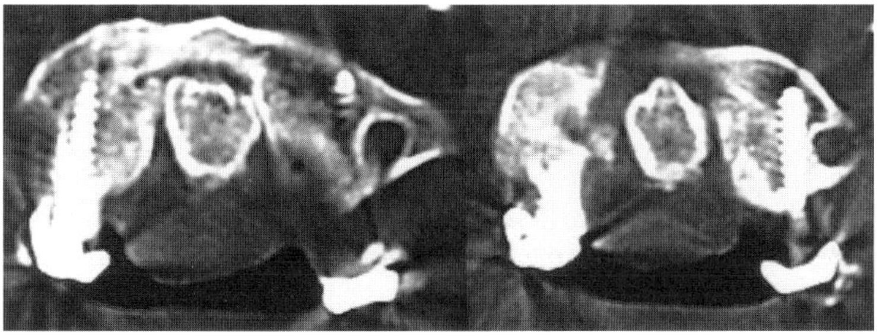

Fig. 3. Axial CT images showing medial angulation of C1 screws and relationship to transverse foramina.

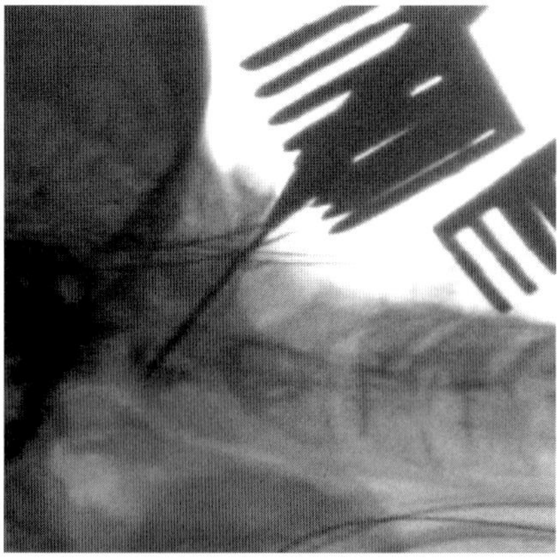

Fig. 4. Intraoperative fluoroscopic image demonstrating C1 screw trajectory toward midpoint of anterior C1 tubercle.

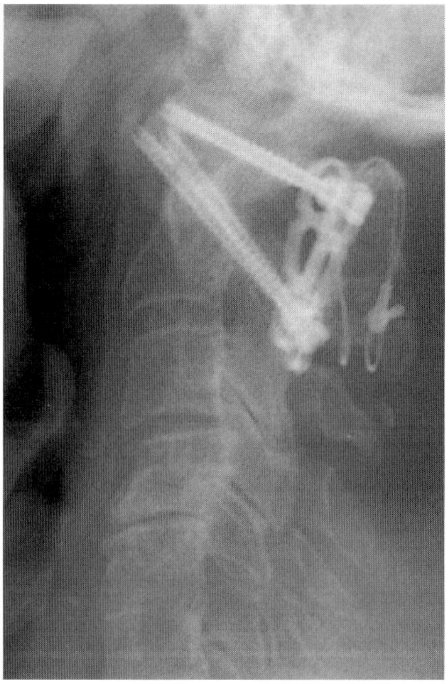

Fig. 5. Completed C1-C2 construct using lateral mass plates and screws.

follow-up radiographs, and 6 patients had delayed postoperative flexion/extension radiographs demonstrating construct stability. In 1 patient a unilateral C1 lateral mass screw was placed after the contralateral lateral mass fractured during drilling. In this patient the polyaxial screw was connected with a rod to a C2 sublaminar hook for atlantoaxial fixation. On follow-up radiographs the screw was noted to be disconnected from the rod, but there was no instability on flexion-extension films and the patient was clinically improved.

Table 1. Case representations

Patient	Age/sex	Presentation	Diagnosis	Treatment	Follow-up	Outcome
1	16/F	Neck pain, neurologically intact	Irreducible type II odontoid fracture	Bilateral C1 LMS, C2 pars screws, polyaxial screw/rod construct; interspinous cable/autograft	6 months	F/E films stable, neurologically intact
2	68/F	Neck pain	Old type II odontoid fracture, nonunion, mobile on F/E films	Bilateral C1 LMS, C2 pars screws, polyaxial screw/rod construct; interspinous cable/autograft	4 months	F/E films stable, clinically improved
3	81/M	Hand numbness, myelopathy	Transverse ligament cyst, irreducible C1-C2 subluxation	C1 laminectomy, unilateral C1 LMS, C2 laminar hook, polyaxial screw/rod construct; lateral autograft arthrodesis	3 months	Rod disconnected from screw, F/E films stable, clinically improved
4	68/M	Hand numbness, neck pain, myelopathy	Transverse ligament cyst, irreducible C1-C2 subluxation	Bilateral C1 LMS, C2 pars screws, plate construct; interspinous cable/autograft	9 months	F/E films stable, symptoms improved
5	74/F	Neck pain, hand numbness, myelopathy	Reducible C1-C2 subluxation, medial R VA	L C1-C2 TAS; R C1 LMS, C2 pars screw, plate construct; interspinous cable/autograft	18 months	Osseous fusion, F/E films stable, symptoms improved
6	46/F	Hand numbness, myelopathy	Transverse ligament cyst, cervicomedullary compression, medial L VA, cervicothoracic kyphosis	Transoral odontoidectomy; posterior atlantoaxial fixation with R C1 LMS, C2 pars screw, plate; interspinous cable/autograft	3 months	F/E films stable, clinically stable

Table 1 (continued)

Patient	Age/sex	Presentation	Diagnosis	Treatment	Follow-up	Outcome
7	34/M	Neck pain, neurologically intact	Irreducible type III odontoid fracture	Bilateral C1, C3 LMS, C2 pars screws, plate construct; interspinous cable/autograft	9 months	Osseous fusion, F/E films stable, neurologically intact
8	72/F	Hand weakness, myelopathy	Congenitally narrow canal at C1, cervicomedullary compression, C1-C2 subluxation, bilateral medial VAs	C1 laminectomy; bilateral C1, C3 LMS, plate construct; C2 sublaminar cables; lateral autograft arthrodesis	3 months	F/E films stable, clinically stable
9	69/F	Neck pain, neurologically intact	Leiomyosarcoma metastasis to R C2 pars, medial L VA	Tumor resection; bilateral C1, C3, C4 LMS, L C2 pars screw, plate construct; lateral autograft arthrodesis	16 months	F/E films stable, neurologically intact, died from diffuse metastases
10	74/M	R hemiparesis, neck pain	Metastatic colon cancer, pathologic C2 burst fracture, spinal cord compression	Occipitocervical fusion to C5 with polyaxial screw/rod system, bilateral C1 LMS	9 days	Died from pneumonia

LMS = Lateral mass screw, TAS = transarticular screw, F/E = flexion/extension, VA = vertebral artery.

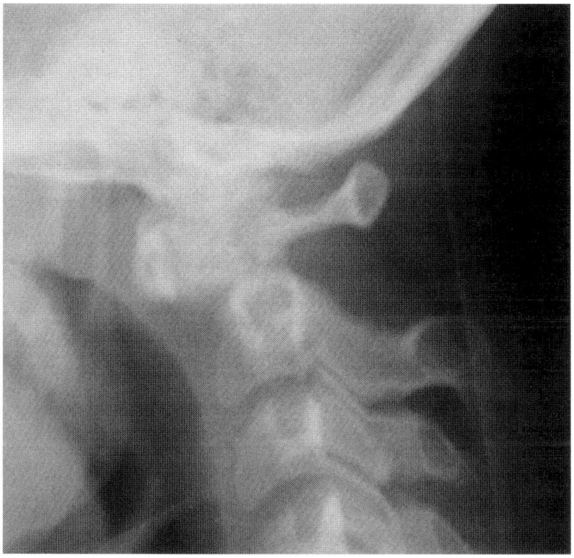

Fig. 6. Patient 1. Preoperative lateral cervical radiograph demonstrating anteriorly displaced type II odontoid fracture.

Illustrative Case: Patient 1

A neurologically intact 16-year-old girl was referred for management of a type II odontoid fracture. She had sustained the fracture 2 months earlier in a motor vehicle accident and had been treated with external immobilization by the referring physician. She was referred when follow-up radiographs showed a 1-cm subluxation at C1-C2 (fig. 6). After 3 days of halo traction, follow-up radiographs demonstrated minimal reduction of the subluxation, and she was taken to the OR for internal fixation. Intraoperative attempts to reduce the fracture under fluoroscopy were unsuccessful. Internal fixation was achieved using a polyaxial screw-rod system with C1 lateral mass screws and C2 pars interarticularis screws, supplemented with interspinous iliac crest autograft and sublaminar cable. The patient was mobilized postoperatively in a hard cervical collar. Postoperative radiographs revealed solid fixation at C1-C2 (fig. 7). The patient is neurologically intact at 6 months' follow-up.

Discussion

We have described a technique to achieve solid fixation of the C1 lateral mass that can be utilized in a variety of instrumentation constructs for varying

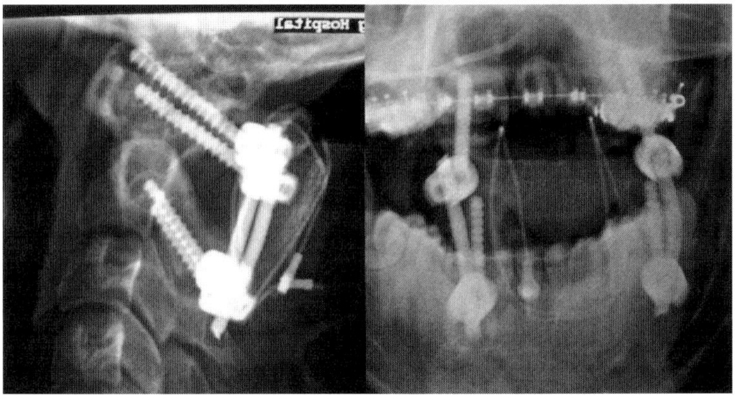

Fig. 7. Patient 1. Postoperative AP and lateral radiographs demonstrating C1-C2 construct with polyaxial screw-rod system and interspinous cable and autograft.

indications. In our experience, the most common indication for the use of C1 lateral mass screws is atlantoaxial instability. Although a variety of techniques exist to treat atlantoaxial instability, certain anatomic factors may preclude their application in specific situations. C1-C2 interspinous fusion techniques using either sublaminar cables or interlaminar clamps in combination with iliac crest autograft require the presence of intact posterior elements. These techniques cannot be applied when the C1 arch or C2 laminae have been disrupted by trauma, neoplasm, or other pathologic processes, or when resection of these elements is necessary to achieve neural decompression. C1-C2 transarticular screw fixation is likewise precluded by a variety of factors. In up to 20% of patients, a medially located or 'high-riding' vertebral artery will preclude safe passage of C1-C2 transarticular screws unilaterally. In 3% of patients, vertebral artery anatomy will preclude passage of screws bilaterally [9, 10]. Irreducible C1-C2 subluxation will likewise preclude optimal placement of C1-C2 transarticular screws. In this case, a screw trajectory traversing the articular surfaces of C1 and C2 cannot be achieved. Severe cervicothoracic kyphosis may preclude C1-C2 transarticular screw placement by obstructing the trajectory of the instruments used to insert the screws. Destruction or erosion of the osseous substrate for screw fixation by trauma, neoplasm, or other pathologic processes will likewise preclude transarticular screw placement. In these situations occipitocervical fusion may be considered as an alternative means to treat atlantoaxial instability. Occipitocervical fusion may be avoided by using C1 lateral mass screws to achieve atlantocervical fixation. By avoiding occipitocervical fixation, patients avoid the risk of intracranial bleeding which may occur with placement of occipital hardware [11]. Additionally, range of motion at the atlantooccipital joint is maintained, reducing morbidity from craniocervical malalignment that may occur following occipitocervical fusion. Clinical studies have also suggested that avoidance of occipitocervical fusion may decrease the incidence of delayed subaxial subluxation [12, 13]. In this series we achieved atlantocervical fixation in 7 patients who demonstrated various anatomic characteristics that precluded traditional methods of atlantoaxial fixation. These patients were all mobilized in hard cervical collars, avoiding postoperative halo vest immobilization.

It is likely that C1 lateral mass screws will also prove to be an extremely useful technique for occipitocervical fixation. C1 lateral mass screws provide additional fixation points for occipitocervical constructs, possibly increasing resistance to construct failure. This additional construct integrity is achieved without fusing additional cervical levels, thus preserving cervical motion segments. In the one patient in this series who underwent occipitocervical fixation, we were able to achieve solid C1 fixation and integration into the occipitocervical construct using C1 lateral mass screws. As the use of polyaxial screw-rod systems for occipitocervical fixation becomes more widespread, we anticipate that C1 lateral mass screws will be used more frequently, since the contourable rods used in these systems will allow C1 screws to be easily incorporated into occipitocervical constructs.

In 6 of the 9 patients in this series who underwent atlantocervical fixation, constructs using C1 lateral mass screws were supplemented with a posterior C1-C2 fusion using sublaminar cable and interspinous autograft. In recent case series, Dickman et al. [4] reported an 86% fusion rate after interspinous fusion with cables and autograft, while Farey et al. [5] reported a 58% fusion rate. In two smaller series, fusion rates of 100% were achieved using the Brooks method of interspinous fusion, but all patients were immobilized in a halo vest for 3 months [14, 15]. It is not clear from this series whether C1 lateral mass screw constructs will increase fusion rates when applied in addition to interspinous fusion techniques, but it seems likely that the additional rigidity conferred by these constructs should result in improved outcomes. The ability of unilateral C1 lateral mass screw constructs to increase fusion rates when applied together with contralateral C1-C2 transarticular screws is also unclear. Song et al. [16] reported a 95% fusion rate after unilateral transarticular screw placement combined with posterior interspinous fusion in a group of patients with high-riding vertebral arteries. In the present series, 1 patient had a unilateral C1 lateral mass screw construct in combination with a contralateral transarticular screw and interspinous fusion. Again, it seems likely that the supplemental fixation provided by the C1 lateral mass screw construct will increase rigidity and result in higher fusion rates.

It is also unclear whether C1 lateral mass screw constructs can be used as a stand-alone method for achieving atlantocervical fusion in the absence of interspinous fusion or unilateral transarticular screw fixation. Harms and

Melcher [2] suggest that temporary C1-C2 constructs using C1 lateral mass screws may be used in selected cases, including rotatory subluxation and young patients with displaced odontoid fractures, allowing preservation of rotation at C1-C2 after instrumentation removal. In addition, they state that C1-C2 fixation with C1 lateral mass screws eliminates the morbidity associated with passage of C1 sublaminar cables. In this series we treated 3 patients with displaced odontoid fractures, adding interspinous cable and autograft to increase construct rigidity and provide additional substrate for bony fusion. We feel that odontoid fractures with irreducible subluxation are best treated with C1-C2 interspinous arthrodesis in addition to instrumentation, to provide optimal rates of long-term fixation. In our experience, passage of C1 sublaminar cables can be performed with minimal morbidity when neural compression is not present. In this series 3 patients were treated with stand-alone constructs because absence of the C1 or C2 laminae precluded interspinous arthrodesis. Two patients had stable radiographs at follow-up, and rod-screw separation occurred in 1 patient with a unilateral construct, although there was no overt radiographic instability. When stand-alone constructs are used, it is important to achieve lateral arthrodesis by decorticating the lateral masses and C1-C2 joint space, with placement of cancellous autograft laterally. In the future, the decision to employ a C1 lateral mass screw construct without interspinous fusion or contralateral transarticular screw fixation should be considered on an individual basis in the context of the pathologic process causing instability, bone quality, and other comorbidities influencing bone fusion, as well as the potential morbidity of the alternative treatment, occipitocervical fusion. Larger studies with long-term follow-up will be necessary to determine the safety and efficacy of C1 lateral mass screw constructs.

To date, only one study has examined the biomechanical characteristics of atlantoaxial constructs using C1 lateral mass screws. Lynch et al. [17] evaluated an atlantoaxial construct with C1 lateral mass screws and C2 pedicle screws with and without supplemental interspinous cable and graft, and compared this construct with atlantoaxial transarticular screws. The C1 lateral mass screw construct was most resistant to lateral bending and axial rotation, and less resistant to flexion and extension. Adding a posterior cable and graft reduced motion slightly. Compared to transarticular screws, the C1 lateral mass screw construct was slightly less rigid, allowing an average of 0.6° more motion. This study suggests that C1 lateral mass screw constructs are a reasonable alternative to transarticular screws for achieving atlantoaxial stabilization.

Harms and Melcher [2] used a specially modified screw at C1 with an unthreaded proximal shaft, in order to reduce the risk of greater occipital nerve irritation as well as screw breakage. In our series we used standard screws with threads along the entire shaft. We did not observe any cases of occipital neuralgia or screw breakage. These results indicate that standard screws may be used at C1. We believe the risk of greater occipital nerve irritation is small as long as there is adequate space caudal to the C1 screw for passage of the nerve. In 1 patient not included in this series, placement of C1 lateral mass screws was planned. However, intraoperatively the C2 nerve roots were found to be much larger than usual, occupying the entire space between the inferior aspect of the C1 dorsal arch and the superior aspect of the C2 pars. In this case, we elected not to place C1 screws, since the risk of C2 irritation was unacceptably high. In this case the alternative would be to place C1 screws directly into the dorsal aspect of the C1 arch, rather than into the inferior surface of the arch. This would place the screw shafts away from the C2 nerve roots. However, this can only be considered when the rostrocaudal dimension of the C1 arch is large enough to accommodate a screw. In addition, the vertebral artery in the C1 groove must be retracted rostrally during drilling, increasing the risk of embolic complications or direct injury to the vertebral artery by the drill, retractor, or other instruments.

The risk of vertebral artery injury must always be assessed when placement of lateral mass screws or transarticular screws is planned. In this small case series, there were no vertebral artery injuries. To minimize this risk, preoperative assessment of the path of the vertebral artery using CT scanning is mandatory prior to placement of C1 lateral mass screws. Magnetic resonance angiography or catheter angiography may be performed to provide additional information concerning the path and patency of the vertebral arteries, although in our experience we have not found this to be necessary. The surgeon must note that the trajectory of the C1 lateral mass screw is very different from that of lateral mass screws placed in the subaxial cervical spine. Particularly important is that the C1 screw is placed with a slight medial angulation to avoid the vertebral artery laterally and the spinal canal medially. We consider the use of intraoperative fluoroscopy or CT-based image guidance mandatory to safely place C1 lateral mass screws. Fluoroscopy allows safe placement of bicortical screws under direct visualization, while CT-based image guidance provides additional three-dimensional information about the vertebral artery and spinal canal. Virtual fluoroscopy may also prove to be a useful adjunct to screw placement.

Conclusion

The placement of C1 lateral mass screws provides a useful alternative method to achieve atlantocervical fixation when anatomic factors preclude the placement of atlantoaxial transarticular screws. This method achieves immediate rigid stabilization of the atlantoaxial joint and obviates the need for halo vest immobilization. This technique may be used in certain cases as an alternative to occipitocervical fusion, and may also be used to increase construct stability when occipitocervical fixation is employed. Evaluation of the course of the vertebral artery with preoperative CT scanning and use of intraoperative fluoroscopy or image guidance are mandatory when using this technique. Placement of C1 lateral mass screws is a technically demanding procedure that may result in grave complications from vertebral artery injury if improperly performed. We thus advocate that this procedure only be performed by surgeons who are highly experienced in the treatment of atlantoaxial instability, and who have an intimate understanding of the anatomy of the region. The uninitiated surgeon can minimize the possibility of complications during C1 lateral mass screw placement by first performing this procedure in a cadaveric setting. Further biomechanical analysis of this technique should be performed to quantify the strength of constructs employing C1 lateral mass screws as compared with other fixation methods. Further clinical studies should be performed to determine the safety and efficacy of this technique.

References

1 Fiore AJ, Haid RW, Rodts GE, Subach BR, Mummaneni PV, Riedel CJ, Birch BD: Atlantal lateral mass screws for posterior spinal reconstruction: Technical note and case series. Neurosurg Focus 2002:12/1:article 5.

2 Harms J, Melcher RP: Posterior C1-C2 fusion with polyaxial screw and rod fixation. Spine 2001;26:2467–2471.

3 Stokes JK, Villavicencio AT, Liu PC, Bray RS, Johnson JP: Posterior atlantoaxial stabilization: New alternative to C1–2 transarticular screws. Neurosurg Focus 2002;12/1:article 6.

4 Dickman CA, Sonntag VK, Papadopoulos SM, Hadley MN: The interspinous method of posterior atlantoaxial arthrodesis. J Neurosurg 1991;74:190–198.

5 Farey ID, Nadkarni S, Smith N: Modified Gallie technique versus transarticular screw fixation in C1-C2 fusion. Clin Orthop 1999;35:126–135.

6 Dickman CA, Sonntag VK: Posterior C1-C2 transarticular screw fixation for atlantoaxial arthrodesis. Neurosurgery 1998;43:275–281.

7 Haid RW, Subach BR, McLaughlin MR, Rodts GE, Wahlig JB: C1-C2 transarticular screw fixation for atlantoaxial instability: A 6-year experience. Neurosurgery 2001;49:65–70.

8 Moskovich R, Crockard HA: Atlantoaxial arthrodesis using interlaminar clamps. Spine 1992;17:261–267.

9 Madawi AA, Casey AT, Solanki GA, Tuite G, Veres R, Crockard HA: Radiological and anatomical evaluation of the atlantoaxial transarticular screw fixation technique. J Neurosurg 1997;86:961–968.

10 Paramore CG, Dickman CA, et al: The anatomic suitability of the C1-2 complex for transarticular screw fixation. J Neurosurg 1996;85:221–224.

11 Vale FL, Oliver M, Cahill DW: Rigid occipitocervical fusion. J Neurosurg 1997;91(suppl 2):144–150.

12 Clark CR, Goetz DD, Menezes AH: Arthrodesis of the cervical spine in rheumatoid arthritis. J Bone Joint Surg Am 1989;71:381–392.

13 Kraus DR, Peppelman WC, Agarwal AK, DeLeeuw HW, Donaldson WF: Incidence of subaxial subluxation in patients with generalized rheumatoid arthritis who had previous occipital cervical fusions. Spine 1991;16(suppl):486–489.
14 Boden SD, Dodge LD, Bohlman HH, Rechtine GR: Rheumatoid arthritis of the cervical spine. A long-term analysis with predictors of paralysis and recovery. J Bone Joint Surg Am 1993;75:1282–1297.
15 McCarron RF, Robertson WW: Brooks fusion for atlantoaxial instability in rheumatoid arthritis. South Med J 1988;81:474–476.
16 Song GS, Theodore N, et al: Unilateral posterior atlantoaxial transarticular screw fixation. J Neurosurg 1997;87:851–855.
17 Lynch JJ, Crawford NR, Chamberlain RH, Bartolomei JC, Sonntag VK: Biomechanics of lateral mass/pedicle screw fixation at C1-2. Proceedings of the 2002 Annual Meeting of the American Association of Neurological Surgeons, Chicago, 2002.

Regis W. Haid, Jr., MD
Department of Neurosurgery, Emory University
1365B Clifton Road, NE, Ste. 6400, Atlanta, GA 30322 (USA)
Tel. +1 404 778 5770, Fax +1 404 778 4472, E-mail regis_haid@emoryhealthcare.org

Haid RW Jr, Subach BR, Rodts GE Jr (eds): Advances in Spinal Stabilization.
Prog Neurol Surg. Basel, Karger, 2003, vol 16, pp 142–153

Cervical Laminoplasty

Adrian T.H. Casey[a,b], *H. Alan Crockard*[a]

[a] Victor Horsley Department of Neurosurgery, National Hospital for Neurology and Neurosurgery, London, and
[b] Spinal Surgery Unit, The Royal National Orthopaedic Hospital, Stanmore, UK

Cervical laminoplasty is very much a Japanese invention. Its popularity in Japan arises from the formidable challenges of anterior decompression for ossification of the posterior longitudinal ligament [1–5]. These anterior multilevel surgeries would be frequently complicated by dural tears as the dura is usually intimately associated with the ossified ligament [1, 6–9]. There was also a significant risk of instrumentation or graft failure [2]. It has been reported that the rate of these complications including cerebrospinal fluid leakage and dislodgment or pseudarthrosis of the strut grafted bone was 24% and the rate of the salvage operation required was 12.5% [10].

In the past, laminectomy has been the most common method to achieve posterior decompression of the cervical spine in these patients. However, the procedure has been complicated by postoperative instability resulting in deformity, particularly kyphosis [11–15], which may exacerbate neurological symptoms.

Kyphosis and instability may leave the spine more vulnerable to cervical spine trauma, especially flexion injuries. In addition, postlaminectomy membranes have been implicated in arachnoiditis and restenosis after simple laminectomy [16, 17]. To avoid the disadvantages of laminectomy, several authors have described the technique of cervical laminoplasty whereby decompression is achieved without removal of the posterior spinal elements, maintaining the biomechanical integrity of the cervical spine and the spinal cord-protective features of the posterior elements [3, 18–25]. This is a more physiological solution. Expansive open-door laminoplasty was first described by Hirabayashi et al. [26] as a development of the air drill laminectomy technique of Kirita [27] and has since been modified by Hirabayashi et al. and many others [3, 18–25, 28]. The authors of this chapter present a modification of the technique using titanium miniplates to stabilize the posterior elements in the open position [22].

Table 1. Indications for expansive cervical laminoplasty

OPLL over multiple levels (with maintained cervical lordosis)
Congenital canal stenosis (with maintained cervical lordosis)
Multilevel cervical spondylosis (with maintained cervical lordosis)
Posterior compression from ligamentous hypertrophy (with maintained cervical lordosis)
As part of a staged anterior and posterior canal expanding procedure

OPLL = Ossification of the posterior longitudinal ligament.

Table 2. Contraindications for expansive cervical laminoplasty

Significant anterior compression
Established absolute kyphosis
Isolated radiculopathy
Loss of anterior column support resulting from tumour, trauma or infection

This method has the advantage of technical simplicity and allows for postoperative magnetic resonance imaging because the use of stainless steel implants is avoided. It has been used in the authors' departments in more than 300 cases now, with good short- and long-term results. The technique is no longer limited to ossification of the posterior longitudinal ligament, which is rare in Caucasians. Its most frequent use is now for multilevel cervical spondylotic myelopathy associated with varying degrees of constitutional canal stenosis. The indications and contraindications are listed in tables 1 and 2.

Kyphosis is a contraindication to laminectomy [29] and probably laminoplasty [30, 31].

There are several technical variations. The two main differences are whether the opening is in the midline (French door) or to one side (open door). Then there are differences in how to keep the door open. Initially the techniques were quite cumbersome and involved suturing or wiring the bony posterior elements to muscle. Inevitably they did not always keep the door as open as it may have been originally at the time of surgery. The Queen Square technique uses titanium miniplates with no bone graft to keep the door open. In our experience this has been a simple and reliable technique. Alternative techniques have used ceramic spacers or bone graft to keep the doors open.

Three types of Z plasty may be performed: on the lamina using the method of Hattori as reported by Oyama et al. [32], between each lamina using the reciprocal method of Tomimura and Morizono [33] and between two segmental laminae using the Chiba University technique [34]. The variety of reported techniques are illustrated in figure 1.

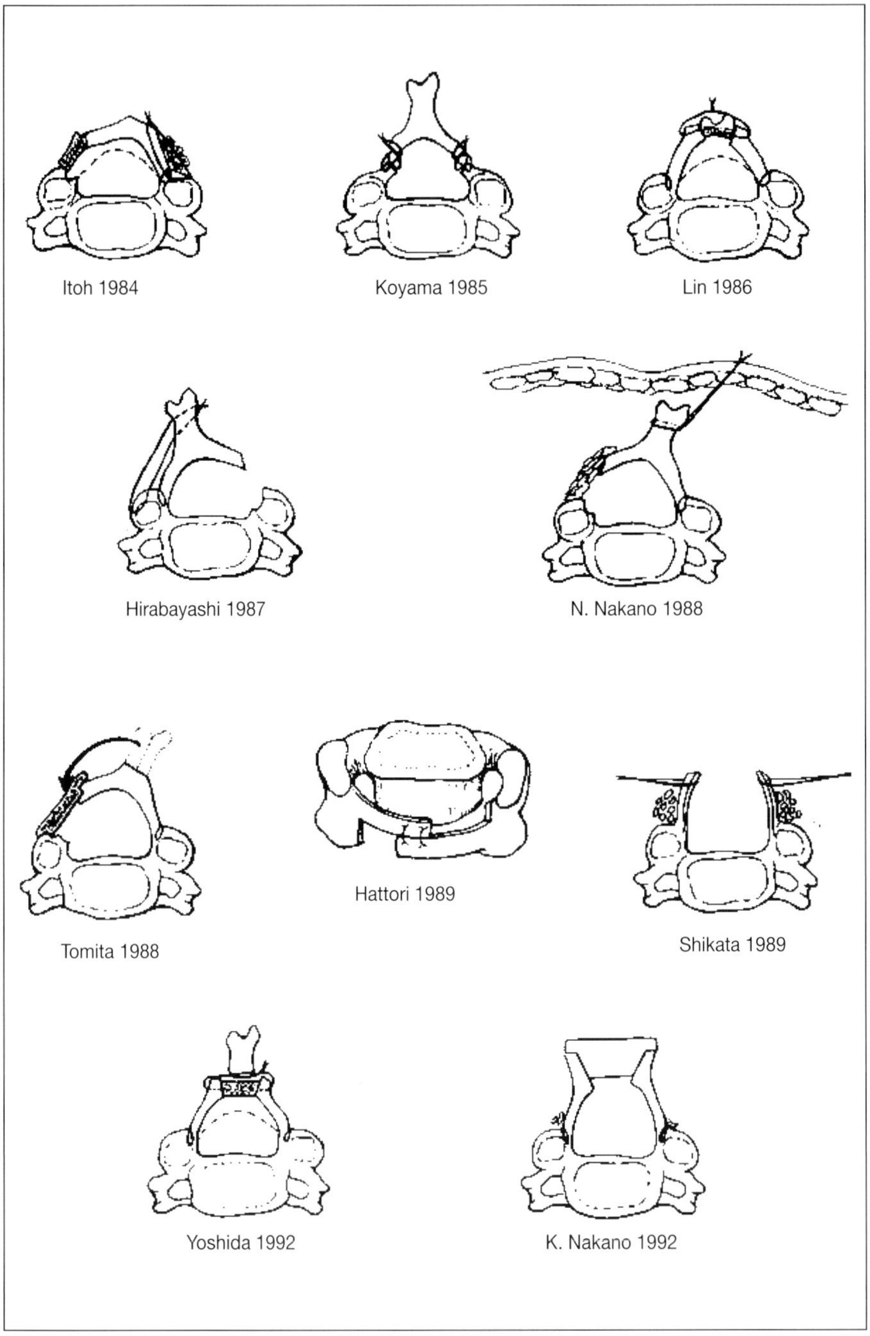

Fig. 1. Different techniques reported.

Tomita et al. have [3] championed the use of their thread wire saw to achieve the opening. This is similar to a very fine Gigli saw. It was developed for en bloc vertebrectomy. This is a clever technical innovation, however it does require sublaminar passage of the wire. This is very much finer than sublaminar wires and indeed cables which have been implicated in neurological deterioration. The majority of the other techniques require a high-speed drill.

Queen Square Technique [22]

Surgical technique (C3–C6): The patient is placed in a prone position with the head slightly flexed secured by Mayfield pins. The body is supported by a Montreal mattress. Somatosensory evoked potentials are recorded. A standard posterior midline approach allows exposure of the cervical laminas from the caudal edge of C2 to the cranial edge of C7 and laterally to the lateral aspect of the facet joints. Care is taken to preserve the facet capsules and soft tissue attachments to the lateral masses. The spinous processes and interspinous ligaments are preserved.

Using a 3-mm spherical cutting burr, two channels are drilled bilaterally. These are placed at the junction of the lamina and the medial aspect of the lateral masses (fig. 2a). Care is taken to avoid damage to the facet joints. Using this technique, the canal is entered laterally, where spinal cord compression is less severe. Inadvertent plunging penetration of the canal is prevented by the shelf created in the medial aspect of the lateral masses. The depth of the channels is increased until the ventral cortex of the lamina is identified. The laminoplasty is opened on the side with clinical evidence of unilateral radiculopathy or with asymmetric canal or foraminal stenosis identified on the preoperative scans. Specific radiculopathies can also be addressed with foraminal decompressions. If there is no unilateral radiculopathy or asymmetric stenosis, either side may be opened.

On the side to be opened, the channel is completed through the ventral cortex of the lamina with a diamond burr or 1-mm Kerrison up-cutting rongeur. Alternatively, the craniotome attachment for the Midas Rex (Midas Rex Pneumatic Tools, Fort Worth, Tex., USA) may be used to transect the lamina on the opening side. This is in fact our most usual technique. There have been no dural tears or neurological deteriorations in our series, using the craniotome attachment to open the door. On the hinge side, the ventral cortex of the lamina is thinned until the posterior elements can be rotated dorsally to effect decompression of the spinal cord (fig. 2b). This is done en bloc because the interspinous ligament and ligamentum flavum are intact from the occiput through C7. Hirabayashi et al. [26] suggest a limited osteotomy of the spinous process of C7 (or most caudal vertebra) to allow a sufficient opening of the door.

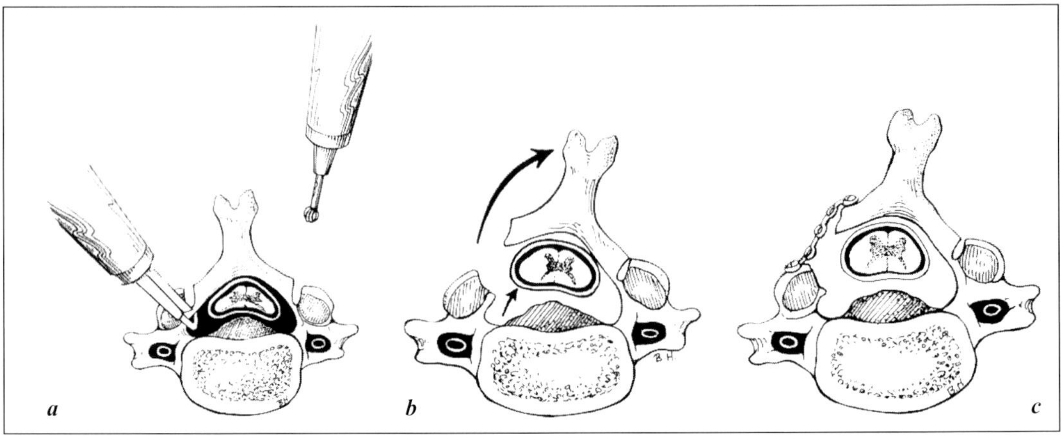

Fig. 2. Operative sequence showing preparation of the bilateral channels for the hinge side (right) and opening side (left) of the laminoplasty (***a***), mobilization and rotation of the posterior elements (***b***), and stabilization of the open-door laminoplasty with titanium miniplates (***c***) [modified from 22].

Release of ligamentum flavum, dural adhesions, and bridging vessels is performed on the opening side as required to elevate the posterior elements. At C2–C3 and C6–C7, partial resection of the intraspinous ligaments on the opening side and partial subperiosteal release of the intraspinous ligaments of C2 and C7 on the hinge side may be necessary to allow adequate mobilization and rotation of the posterior elements, achieving full decompression (fig. 2b). Vigorous epidural bleeding is occasionally encountered on release of the stenotic canal. This can be controlled with bipolar coagulation and haemostatic material. After adequate decompression, the dura is typically pulsatile, indicating satisfactory decompression. When the open door has been adequately mobilized, it is stabilized with titanium miniplates (Lehbinger, Freiburg, Germany).

Hirabayashi et al. [35] unflex the neck prior to fixing their laminoplasty. This they claim helps maintain and secure cervical lordosis. We most often use a straight five-hole plate bent into sigmoid shape/open Z configuration (fig. 2c) to allow one hole for fixation into the lamina and 2 screws into the corresponding lateral mass. Longer or shorter plates can be fashioned as needed to achieve adequate opening. The plates are held in position with 2 or 3 screws 5–9 mm in length. An attempt is made to angle the screws away from the facet joints. We typically use one plate per level, if possible, to distribute the forces over multiple fixation points (fig. 3). No formal attempt is made to graft bone to the operative site. However, on the hinge side, where the adjacent lamina and lateral masses are still connected, the dorsal cortex of these structures are

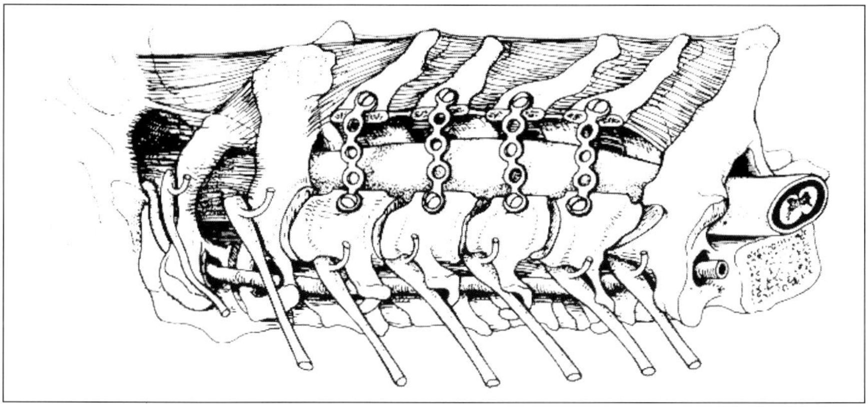

Fig. 3. Schematic diagram showing the orientation of the titanium miniplates in a C3–C6 laminoplasty and adjacent anatomic structures.

brought into contact as the hinge side trough is closed during elevation and rotation of the posterior elements into the open position. This is analogous to a green stick fracture. The morbidity associated with harvesting bone graft is avoided. A soft collar is used to facilitate patient comfort while mobilizing during the first few days after surgery. No other external orthosis is used after surgery.

Discussion

Anterior and posterior decompression are established techniques in the management of multilevel cervical canal stenosis resulting in myeloradiculopathy. Anterior cervical discectomy and fusion immobilize segments of the cervical spine and result in high mechanical demands on the adjacent intervertebral segments. Over the patient's lifetime, abnormal mechanical stresses can produce significant radiographic and clinical evidence of deterioration. Hilibrand et al. [36] in a consecutive series of 374 patients reported that symptomatic adjacent-segment disease occurred at a relatively constant incidence of 2.9%/year (range 0.0–4.8%/year) during the 10 years after the operation. Survivorship analysis predicted that 25.6% of the patients (95% confidence interval, 20–32%) who had an anterior cervical arthrodesis would have new disease at an adjacent level within 10 years after the operation. However, contrary to their hypothesis, they found that the risk of new disease at an adjacent level was significantly lower following a multilevel arthrodesis than it was following a single-level arthrodesis ($p = 0.001$).

Nonetheless there is an intellectual reluctance to perform a multilevel trench procedure with fusion in a young patient. The incidence of complications for anterior multilevel corpectomy has been reported to be high even in expert hands. Saunders et al. [37] did a retrospective analysis of 31 cases of cervical spondylotic myelopathy treated by four-level subaxial cervical corpectomy. Three patients died within 3 weeks of surgery (9.7%). Delayed radiculopathy occurred in 4 patients after surgery, 3 had acute graft complications, and 1 had pseudomeningocoele, resulting in a morbidity rate of 25.8%. There were no cases of infection or increasing myelopathy. In another series by these authors, on 40 cases of cervical corpectomy, they reported a perioperative complication rate of 47.5%, with a 7.5% incidence of persistent sequelae [37–39]. Fessler et al. [40] have reported their extensive experience of cervical corpectomy in a retrospective series of 93 cases over 10 years with a lower complication rate. In another more recent series Edwards et al. [41] have attempted to compare the neurological outcome and complications of cervical corpectomy and cervical laminoplasty. Medical records of all patients treated for multilevel cervical myelopathy with either multilevel corpectomy or laminoplasty between 1994 and 1999 at the Emory Spine Center were reviewed. From a pool of 38 patients meeting stringent inclusion and exclusion criteria, 13 patients who underwent multilevel corpectomy were blindly matched with 13 patients who underwent laminoplasty based on known prognostic criteria. Improvement in function averaged 1.6 Nurick grades after laminoplasty and 0.9 grades after multilevel corpectomy ($p > 0.05$). Subjective improvements in strength, dexterity, sensation, pain, and gait were similar for the two operations. The prevalence of axial discomfort at the latest follow-up was the same for each cohort, but the analgesic requirements tended to be greater for patients who underwent multilevel corpectomy. This is the opposite finding to the larger study of Hosono et al. [42] on pain. Sagittal motion from C2 to C7 decreased by 57% after multilevel corpectomy and by 38% after laminoplasty. One complication (C6–C7 herniated nucleus pulposus requiring anterior discectomy with fusion) occurred in the laminoplasty group [41]. Multilevel corpectomy complications included the progression of myelopathy, non-union, persistent dysphagia, persistent dysphonia, and subjacent motion segment ankylosis.

An alternative posterior decompressive procedure to laminoplasty is cervical laminectomy with posterior fixation/fusion. Today this would be performed using the lateral mass screw/rod system. This will also prevent postoperative kyphus. It will more reliably immobilize the spine. Adams and Logue [43, 44] have shown that one of the reasons for delayed deterioration following cervical laminectomy is hypermobility. Screw/rod fixation is therefore an attractive option. However the extra rigidity is probably not required as Herkowitz [45, 46] concluded from his 'biomechanical study' that stability of the cervical spine after laminoplasty was not significantly different from that of the intact control. Laminoplasty affords some rigidity, but still preserves motion [47]. The long-term effects of laminoplasty on cervical movement and alignment were investigated by radiography and CT scans in a study of 56 patients with multi-segmental myelopathy who had undergone a C3 to C7 open-door laminoplasty. Follow-up averaged 5.8 years. Satisfactory neurological improvement occurred in 73%. Cervical flexion decreased by 35% and extension by 57%; the decrease of both movements was statistically significant. Decreased vertebral slip as well as slightly reduced lordosis was seen after operation.

Cervical laminectomy and laminoplasty have been compared in a retrospective study [48]. This is another study from Emory, with similar design principles to the corpectomy/laminoplasty study described above (an independent matched cohort analysis), involving 13 patients in each arm. Both objective improvement in patient function (Nurick score) and the number of patients reporting subjective improvement in strength, dexterity, sensation, pain, and gait tended to be greater in the laminoplasty cohort [48]. Whereas no complications occurred in the laminoplasty cohort, there were 14 complications in 9 patients that underwent laminectomy with fusion. Complications included progression of myelopathy, non-union, instrumentation failure, development of a significant kyphotic alignment, persistent bone graft harvest site pain, subjacent degeneration requiring reoperation, and deep infection. The marked difference in complications and functional improvement between these matched cohorts suggests that laminoplasty may be preferable to laminectomy with fusion, as a posterior procedure for multilevel cervical myelopathy [48]. Similar findings were found in a less well-controlled study by Herkowitz [49]. In this retrospective study he compared the results and complications of 45 patients with at least a 2-year follow-up, who had undergone anterior fusion, cervical laminectomy, or cervical laminoplasty for the surgical management of multiple level cervical radiculopathy due to cervical spondylosis. Eighteen patients (58 levels) underwent anterior fusion, 12 patients (38 levels) had a cervical laminectomy, and 15 patients (57 levels) underwent a cervical laminoplasty. In another study by Baisden et al. [50], radiographic and biomechanical results in the goat model revealed that laminoplasty was superior to laminectomy in maintaining cervical alignment and preventing postoperative spinal deformities. Quite how this relates to humans is debatable.

Complications

There are two notable complications with cervical laminoplasty – radiculopathy and pain. These have been the subject of several studies [51]. C5,C6 radicular pain and/or paresis are the most frequent complications that occur in approximately 5–10% of the patients in the series of Hirabayashi et al. [35] of 350 patients although most complications resolve spontaneously within 2 years. Of 365 patients who had undergone laminoplasty, 20 patients (5.5%) developed postoperative radiculopathy. Using data from postoperative computed tomography scans and other sources, these patients were compared with 211 patients with no radiculopathy, who had undergone laminoplasty during the same period, to identify risk factors related to patient characteristics and surgical techniques. Of various risk factors studied, the narrowest level of the spinal canal, preoperative symptomatic severity, flatness of the spinal cord assessed by computed tomography myelopathy at C4–C5, cervical curvature, anterior protrusion of the superior articular process as assessed by computed tomography scan, laterality of the osteophytes, and ossification of the posterior longitudinal ligament could not significantly discriminate between patients with and without postoperative radiculopathy. The angle of lamina as measured by using computed tomography scans obtained after expansion in the patients with radiculopathy was greater on both the opened and hinged sides and was significantly greater than the angle in patients without radiculopathy ($p < 0.05$). The incidence of radiculopathy on both the opened and hinged sides was significantly higher in patients in whom the bony gutter had been cut on the lateral side of the medial aspect of the zygapophyseal joint. An alternative theory is that too radical a decompression allows slumping backwards of the spinal cord, putting traction on the anatomically vulnerable C5 nerve root. This is the theory espoused for C5 radiculopathy following the trench corpectomy procedure. Here it now recommended limiting the decompression to 15 mm from right to left. Friction heat generated by drilling on the open and hinge sides, traumatic use of Kerrison rongeurs, and a drop of the hinge into the canal are also by some considered as causes of such injury. However, these types of trauma during the operation are likely to damage the posterior root rather than the anterior root; therefore, the sensory disturbance is expected to be stronger. Nevertheless, in most cases, sensory disturbance at C5 or C6 was absent. This lends credence to the tethering action on the anterior root [35].

Pain

There is an increasing recognition that this is quite a painful procedure in the short term, mainly with pain in the trapezius region. In the long run a fair number of patients experience neck pain. This has been studied by Hosono et al. [42]. Ninety-eight patients had surgery for their disability secondary to cervical spondylotic myelopathy. Of those patients, 72 had laminoplasty and 26 had anterior interbody fusion. The presence or absence of axial symptoms was investigated before and after surgery. The duration, severity, and laterality of symptoms were also recorded. The prevalence of postoperative axial symptoms was significantly higher after laminoplasty than after anterior fusion (60 vs. 19%; $p < 0.05$). In 18 patients (25%) from the laminoplasty group, the chief complaints after surgery were related to axial symptoms for more than 3 months, whereas in the anterior fusion group, no patient reported having such severe pain after surgery. In this group shoulder pain developed exclusively on the hinged side.

In conclusion, open door expansive laminoplasty is a versatile, easy and effective method for achieving multilevel decompression of the cervical spine affected by ossification of the posterior longitudinal ligament or cervical spondylosis [51].

References

1 Banerji D, Acharya R, Behari S, Chhabra DK, Jain VK: Corpectomy for multi-level cervical spondylosis and ossification of the posterior longitudinal ligament. Neurosurg Rev 1997;20/1: 25–31.

2 Epstein NE: Reoperation rates for acute graft extrusion and pseudarthrosis after one-level anterior corpectomy and fusion with and without plate instrumentation: Etiology and corrective management. Surg Neurol 2001;56/2:73–81.

3 Tomita K, Kawahara N, Toribatake Y, Heller JG: Expansive midline T-saw laminoplasty (modified spinous process-splitting) for the management of cervical myelopathy. Spine 1998;23/1:32–37.

4 Nakano N, Nakano T: Clinical results following enlargement of the cervical spinal canal by means of laminoplasty. Nippon Seikeigeka Gakkai Zasshi 1988;62:1139–1147.

5 Morimoto T, Uranishi R, Nakase H, Kawaguchi S, Hoshido T, Sakaki T: Extensive cervical laminoplasty for patients with long segment OPLL in the cervical spine: An alternative to the anterior approach. J Clin Neurosci 2000;7/3:217–222.

6 Kojima T, Waga S, Kubo Y, Kanamaru K, Shimosaka S, Shimizu T: Anterior cervical vertebrectomy and interbody fusion for multi-level spondylosis and ossification of the posterior longitudinal ligament. Neurosurgery 1989;24:864–872.

7 Onari K, Akiyama N, Kondo S, Toguchi A, Mihara H, Tsuchiya T: Long-term follow-up results of anterior interbody fusion applied for cervical myelopathy due to ossification of the posterior longitudinal ligament. Spine 2001;26:488–493.

8 Sridhar K, Ramamurthi R, Vasudevan MC, Ramamurthi B: Surgery for ossification of the posterior longitudinal ligament of the cervical spine. Neurol India 2001;49/2:116–123.

9 Epstein NE: Identification of ossification of the posterior longitudinal ligament extending through the dura on preoperative computed tomographic examinations of the cervical spine. Spine 2001; 26/2:182–186.

10 Shinomiya K, Okamoto A, Kamikozuru M, Furuya K, Yamaura I: An analysis of failures in primary cervical anterior spinal cord decompression and fusion. J Spinal Disord 1993;6/4:277–288.

11 Callahan RA, Johnson RM, Margolis RN, Keggi KJ, Albright JA, Southwick WO: Cervical facet fusion for control of instability following laminectomy. J Bone Joint Surg Am 1977;59:991–1002.

12 Fager CA: Laminectomy and kyphotic deformity. J Neurosurg 2001;95(suppl 1):157–158.

13 Herman JM, Sonntag VK: Cervical corpectomy and plate fixation for postlaminectomy kyphosis. J Neurosurg 1994;80:963–970.

14 Zdeblick TA, Bohlman HH: Cervical kyphosis and myelopathy. Treatment by anterior corpectomy and strut-grafting. J Bone Joint Surg Am 1989;71/2:170–182.

15 Yonenobu K, Hosono N, Iwasaki M, Asano M, Ono K: Neurologic complications of surgery for cervical compression myelopathy. Spine 1991;16:1277–1282.

16 Skowronski J, Bielecki M: The results of laminectomy and laminoplasty in cervical myeloradiculopathy. Rocz Akad Med Bialymst 1992;37:71–73.

17 Yonenobu K, Wada E, Suzuki S, Kanazawa A: The dorsal approach in degeneratively changed cervical spine. Orthopäde 1996;25:533–541.
18 Kawai S, Sunago K, Doi K, Saika M, Taguchi T: Cervical laminoplasty (Hattori's method). Procedure and follow-up results. Spine 1988;13:1245–1250.
19 Lee TT, Manzano GR, Green BA: Modified open-door cervical expansive laminoplasty for spondylotic myelopathy: Operative technique, outcome, and predictors for gait improvement. J Neurosurg 1997;86/1:64–68.
20 Ishibashi K: Expansive laminoplasty by sagittal splitting of the spinous process for cervical myelopathy: Correlation of clinical results with morphological changes in the cervical spine. Kurume Med J 2000;47/2:135–145.
21 Morimoto T, Yamada T, Okumura Y, Kakizaki T, Kawaguchi S, Hiramatsu K, et al: Expanding laminoplasty for cervical myelopathy-spinous process roofing technique. Acta Neurochir 1996; 138:720–725.
22 O'Brien MF, Peterson D, Casey AT, Crockard HA: A novel technique for laminoplasty augmentation of spinal canal area using titanium miniplate stabilization. A computerized morphometric analysis. Spine 1996;21:474–484.
23 Gillett GR, Erasmus AM, Lind CR: CG-clip expansive open-door laminoplasty: A technical note. Br J Neurosurg 1999;13:405–408.
24 Hirabayashi K, Bohlman HH: Multilevel cervical spondylosis. Laminoplasty versus anterior decompression. Spine 1995;20:1732–1734.
25 Wang JM, Roh KJ, Kim DJ, Kim DW: A new method of stabilising the elevated laminae in open-door laminoplasty using an anchor system. J Bone Joint Surg Br 1998;80:1005–1008.
26 Hirabayashi K: Expansive open-door laminoplasty for cervical spondylotic myelopathy. Jpn J Surg 1978;32:1159–1163.
27 Kirita Y: Posterior decompression for cervical spondylosis and ossification of the posterior longitudinal ligament. Shujutsu 1976;30:287–302.
28 Nakano K, Harata S, Suetsuna F, Araki T, Itoh J: Spinous process-splitting laminoplasty using hydroxyapatite spinous process spacer. Spine 1992;17(suppl 3):S41–S43.
29 Batzdorf U, Batzdorff A: Analysis of cervical spine curvature in patients with cervical spondylosis. Neurosurgery 1988;22:827–836.
30 Matsunaga S, Sakou T, Nakanisi K: Analysis of the cervical spine alignment following laminoplasty and laminectomy. Spinal Cord 1999;37/1:20–24.
31 Fujimura Y, Nishi Y: Atrophy of the nuchal muscle and change in cervical curvature after expansive open-door laminoplasty. Arch Orthop Trauma Surg 1996;115/3–4:203–205.
32 Oyama M, Hattori S, Noriwaki N: A new method of cervical laminectomy. Chubu Nippon Seikeigeka Gakkai Zasshi 1984;16:792–794.
33 Tomimura KS, Morizono Y: Osteoplastic enlargement of the cervical canal for cervical spondylosis. Rinsho Seikeigeka 1984;19:491–497.
34 Watanabe TI, Goto S: Expansive laminoplasty (Chiba modification) for cervical myelopathy. Shujutsu 1987;41:519–527.
35 Hirabayashi K, Toyama Y, Chiba K: Expansive laminoplasty for myelopathy in ossification of the longitudinal ligament. Clin Orthop 1999;359:35–48.
36 Hilibrand AS, Carlson GD, Palumbo MA, Jones PK, Bohlman HH: Radiculopathy and myelopathy at segments adjacent to the site of a previous anterior cervical arthrodesis. J Bone Joint Surg Am 1999;81:519–528.
37 Saunders RL, Pikus HJ, Ball P: Four-level cervical corpectomy. Spine 1998;23:2455–2461.
38 Saunders RL, Bernini PM, Shirreffs TG Jr, Reeves AG: Central corpectomy for cervical spondylotic myelopathy: A consecutive series with long-term follow-up evaluation. J Neurosurg 1991; 74/2:163–170.
39 Saunders RL: Anterior reconstructive procedures in cervical spondylotic myelopathy. Clin Neurosurg 1991;37:682–721.
40 Fessler RG, Steck JC, Giovanini MA: Anterior cervical corpectomy for cervical spondylotic myelopathy. Neurosurgery 1998;43/2:257–265.
41 Edwards CC 2nd, Heller JG, Murakami H: Corpectomy versus laminoplasty for multilevel cervical myelopathy: An independent matched cohort analysis. Spine 2002;27/11:1168–1175.

42 Hosono N, Yonenobu K, Ono K: Neck and shoulder pain after laminoplasty. A noticeable complication. Spine 1996;21:1969–1973.

43 Adams CB, Logue V: Studies in cervical spondylotic myelopathy. II. The movement and contour of the spine in relation to the neural complications of cervical spondylosis. Brain 1971;94:568–586.

44 Adams CB, Logue V: Studies in cervical spondylotic myelopathy. III. Some functional effects of operations for cervical spondylotic myelopathy. Brain 1971;94:587–594.

45 Herkowitz HN: The surgical management of cervical spondylotic radiculopathy and myelopathy. Clin Orthop 1989/239:94–108.

46 Herkowitz HN: Cervical laminoplasty: Its role in the treatment of cervical radiculopathy. J Spinal Disord 1988;1/3:179–188.

47 Baba H, Maezawa Y, Furusawa N, Imura S, Tomita K: Flexibility and alignment of the cervical spine after laminoplasty for spondylotic myelopathy. A radiographic study. Int Orthop 1995;19/2:116–121.

48 Heller JG, Edwards CC 2nd, Murakami H, Rodts GE: Laminoplasty versus laminectomy and fusion for multilevel cervical myelopathy: An independent matched cohort analysis. Spine 2001;26:1330–1336.

49 Herkowitz HN: A comparison of anterior cervical fusion, cervical laminectomy, and cervical laminoplasty for the surgical management of multiple level spondylotic radiculopathy. Spine 1988;13:774–780.

50 Baisden J, Voo LM, Cusick JF, Pintar FA, Yoganandan N: Evaluation of cervical laminectomy and laminoplasty. A longitudinal study in the goat model. Spine 1999;24:1283–1289.

51 Uematsu Y, Tokuhashi Y, Matsuzaki H: Radiculopathy after laminoplasty of the cervical spine. Spine 1998;23:2057–2062.

Professor Alan Crockard, DSc FRCS, FRCS (Ed)
Department of Surgical Neurology
National Hospital for Neurology and Neurosurgery
Box 3, Queen Square, London WC1N 3BG (UK)
Tel. +44 20 7829 8714, Fax +44 20 7813 1138
E-Mail alan.crockard@uclh.org, A.Crockard@ion.ucl.ac.uk

Haid RW Jr, Subach BR, Rodts GE Jr (eds): Advances in Spinal Stabilization.
Prog Neurol Surg. Basel, Karger, 2003, vol 16, pp 154–164

Cervical Pedicle Screws: Advances in Spinal Stabilization

Jay Y. Chun[a], *Praveen V. Mummaneni*[b], *Barry D. Birch*[c], *Rick C. Sasso*[d]

[a] Department of Neurosurgery, University of California, San Francisco, Calif.,
[b] Department of Neurosurgery, Emory University, Atlanta, Ga.,
[c] Department of Neurosurgery, The Mayo Clinic, Scottsdale, Ariz., and
[d] Indiana Spine Group, Indianapolis, Ind., USA

Since Hadra [8] first used silver wires to internally fixate the cervical spine in 1891, cervical spinal fixation has undergone significant transformation. Posterior instrumentation systems have evolved from wires to facet screws, lateral mass plates, and ultimately to cervical pedicle screws. These advances in cervical stabilization techniques have been accompanied by innovative spine image guidance systems to assist with appropriate placement.

Transpedicular fixation of the cervical spine poses a particular challenge to surgeons due to the close proximity of the cervical pedicle to the spinal cord, nerve roots and the vertebral arteries. Nevertheless, possible biomechanical advantages afforded by cervical pedicle screws over lateral mass screws and posterior cervical wires are the primary factor in the continuing study and advancement in pedicle screw application for cervical spine fixation.

Anatomy

Due to the small margin of error allowed for ideal cervical pedicle screw placement, even small miscalculations can result in a vascular or neural injury. Therefore, intimate knowledge of the cervical pedicles is important.

Pedicle Measurement Studies

It should be noted that some surgeons feel that C2 does not have a true pedicle but rather has a large elongated pars; we disagree with this. Panjabi et al. [17]

Table 1. Pedicle dimensions

	C2	C3	C4	C5	C6	C7	T1
Panjabi et al. [17], 1991							
Width, mm	7.7	5.8	5.7	6.1	6.3	6.6	
Height, mm	9.4	7.6	7.4	6.7	7.1	7.5	
Cross-sectional area, mm^2	32.3	24.2	24.7	23.8	24.5	30.4	
Rampersaud et al. [24], 2001							
Width, mm	7.4	4.9	4.8	5.1	5.4	6.5	8.0
Height, mm	8.0	6.2	6.8	6.5	6.4	7.1	9.4

in 1991 were among the first to understand the three-dimensional anatomy of the cervical pedicle and to propose that the cervical pedicle could tolerate pedicle screw placement. In their cadaveric study of 12 cervical spines, Panjabi et al. systematically demonstrated that both the width and height of the cervical pedicle was the greatest at C2 (C2 width and height were on the average 7.7 and 9.4 mm, respectively) (table 1). In addition, they demonstrated that the cross-sectional area of the C2 pedicle was the greatest of all the cervical pedicles. From C3–C7, the pedicle angles to the transverse plane ranged from an average of 9.2° below to 13.4° above the transverse plane. In the sagittal plane, there was a decrement of the pedicle angle from an average of 41.6° at C3 to 33.1° at C7.

Other cadaveric studies have also demonstrated the feasibility of placing screws within the cervical pedicle. An et al. [6] in 1991 utilized a cadaveric study to investigate the pedicle anatomy from C7–T2. In terms of C7 pedicle anatomy, they demonstrated that the medial angulation averaged 34° at C7, while the mediolateral and superoinferior outer pedicle diameters were on average 6.9 and 7.5 mm, respectively. The pedicle distances (from the entry point to the posterior vertebral body line) measured 9.1 mm on average. An et al. recommended that for pedicle screw placement, the entry point should be 1 mm inferior to the midpoint of the facet with a 25–30° medial angle.

Shin et al. [19] further defined the cervical pedicle anatomy by addressing cross-sectional variability of the cervical pedicles. They demonstrated that the medial pedicle walls are consistently thicker than the lateral pedicle walls and that there was a substantial variability in the composition and shape of the cervical pedicle cross section.

Both Xu et al. [23] and Ugur et al. [22] expanded on prior anatomical studies by evaluating the relationship between the cervical pedicles and the adjacent neural structures. These studies showed that there was no gap between the pedicle and the superior portion of the nerve root and between the pedicle and the thecal sac from C3 to C7. The average distances between the pedicle and the

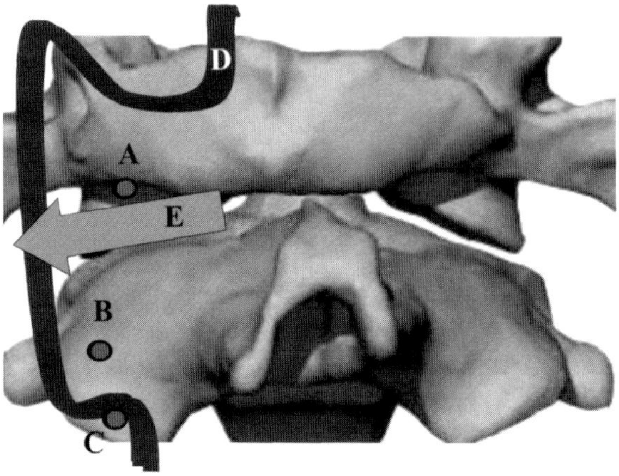

Fig. 1. Entry point of C2 pedicle screw (B) is 2 mm superior and 1–2 mm lateral to the C2 pars screw entry point. The C2 pedicle screw is angled more medially (C). A = C1 lateral mass screw entry point; D = vertebral artery; E = C2 nerve root exit.

inferior nerve root margins ranged from 1.4 to 1.6 mm. Consequently, both studies concluded that the risk of neurological injuries may be higher in screw penetration of the medial or superior cortex of the pedicle rather than in screw penetration of the inferior cortex of the pedicle (fig. 1).

Technique Studies

Ludwig et al. [15] compared the accuracy of three different techniques for placing pedicle screws in cadaveric specimens. With screws placed based on morphometric data alone, 12.5% of the screws were placed entirely within the pedicle; 21.9% had a noncritical breach, and 65% had a critical breach ('critical': encroachment of vertebral artery, nerve root or spinal cord by the screw, 'noncritical': violation of the pedicle cortex without injury to surrounding vital structure). In the second technique (laminoforaminotomy), 45% of the screws were within the pedicle; 15.4% had a noncritical breach, and 39.6% had a critical breach. In the third technique (computer-assisted surgical guidance system), 76% of the screws were placed entirely within the pedicle; 13.4% had a noncritical breach, and 10.6% had a critical breach.

Biomechanical Studies

Once the feasibility of screw placement within the cervical pedicle was demonstrated, biomechanical studies were required to justify the use of cervical pedicle screw fixation in light of the technically challenging nature of pedicle screw placement. Kotani et al. [13] in 1994 compared the biomechanical stability of seven different cervical fixation methods, including transpedicular screw fixation. They demonstrated that the three-column fixation of the cervical spine using cervical pedicle screws offered increased stability over other posterior cervical fixation systems. Even when both the anterior and middle columns were compromised, the stability provided by cervical pedicle fixation was similar to combined anterior plate and posterior triple wiring in one-level fixation.

Additionally, Jones et al. [10] in 1997 demonstrated in cadaveric specimens that cervical pedicle screws had a significantly higher pullout strength than lateral mass screws. The load failure mean for cervical pedicle screws was 677 N in contrast to 355 N for lateral mass screws.

Kowalski et al. [14] in 2000 further evaluated the pullout strengths of pedicle screws. They compared the 'standard' method of pedicle screw placement (decortication of the lateral mass and passage of a hand drill prior to tapping) to the Abumi insertion method (decortication of the entire lateral mass, which provides a direct view of the pedicle introitus). There was no significant difference in the mean pullout resistance between the Abumi (696 N) and standard (636.5 N) insertion techniques ($p = 0.41$).

These studies demonstrated that cervical pedicle screw constructs are biomechanically stronger than lateral mass screw or wire fixation systems.

Clinical Studies

In 1989 Roy-Camille [25] described the technique and the indication for the placement of a transpars screw at C2 for Hangman's fractures. For C2, he recommended drilling approximately 15° in the medial direction and 35° in the superior direction.

Abumi et al. [1] in 1994 was the first to report placement of pedicle screws in the subaxial spine. Thirteen patients with fractures/dislocation of the middle and lower cervical spine underwent transpedicular screw fixation. The angle of the cervical pedicle screws of Abumi et al. ranged from 25 to 45° medial to the midline in the transverse plane. All patients had solid fusion without loss of correction at an average of 22 months' follow-up. Despite three cortical breaches of the 52 screws that were placed, no neurological or vascular complications were observed. This study demonstrated that safe and successful placement of cervical pedicle screws was possible.

Abumi and Kaneda [2] further utilized pedicle screw fixation for nontraumatic lesions of the cervical spine. They analyzed the clinical results in 45 patients and demonstrated that the solid fusion was obtained in all patients except 8 patients who did not receive bone graft. There was one case of transient radiculopathy.

Abumi et al. [3] in 2000 followed this study with another large retrospective study analyzing the complications associated with pedicle screw fixation of the cervical spine. Seven hundred twelve screws were inserted into the cervical pedicles, and the locations of 669 screws were radiologically evaluated in 180 consecutive patients. Forty-five screws (6.7%) were found to penetrate the pedicle, and 2 of the 45 screws caused a postoperative radiculopathy. Abumi et al. concluded that the incidence of clinically significant complications caused by cervical pedicle screw insertion was extremely low.

Since then other studies have reported successful placement of pedicle screws in the cervical spine. Albert et al. [5] demonstrated successful use of C7 pedicle screws in 21 patients. Pedicle screws were placed after direct palpation of the pedicle with a right angle nerve hook after laminoforaminotomy at C7. There were no neurological complications related to pedicle screw placement and no failures of fixation or complications at 1-year follow-up.

More recently, Harms and Melcher [9] in 2001, Mummaneni et al. [16] in 2002, and Fiore et al. [7] in 2002 demonstrated a novel technique of atlantoaxial stabilization using lateral mass fixation at C1 and C2 pars screw fixation with minipolyaxial screws and rods. No neural or vascular damage related to this technique was observed in these studies. The early clinical and radiologic follow-up data indicated solid fusion in all patients.

Surgical Technique

For posterior cervical pedicle screw (and lateral mass screw) fixation, we prefer to use a polyaxial screw-rod system (VERTEX, Medtronic Sofamor Danek, Memphis, Tenn., USA). This system is more versatile than standard lateral mass plating systems and allows for more varied screw entry points and screw angles because the screw placement is not dependent on the predetermined plate entry holes.

C2 Pars Screw Placement

We recommend a screw entry point 3 mm superior and 3 mm lateral to the C2/3 facet joint. We drill approximately 15° in the medial direction and 35° in the superior direction with direct visualization and palpation of the medial and superior aspect of the C2 pars with a Penfield 4 to decrease the chance of cortex violation (fig. 2–4). We use a handheld drill to create the screw pathway. We then tap and place a polyaxial VERTEX screw.

2 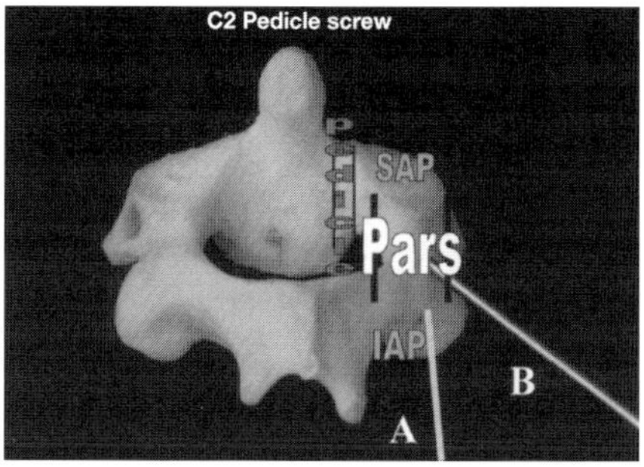

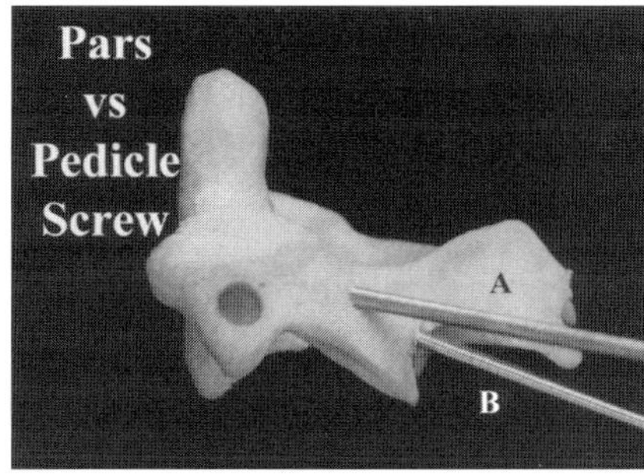 3

Fig. 2. A C2 pars screw (A) has a higher risk of vertebral artery injury than a C2 pedicle screw (B) because the vertebral artery runs occasionally through the inferior portion of the pars of C2. SAP = Superior articulating process; IAP = inferior articulating process.

Fig. 3. The trajectory of a C2 pedicle screw (A) and the trajectory of a C2 pars screw (B) are shown.

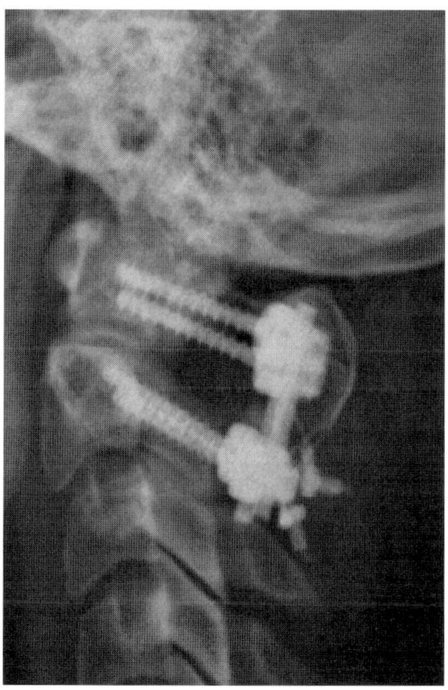

Fig. 4. Lateral cervical x-ray shows C1 lateral mass screws and C2 pars screws.

C2 Pedicle Screw Placement

The entry point for C2 pedicle screws is 1–2 mm superior and 1–2 mm more lateral than that of the C2 pars screw. We expose and palpate the medial portion of the C2 pars to guide our medial trajectory, which is approximately 25°

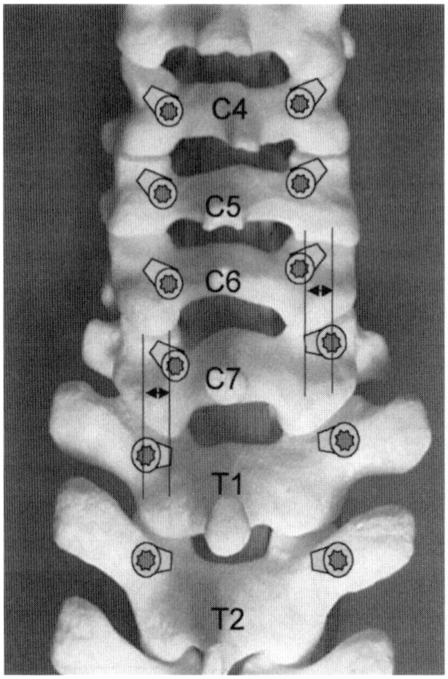

Fig. 5. The difference in the angulation of pedicle screws versus lateral mass screws in the subaxial spine is shown.

(this is more medial angulation than the pars screw as the entry point is more lateral). We also angle approximately 25° in the superior direction. We use fluoroscopy or image guidance to help with screw trajectory.

Since the vertebral artery occasionally runs within the inferior pars of C2, the entry point of the C2 pedicle screw is safer than the entry point of the C2 pars screw because the C2 pedicle screw entry point is more superior than the entry point of the C2 pars screw.

Violation of the medial pedicle wall is unlikely with a C2 pedicle screw because the bone here is cortical and quite strong. We prefer to use the tap from the VERTEX set to enter and create a screw pathway because the tap is less likely to create a cortical wall breach than is the drill.

C3–C6 Pedicle Screw Placement

The entry point of C3–C6 pedicle screws is slightly lateral to the center of the facet and close to the posterior margin of the superior articular surface. After decorticating the lateral mass, the pedicle can then be probed to validate screw trajectory. The tap from the VERTEX (Medtronic Sofamor Danek) instrumentation set is particularly good for this maneuver because it is delicate with fine cutting edges and has a tendency to be 'sucked down the pedicle' (fig. 5–8).

6

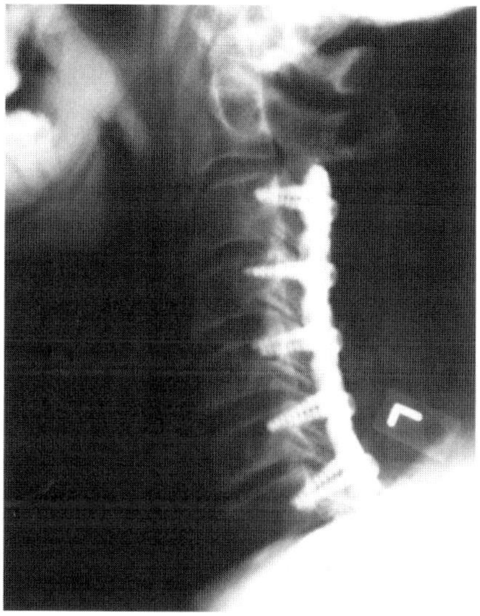

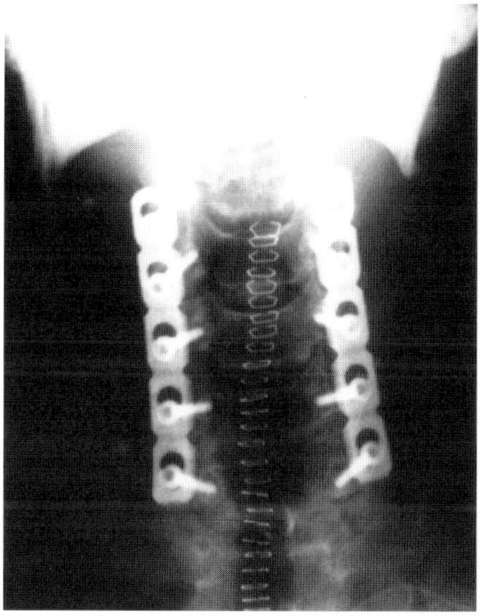

7

Fig. 6. Lateral cervical spine x-ray of subaxial pedicle screws.
Fig. 7. Anterior-posterior cervical spine x-ray of subaxial pedicle screws.

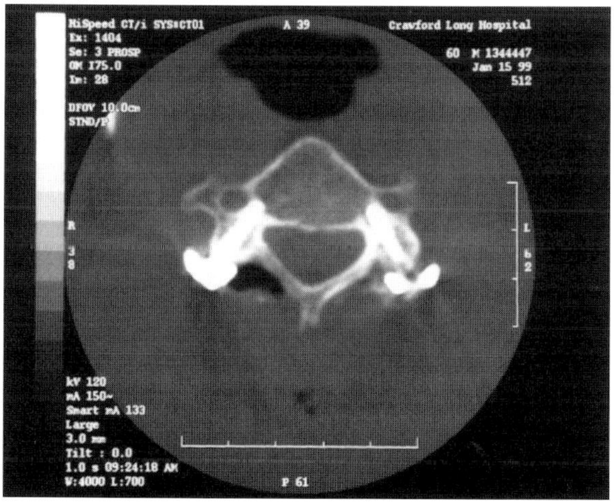

Fig. 8. Axial CT of cervical pedicle screws.

Laminotomies are not routinely performed to identify the medial aspect of the C3–C6 pedicle unless prior facetectomy or laminotomy has been performed for decompressive purposes. Image guidance with Stealth is helpful for appropriate screw placement. Based on measurements from preoperative CT images, the intended angle of the pedicle screw (usually 30–40° medial to the midline in the transverse plane) can be determined, and this is confirmed intraoperatively with image guidance.

C7 and T1 Pedicle Screw Placement

For C7 and T1 pedicle screw placement, we prefer to create laminoforaminotomies at C6–C7 and at C7–T1, respectively. This window allows for direct palpation of the medial, superior, and inferior walls of the pedicle with a right angle nerve hook (fig. 8).

We use a 2-mm burr to establish an entry point that is based on the direct palpation of the medial wall of the pedicle. We then use the tap from the VERTEX instrumentation system to cut and tap the pedicle. The VERTEX tap has a tendency to be 'sucked down' the pedicle with minimal downward force.

If the pedicle is sclerotic, then a drill with an automatic stop at 18 mm can be used instead. It is especially important to sound the pedicle through the laminoforaminotomy when using the drill as perforations are more likely with this instrument than with the VERTEX tap.

If a cortical perforation is made at C7 or T1, the safest place to perforate the pedicle is directly lateral to it since the vertebral artery is not present at C7 or T1. The important structures are the thecal sac medially and the nerve roots superior and inferior to the pedicle. The lateral cortex of the pedicle is a relatively 'safe zone'. In fact, at T1, a lateral cortical penetration may be performed and a longer screw used to fixate the end of the screw into the costotransverse junction, which can increase the pullout strength of the screw [7].

Image Guidance Technology

Safe placement of cervical pedicle screws requires knowledge of the three-dimensional anatomical structure of the pedicles and entry points, and the pedicles' relationship to neural and vascular structures. Given the wide variability of cervical pedicle dimensions and questionable reliability of topographical surface anatomy, greater reliance on visualization/palpation of pedicle and/or image guidance is preferred.

Ludwig et al. [15] in 2000 investigated comparative accuracy of three different techniques of pedicle screw placement in cadaveric specimens. They compared screw placement using morphometric data versus laminoforaminotomy versus image guidance. They showed that the computer-assisted, image-guided placement had the lowest error rate.

It is our preference to use image guidance for pedicle screw placement from C3–C6. For C2, C7, and T1 it has been our experience that anatomic landmarks and medial pedicle wall palpation with a Penfield 4 are adequate for accurate screw placement.

Conclusion

The purpose of posterior cervical fixation is to provide adequate fixation to resist deforming forces until solid bony fusion occurs. To this end, lateral mass plating has been widely utilized. The procedure has been shown to be relatively easy and complications are minimal. Unfortunately, there are circumstances, such as when lateral masses are eroded or not available, that require an alternative fixation technique. Under these circumstances, cervical pedicle screws may be a viable alternative for fixation.

The biomechanical advantages of cervical pedicle screws have been demonstrated. Nevertheless, current data seems to indicate that unless one is intimately familiar with cervical pedicle anatomy and is well versed in cervical pedicle screw placement, this fixation option should be performed sparingly.

Use of image guidance for accurate cervical pedicle screw placement seems promising, and we have successfully utilized the Stealth system for this purpose.

References

1 Abumi K, Itoh H, Taneichi H, Kaneda K: Transpedicular screw fixation for traumatic lesions of the middle and lower cervical spine: Description of the techniques and preliminary report. J Spinal Disord 1994;7:19–28.

2 Abumi K, Kaneda K: Pedicle screw fixation for nontraumatic lesions of the cervical spine. Spine 1997;22:1853–1863.

3 Abumi K, Kaneda K, Shono Y, Fujiya M: One-stage posterior decompression and reconstruction of the cervical spine by using pedicle screw fixation systems. J Neurosurg 1999;90:19–26.

4 Abumi K, Shono Y, Ito M, Taneichi H, Kotani Y, Kaneda K: Complications of pedicle screw fixation in reconstructive surgery of the cervical spine. Spine 2000;25:962–969.

5 Albert TJ, Klein GR, Joffe D, Vaccaro AR: Use of cervicothoracic junction pedicle screws for reconstruction of complex cervical spine pathology. Spine 1998;23:1596–1599.

6 An HS, Gordin R, Renner K: Anatomic considerations for plate-screw fixation of the cervical spine. Spine 1991;16:S548–S551.

7 Fiore A, Haid R, Rodts G, Subach B, Mumanneni P, Reidel C, Birch B: Atlantal lateral mass screws for posterior spinal reconstruction. Neurosurg Focus 2002;12/1:1–6.

8 Hadra BE: The classic: Wiring of the vertebrae as a means of immobilization in fracture and Potts' disease. Berthold E. Hadra. Med Times and Register, Vol22, May 23, 1891. Clin Orthop 1975; 112:4–8.

9 Harms J, Melcher RP: Posterior C1–C2 fusion with polyaxial screw and rod fixation. Spine 2001;26:2467–2471.

10 Jones EL, Heller JG, Silcox DH, Hutton WC: Cervical pedicle screws versus lateral mass screws. Anatomic feasibility and biomechanical comparison. Spine 1997;22:977–982.

11 Karaikovic EE, Daubs MD, Madsen RW, Gaines RW Jr: Morphologic characteristics of human cervical pedicles. Spine 1997;22:493–500.
12 Karaikovic EE, Yingsakmongkol W, Gaines RW Jr: Accuracy of cervical pedicle screw placement using the funnel technique. Spine 2001;26:2456–2462.
13 Kotani Y, Cunningham BW, Abumi K, McAfee PC: Biomechanical analysis of cervical stabilization systems. An assessment of transpedicular screw fixation in the cervical spine. Spine 1994;19: 2529–2539.
14 Kowalski JM, Ludwig SC, Hutton WC, Heller JG: Cervical spine pedicle screws: A biomechanical comparison of two insertion techniques. Spine 2000;25:2865–2867.
15 Ludwig SC, Kowalski JM, Edwards CC 2nd, Heller JG: Cervical pedicle screws: Comparative accuracy of two insertion techniques. Spine 2000;25:2675–2681.
16 Mummaneni P, Haid R, Traynelis V, Sasso R, Subach B, Fiore A, Rodts G: Posterior cervical fixation using a new polyaxial screw and rod system: Technique and surgical results. Neurosurg Focus 2002;12:1–5.
17 Panjabi MM, Duranceau J, Goel V, Oxland T, Takata K: Cervical human vertebrae. Quantitative three-dimensional anatomy of the middle and lower regions. Spine 1991;16:861–869.
18 Roy-Camille R, Saillant G, Berteaux D, Bisserie M: Severe strains of the cervical spine operated on by a posterior approach. Rev Chir Orthop Reparatrice Appar Mot 1978;64:677–684.
19 Shin EK, Panjabi MM, Chen NC, Wang JL: The anatomic variability of human cervical pedicles: Considerations for transpedicular screw fixation in the middle and lower cervical spine. Eur Spine J 2000;9:61–66.
20 Smith MD, Anderson P, Grady MS: Occipitocervical arthrodesis using contoured plate fixation. An early report on a versatile fixation technique. Spine 1993;18:1984–1990.
21 Stanescu S, Ebraheim NA, Yeasting R, Bailey AS, Jackson WT: Morphometric evaluation of the cervico-thoracic junction. Practical considerations for posterior fixation of the spine. Spine 1994;19:2082–2088.
22 Ugur HC, Attar A, Uz A, Tekdemir I, Egemen N, Caglar S, Genc Y: Surgical anatomic evaluation of the cervical pedicle and adjacent neural structures. Neurosurgery 2000;47:1162–1168.
23 Xu R, Kang A, Ebraheim NA, Yeasting RA: Anatomic relation between the cervical pedicle and the adjacent neural structures. Spine 1999;24:451–454.
24 Rampersaud YR, Simon DA, Foley KT: Accuracy requirements for image-guided spinal pedicle screw placement. Spine 2001;26:352–359.
25 Roy-Camille R, Salient G, Mazel C: Internal fixation of the unstable cervical spine by posterior osteosynthesis with plates and screws; in The Cervical Spine Research Society (ed): The Cervical Spine, ed. 2, Philadelphia, Lippincott, 1989, pp 390–493.

Jay Y. Chun, MD, PhD
UCSF, Department of Neurosurgery
505 Parnassus Ave., M-779, Box 0112
San Francisco, CA 94143 (USA)
Tel. +1 415 753 1772, E-Mail chunj@neurosurg.ucsf.edu

Haid RW Jr, Subach BR, Rodts GE Jr (eds): Advances in Spinal Stabilization.
Prog Neurol Surg. Basel, Karger, 2003, vol 16, pp 165–175

Cervical Lateral Mass Advances

Praveen V. Mummaneni[a], *Vincent C. Traynelis*[b], *Rick C. Sasso*[c]

[a] Department of Neurosurgery, Emory University, Atlanta, Ga.,
[b] Division of Neurosurgery, University of Iowa, Iowa City, Iowa, and
[c] Department of Orthopaedic Surgery, Indiana University School of Medicine, Indianapolis Neurosurgical Group, Indianapolis, Ind., USA

Posterior cervical fixation utilizing lateral mass plates has been shown to be a safe and efficacious method to achieve cervical fusion [1–3]. Lateral mass plating is biomechanically superior to laminar wiring or clamping in limiting cervical motion [4–7]. In addition, unlike posterior laminar wiring or clamping, lateral mass plating does not require the presence of the posterior elements.

However, lateral mass plates have numerous drawbacks. They are difficult to contour, and the screw positions are dictated by the fixed plate entry holes. In addition, the screw trajectories are divergent from the plate entry holes, and the connection of the screw to the plate is not rigid. There is no space to pack autograft bone under the screw-plate connection. Screws placed medially or laterally cannot be captured by the plate. Successive screws cannot be compressed or distracted because of the fixed plate hole distances. Moreover, if the plate needs to be revised, the screws must be removed. Finally, most of the systems currently available do not easily allow for extension of fusion up to the occiput or down to the thoracic spine [8].

The ideal posterior cervical instrumentation system will address these shortfalls from the lateral mass plate systems. Currently, there are three commercially available systems that address the problems of lateral mass plates. These systems do allow for initial screw placement with subsequent rod contouring. The three systems are Starlock/Cervifix (Synthes USA, Paoli, Pa., USA), SUMMIT (DePuy Acromed, Raynham, Mass., USA), and VERTEX (Medtronic Sofamor Danek, Memphis, Tenn., USA).

Instrumentation

The three systems that allow for initial screw placement with subsequent rod attachment differ from each other in several ways.

Starlock/Cervifix Systems (Synthes)

Unlike the VERTEX and SUMMIT systems, the Starlock/Cervifix systems do not have polyaxial screw heads. These systems require the use of an intervening closed-loop eyebolt to connect the screw to the rod and, as a result, the connection of the rod to the screw is not a locked, rigid attachment.

Starlock and Cervifix are two instrumentation sets from Synthes that have interchangeable hardware. Cervifix is more restrictive than Starlock because it requires the surgeon to place the lateral mass screws through closed loop eyebolts, which are already mounted on a rod. The closed-loop eyebolts have the capability of sliding up and down the rod, thus enabling the screws to be placed variably in the sagittal plane [9]. Starlock is an improved version of this system that requires attaching closed-loop eye bolts to standard lateral mass screws and then subsequently threading the rod through the closed-loop eyebolts. However, the threading of a contoured rod through closed-loop eyebolts can be tedious and sometimes impossible [9].

Both the Starlock and Cervifix systems have features that distinguish them from standard lateral mass plate systems. They both have occipital plate extensions to accommodate occipitocervical fusions and laminar hooks for use when lateral mass screw attachment is not possible. It is possible to accommodate thoracic pedicle screws into the systems with appropriate rod contouring and attachment of the closed-loop eyebolts to upper thoracic pedicle screws. Starlock/Cervifix are also compatible with the thoracic hook and rod system marketed by Synthes, and can be attached to a separate thoracic instrumentation system via an adaptive connector.

VERTEX System (Medtronic Sofamor Danek)

The VERTEX system allows for initial polyaxial screw placement with subsequent multiplanar rod contouring and attachment with or without offset connectors. The capability of direct connection of the polyaxial screw to the rod allows for a locked, rigid attachment of the rod to the screw. This is biomechanically a sounder construct than the closed-loop eyebolt connection in the Starlock/Cervifix system.

The novel VERTEX polyaxial screw heads are especially useful for facilitating rod attachments in patients with severely abnormal cervical curvatures. The polyaxial screw heads lock to the rod via top loading locking cap screws that fit inside the screw head. The VERTEX system's polyaxial screw heads are very low profile as a result of this attachment scheme [10].

The VERTEX system is easily adaptable for occipital and thoracic extensions. It consists of 6- to 10-mm titanium occipital screws (which are not polyaxial) and 14- to 18-mm titanium polyaxial cervicothoracic screws. In addition, noncannulated 40–50 mm transarticular titanium polyaxial screws are available for C1/C2 fusion. The system's titanium rods are malleable in three dimensions, and there is an available rod with an occipital plate on one end to allow for occipitocervical fusions.

With the VERTEX system, occipitocervical fusion can be performed, but the nonpolyaxial occipital screws must be placed through the apertures in the occipital plates. The polyaxial cervicothoracic screws, however, are placed independently of the rod system. These polyaxial 14- to 18-mm screws are ideal for placement in the C1 lateral mass, C2 pars, C3–7 lateral masses, and upper thoracic pedicles [10, 11]. The contoured rods are then linked either directly to the polyaxial screw heads with a locking cap screw or are linked via an offset connector.

SUMMIT System (DePuy Acromed)

The SUMMIT system shares many of the features of the VERTEX system. SUMMIT polyaxial screw heads are placed independently of the rod and are then connected directly to the rod through a rigid locked connection. Recently, an adaptive occipital extension has been made available, and an extension into the thoracic spine is also possible.

However, the SUMMIT polyaxial screw heads are higher profile than are the VERTEX screws, and the locking cap fits around the polyaxial screw head instead of within it, thus further increasing the profile of the system. Consequently, thin patients who have the SUMMIT system implanted in the posterior cervical spine may experience discomfort from the higher profile instrumentation. In addition, in our experience, the higher profile of the polyaxial screw heads of the SUMMIT system makes it more difficult to fit the contoured rod into the screw heads in severely spondylotic patients whose lateral masses are very close together as a result of their hyperlordosis.

Surgical Technique for Placement of Posterior Cervical Instrumentation

Exposure

A standard midline posterior cervical exposure is performed to reveal the lateral aspects of the cervical facets. The exposure is extended for one to two levels below the inferior end of the planned arthrodesis to allow for optimal screw placement. In patients with marked degenerative changes, the osteophytes on the dorsal facets are removed to provide better visualization, to help define the anatomy of the facets, and to provide a suitable surface to allow the polyaxial screw heads to rotate. However, care should be taken to preserve, where possible, the posterior cortex of the articular mass in order to provide for better screw purchase.

In cases where posterior cervical decompression is necessary, we drill and tap pilot holes for the cervical lateral mass screws prior to performing the full laminectomies in order to preserve the normal anatomic landmarks for the screw trajectories. In addition, the lamina serve to protect the neural elements during screw hole preparation.

For occipitocervical fusions, we expose the suboccipital area up to the inion.

For cervicothoracic fusions, we expose the thoracic transverse processes. At C7 and T1, when canal decompression is not necessary, at least minimal laminoforaminotomies are performed to expose the medial walls of the C7 and T1 pedicles to help guide C7 and T1 pedicle screw placement.

Screw Placement (VERTEX System)

We prefer to use the VERTEX system for posterior occipitocervicothoracic arthrodesis. This system has the advantage of having low profile polyaxial screw heads that can attach either directly or via an offset connector to the rod.

After the exposure is completed, we turn our attention to cervical polyaxial screw placement. Initially, we perforate the posterior cortices of the lateral masses with a high-speed drill. Our screw trajectories for C3–7 are based on the guidelines set by Haid, Papadopoulos, and Sonntag (unpubl. data, presented at the American Association of Neurological Surgeons Annual Meeting, 1991) and further elucidated by McCafferty et al. [12]. Entry points are 1 mm medial to the center of the lateral mass and trajectories are 20–30° cephalad and 20–30° lateral (fig. 1, 2). We 'normalize' the entry point and screw trajectory at each lateral mass to allow for changes in the orientation of the lateral masses secondary to accentuated cervical lordosis or kyphosis and to allow for each patient's unique pathoanatomy.

Some surgeons elect to place screws with the assistance of fluoroscopy or image guidance. However, we do not routinely use fluoroscopy or image guidance (except for screw placement into C1 and C2). Consequently, attention to the patient's unique cervical anatomy is of paramount importance for us.

For screw placement into the lateral mass of C1, we utilize the technique described by Harms and Melcher [13] and refined by Fiore et al. [11]. The screw entry point is at the junction of the posterior arch of C1 and the center of the posterior, inferior C1 lateral mass. The C2 nerve root is gently retracted inferiorly with a Penfield 4 to expose the screw entry point. The screw trajectory is parallel to the plane of the C1 lamina and is aimed straight anterior from

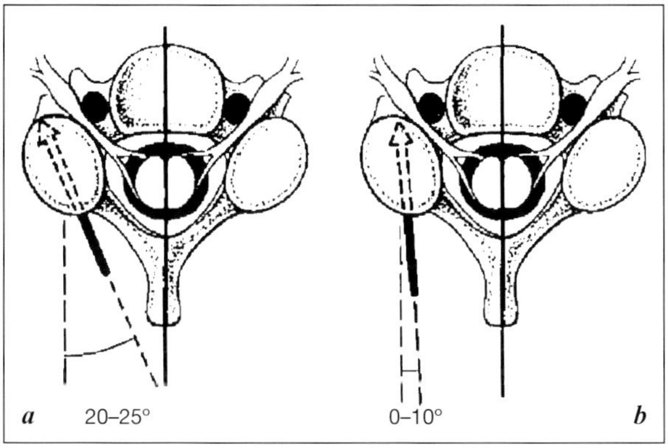

Fig. 1. Illustration of the lateral mass screw trajectory in the axial plane. ***a*** Appropriate angle. ***b*** The screw trajectory puts the nerve root at risk.

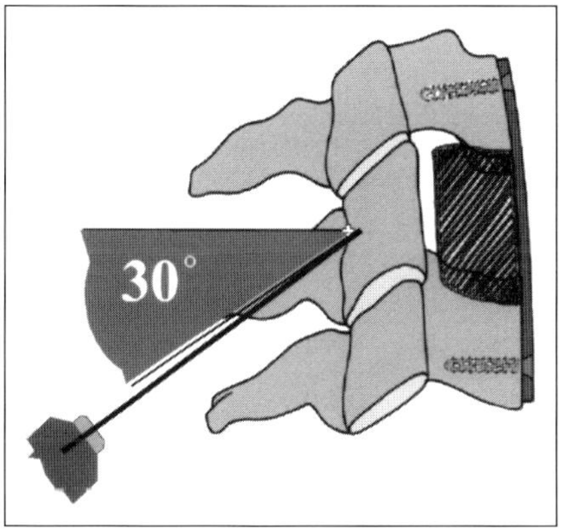

Fig. 2. Lateral mass screw trajectory in the sagittal plane.

the entry point. Screw depth is guided by lateral fluoroscopy and can be estimated by preoperative Stealth CT planning.

For screw placement into the C2 pars, we pay close attention to the preoperative CT to assess the course of the vertebral artery. In addition, we palpate the medial pars with a blunt probe to help guide our screw trajectory. We utilize a screw entry point 3 mm superior and lateral ('3 mm up and out') to the medial aspect of the C2/3 facet joint. The screw trajectory is 10–15° medial and 35° cephalad. We typically use 4-mm width and 16-mm length screws for the C2 pars [10, 11].

For C1/2 transarticular screw placement, the entry point and trajectory are the same as for C2 pars screws; the screw length, however, is longer (up to 50 mm in some cases) [14, 15]. We prefer to use lateral fluoroscopy for guidance when placing C1/2 transarticular screws.

Screw placement at C7 is dependent on the bony anatomy. We scrutinize the preoperative CT scan to assess if the patient's C7 lateral mass has a typical cervical anatomy or has a transitional thoracic anatomy with a well-formed pedicle. When the C7 anatomy is transitional, we prefer to place a C7 pedicle screw.

For pedicle screw placement at C7 or in the upper thoracic spine, we expose and palpate the medial walls of the pedicles and utilize an entry point 1 mm below the center of the facet joint. Our screw trajectory is typically 25–30° medial while maintaining a perpendicular angle in the sagittal plane [10]. We have found it useful to use the drill to create a small pilot hole for entry of the tap into the pedicle. We then use the 4.0-mm tap from the VERTEX set to create the screw path and simultaneously tap the pedicle. This instrument is delicate and particularly useful to find an appropriate trajectory into the C7 and thoracic pedicles. It has a tendency to be 'sucked down' the pedicle with gentle manipulation in experienced hands.

In the thoracic spine, pedicle screws also can be placed laterally into the costotransverse joint to achieve greater cortical purchase [16].

After polyaxial screw placement, the appropriate posterior decompressions are performed based on the patient's symptoms. In addition, the facet joints to be fused are stripped of cartilage and decorticated with a high-speed drill and packed with autograft.

The final step is rod contouring and attachment. A rod template is used to estimate the rod length and rod contour required. A small endotracheal tube stylet is particularly good for use as a rod template. The titanium rods are then measured, cut, contoured, and directly attached to the polyaxial screw heads with locking cap screws. In cases where the patient's pathoanatomy requires significantly different lateral or medial screw positions at successive levels, we utilize small offset connectors in order to facilitate rod attachment.

When occipitocervical fusions are planned, we utilize a specialized rod with an occipital plate on the cephalad end. The rod and occipital plate are contoured based on the rod trial. We position the occipital plate near the midline occipital keel to provide for the most bony purchase for the occipital screws. The occipital screws are not polyaxial and must be placed through the apertures in the occipital plates. Ideally six occipital screws (three on each side) should be placed near the midline of the suboccipital bone. This has been shown to be the most biomechanically favorable position for suboccipital fixation [17] (fig. 3).

After the instrumentation construct is placed, but before final tightening of the construct, we compress, distract, or laterally rotate each successive segment as needed to restore normal cervical lordosis and sagittal balance. Autograft is then packed over the tops of the fusion sites.

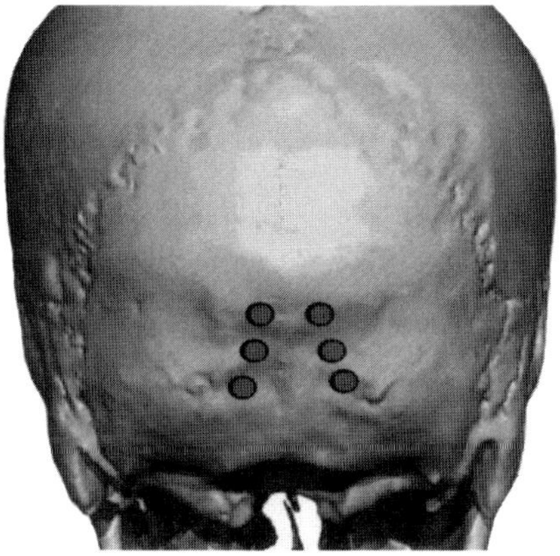

Fig. 3. Optimal screw placement positions for occipital fixation.

Discussion and Conclusion

Lateral mass plating has been shown to be an effective method of achieving posterior cervical arthrodesis and stabilization [3]. Reported complication rates are low. Injuries to the cervical spinal cord or vertebral artery have not been reported in recent large published series on lateral mass plating [3, 5, 18–20]. The reported rate of radiculopathy from malpositioned screws has ranged from 0 to 6% of patients [3, 5, 18–20].

However, lateral mass plates are of limited use when fusing from the occiput to the thoracic spine in patients with abnormal cervical anatomy because of their lack of malleability and their predetermined screw hole trajectories. The Starlock/Cervifix systems overcome some of these problems but are suboptimal because they require threading of a contoured rod through closed loop eyebolts, which is not a rigid connection and which can be tedious and sometimes impossible [9].

The ideal posterior cervical instrumentation system will allow for initial screw placement with subsequent multiplanar rod contouring and attachment via a rigid connection with a locking cap screw. In addition, offset connectors are needed to allow for screw capture at any distance laterally away from the rod (as is the case with C7 and T1 pedicle screws (fig. 4). Finally, the system should be low profile so that the polyaxial screw heads will not be crowded in cases with cervical hyperlordosis.

The new VERTEX and SUMMIT posterior polyaxial cervical screw and rod systems satisfy many of the criteria for the ideal posterior cervical instrumentation system. They have the versatility to accommodate occipitocervical fusions with C1 lateral mass screws and C2 pars screws. In addition, they allow

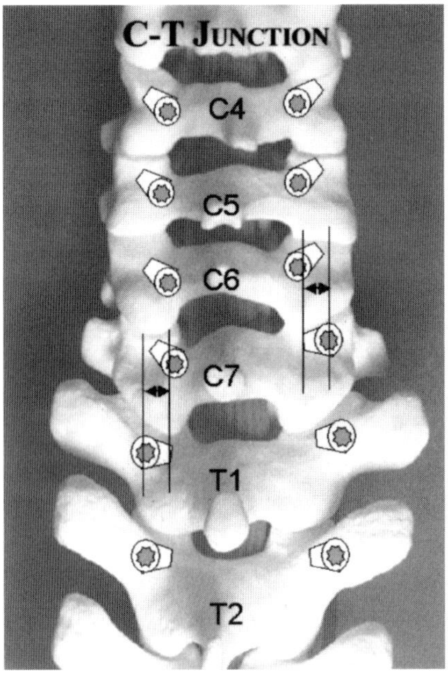

Fig. 4. Different screw trajectory and entry point needed for C7 and T1 pedicle screws as compared to cervical lateral mass screws.

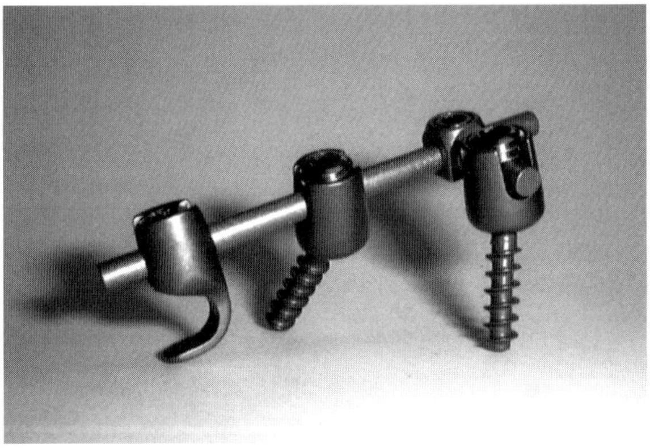

Fig. 5. Photograph of the VERTEX system. Note the polyaxial screw heads, the offset connector, and the laminar hook.

for lateral mass fixation from C3–7 as well as pedicle fixation and laminar hook placement in the lower cervical and upper thoracic spine without the limitations inherent in placing screws through holes in lateral mass plates (fig. 5–8). Finally, the rods are easily contoured and attached directly and rigidly to the polyaxial screw heads.

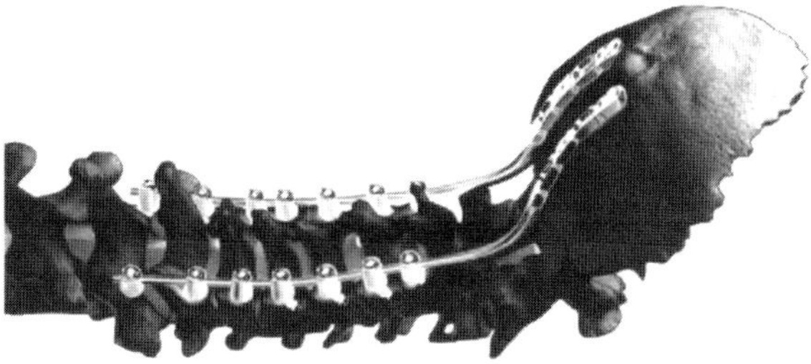

Fig. 6. Photograph of occipitocervicothoracic fixation in a saw bone model utilizing the VERTEX system.

7 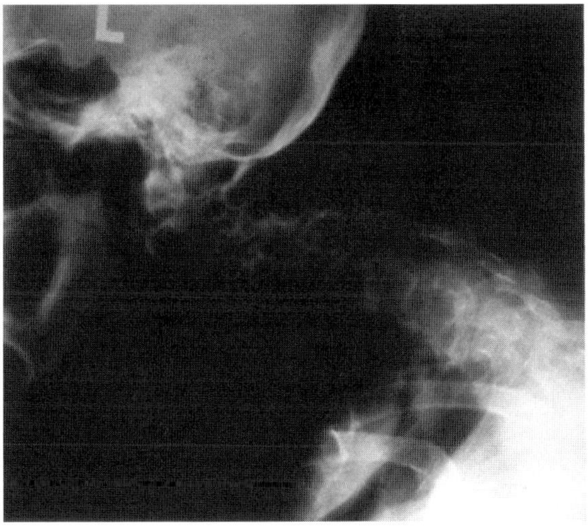 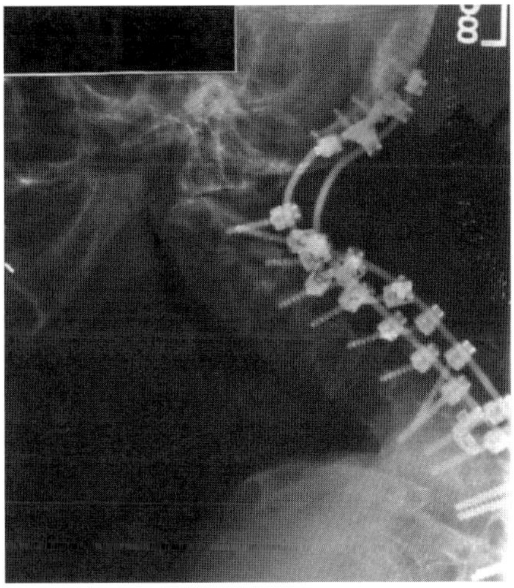 8

Fig. 7. Preoperative x-ray in a severely kyphotic and myelopathic patient.

Fig. 8. Postoperative x-ray in the same patient following posterior cervical decompression and occipitocervicothoracic fusion with the VERTEX system.

The VERTEX system has advantages over the SUMMIT system. VERTEX is lower profile than the SUMMIT system and more easily accommodates complex cervical curvatures and spondylosis as a result. In addition, VERTEX has top-loading offset connectors to easily accommodate cervicothoracic pedicle screws.

Further studies will be required to establish long-term results and fusion rates with the cervical screw-rod systems.

Acknowledgments

We are grateful to Drew Imhulse for assistance with the radiographic images in the figures.

Disclosure Statement

The following authors are consultants for Medtronic Sofamor Danek: Vincent C. Traynelis, MD and Rick C. Sasso, MD.

References

1 Anderson PA, Henley MB, Grady MS, Montesano PX, Winn HR: Posterior cervical arthrodesis with AO reconstruction plates and bone graft. Spine 1991;16(suppl 3):S72–S79.
2 Fehlings MG, Cooper PR, Errico TJ: Posterior plates in the management of cervical instability: Long-term results in 44 patients. J Neurosurg 1994;81:341–349.
3 Graham AW, Swank ML, Kinard RE, Lowery GL, Dials BE: Posterior cervical arthrodesis and stabilization with a lateral mass plate: Clinical and computed tomographic evaluation of lateral mass screw placement and associated complications. Spine 1996;21:323–329.
4 Gill K, Paschal S, Corin J, Ashman R, Bucholz RW: Posterior plating of the cervical spine: A biomechanical comparison of different posterior fusion techniques. Spine 1988;13:813–816.
5 Heller JG, Silcox DH 3rd, Sutterlin CE 3rd: Complications of posterior cervical plating. Spine 1995;20:2442–2448.
6 Sutterlin CE, McAfee PC, Warden KE, Rey RM, Farey ID: A biomechanical evaluation of cervical spinal stabilization methods in a bovine model: Static and cyclical loading. Spine 1988;13: 795–802.
7 Ulrich C, Woersdoerfer O, Kalff R, Claes L, Wilke HJ: Biomechanics of fixation systems to the cervical spine. Spine 1991;16(suppl 3):S4–S9.
8 Smith MD, Anderson P, Grady MS: Occipitocervical arthrodesis using contoured plate fixation: An early report on a versatile fixation technique. Spine 1993;18:1984–1990.
9 Horgan MA, Kellogg JX, Chesnut RM: Posterior cervical arthrodesis and stabilization: An early report using a novel lateral mass screw and rod technique. Neurosurgery 1999;44:1267–1272.
10 Mummaneni PV, Haid RW, Traynelis VC, Sasso RC, Subach BR, Fiore AJ, Rodts GE: Posterior cervical fixation using a new polyaxial screw and rod system: Technique and surgical results. Neurosurg Focus 2002;12/1:1–5.
11 Fiore AJ, Haid RW, Rodts GE, Subach BR, Mummaneni PV, Riedel CJ, Birch BD: C1 lateral mass screws for posterior spinal reconstruction: Technical note and case series. Neurosurg Focus 2002;12/1:1–6.
12 McCafferty RR, Haid RW, Martin G, Rodts GE: Techniques for lateral mass plating of the posterior cervical spine in patients with cervical spinal stenosis. Tech Neurosurg 1999;5/2:101–105.
13 Harms J, Melcher RP: Posterior C1–C2 fusion with polyaxial screw and rod fixation. Spine 2001;26:2467–2471.
14 Haid RW Jr: C1–C2 transarticular screw fixation: Technical aspects. Neurosurgery 2001;49: 71–74.
15 Haid RW Jr, Subach BR, McLaughlin MR, Rodts GE Jr, Wahlig JB Jr: C1–C2 transarticular screw fixation for atlantoaxial instability: A 6-year experience. Neurosurgery 2001;49:65–68.
16 Youkilis AS, Quint DJ, McGillicuddy JE, Papadopoulos SM: Stereotactic navigation for placement of pedicle screws in the thoracic spine. Neurosurgery 2001;48:771–778.
17 Oda I, Abumi K, Sell LC, Haggerty CJ, Cunningham BW, McAfee PC: Biomechanical evaluation of five different occipito-atlanto-axial fixation techniques. Spine 1999;24:2377–2382.

18 Schultz KD Jr, McLaughlin MR, Haid RW Jr, Comey CH, Rodts GE Jr, Alexander J: Single-stage anterior-posterior decompression and stabilization for complex cervical spine disorders. J Neurosurg 2000;93(suppl 2):214–221.
19 Swank MA, Sutterlin CE 3rd, Bossons CR, Dials BE: Rigid internal fixation with lateral mass plates in multilevel anterior and posterior reconstruction of the cervical spine. Spine 1997;22: 274–282.
20 Wellman BJ, Follett KA, Traynelis VC: Complications of posterior articular mass plate fixation of the subaxial cervical spine in 43 consecutive patients. Spine 1998;23:193–200.

Praveen V. Mummaneni, MD
Clinical Instructor/Complex Spine Fellow
Department of Neurosurgery, The Emory Clinic
1365 Clifton Road, Building B, Suite 6400, Atlanta, GA 30322 (USA)
Tel. +1 404 686 8101, Fax +1 404 686 4805, E-Mail vmum@aol.com

Haid RW Jr, Subach BR, Rodts GE Jr (eds): Advances in Spinal Stabilization.
Prog Neurol Surg. Basel, Karger, 2003, vol 16, pp 176–187

Interbody Carbon Fiber

Rudolf Bertagnoli

Klinikum St. Elisabeth, Spinal Department, Straubing, Germany

The fusion of spinal segments is one of the major goals in surgical treatment of degenerative disc disease (DDD). To obtain the best biomechanical support and fusion rates, interbody fusion is the preferred method. The main advantages of implants made of carbon fiber reinforced plastic (CFRP) are the radiolucency and the fact that there is no distortion on CT and MRI. The surgeon can chronologically follow the biological reaction in the fusion section and can clearly detect bony fusion. Regions which are hidden using metal implants could now be analyzed on standard radiographs. In implants made of CFRP matrix materials such as thermoset epoxy resin systems (EPN/DDS) or thermoplastic systems PEAK (PEKEKK™, PEEK™, ULTRAPEK™) are used. The first ones have been clinically used since 1988 following detailed in vitro and in vivo tests starting 1975 according to ISO 10993-1 [1]. In the spine these implant materials have been used since 1993 [2].

These CFRP implants are manufactured using a special fiber winding process of carbon fiber roving which is impregnated with resin and laid on a rotating rod. Due to that and to the design-adapted machining processes the properties of the material could be chosen for each kind of implant design. Hardening, tempering, and machining lead to the final implant geometry and must be controlled.

Interbody fusion with cage support is an ideal situation for the application of resorbable biomaterials [3, 4]. To monitor the production of the new bone masses and to determine the degree of bone fusion, cages made from carbon composite materials are superior to metallic cages due to their radiolucent characteristics.

In the literature some mechanical and in vitro tests performed on CFRP implants could be found: Brantigan et al. [5], Ciapetta et al. [6] (vertebra replacement), Jost et al. [7], Kandziora et al. [8] (80 cervical spines of sheep with different cage designs), Shono et al. [9] (18 calf spines in compression and rotation), and Steinhauser et al. [10] (static and dynamic compression and shear

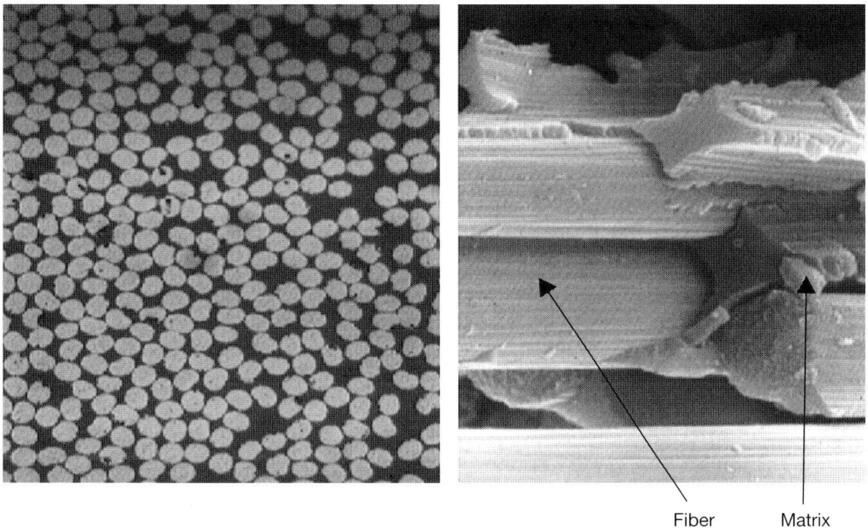

Fig. 1. Cross section and SEM (artificial fracture) of CFRP implants: carbon fiber with a diameter of $\approx 5\ \mu m$ surrounded by matrix material.

testing) all showed very good results. The first animal tests of CFRP implants as interbody lumbar fusion devices were done by Brantigan et al. [5]; they reported 100% fusion after 6, 12 and 24 months in 27 Spanish goats. A summary of clinical experience with CFRP cages is shown in table 1. In all cases high fusion rates were detected with no device-related complications. One case report showed infection and a broken CFRP cage (see table 1) [17].

Material and Methods

Mechanical Tests

To test the axial compression and shear behavior the spinal implants were loaded between two parallel stainless steel plates according to ASTM F2077-00. An axial force rate of 500 N/min was used for quasistatic testing. The loading was stopped when a permanent failure of the specimen occurred or a displacement of 3.0 mm was reached.

For dynamic testing the specimens were tested under cyclic fatigue using a sinusoidal loading waveform at a constant frequency of 5 Hz (lumbar) and 12 Hz (cervical), with an R ratio (Pmin/Pmax) of 0.1. The maximum load cycle was 5,000,000 cycles and a displacement limit error of 3 mm was established.

To determine the pull-out strength, the implants were placed in between two blocks made of Rohacell RC 300WL with mechanical properties comparable to cancellous bone. An axial preload of 100 N was applied. The instrument intended for clinical use was attached

Table 1. Summary of the clinical experience with CFRP cages

Location	Cases	Follow-up	Results	Ref. No.
Lumbar (PLIF)	71	28 months	90% fusion rate, 66% overall satisfaction rate	11
Lumbar (PLIF)	11	6–48 months	90% fusion rate after 48 months	12
Lumbar (PLIF)	221	24 months	98.9% fusion rate, 86% clinical success	13
Lumbar (PLIF)	51	12 months	86% fusion rate (89% of levels)	14
Lumbar (L4–L5)				15
Bilateral	83	12–24 months	>97% fusion rate	
Unilateral	80		100% fusion rate	
Lumbar (ALIF and PLIF), cervical	70	3–12 months	>98% fusion rate	2
Cervical	19	12–21 months	100% fusion rate	16
Lumbar (PLIF)	1	4 week to 25 months	Case report of infection and broken CFRP cage	17

PLIF = Posterior lumbar interbody fusion; ALIF = anterior lumbar interbody fusion.

according to the procedure defined by the manufacturer. A constant deflection rate of 5 mm/min was used. All tests were performed dry at room temperature.

To determine the ultimate torque load, the implants were placed in between two blocks made of Rohacell RC 300WL with mechanical properties comparable to cancellous bone. Prior to testing, an axial preload of 1,000 N was applied to enable settlement of the contact area. The upper as well as the lower block were fixed versus the torsion measurement system. A constant axial preload of 100 N was applied during the test. Torsion was applied at a constant rate of about 100°/min.

All static tests were performed dry at room temperature. The dynamic tests were performed under Ringer solution at 37°C temperature and all specimens were preconditioned.

Clinical Experience

The fusion devices to be assessed at the postoperative evaluation were the CORNERSTONE-SR C (lordotically shaped anterior cervical interbody fusion device, Medtronic Sofamor Danek) and UNION or UNION-L (lordotically shaped anterior or lateral lumbar interbody fusion device, Medtronic Sofamor Danek) spinal fusion cages.

The implant system CORNERSTONE-SR C consists of a basic body (12 × 13 mm), various heights of 4–8 mm (10–16 mm) and two lines of fins (see fig. 2). The anterior retroperitoneal implant system UNION or UNION-L consists of a basic body (24 × 26 or 26 × 31 mm, respectively) with two chambers, various heights of 10–16 mm and three lines of fins (see fig. 2). For both types of implants x-ray contrasts are layers of $BaSO_4$ embedded into the CFRP material. Prior insertion of the implant the fins must be prepared in the bone with a special instrument.

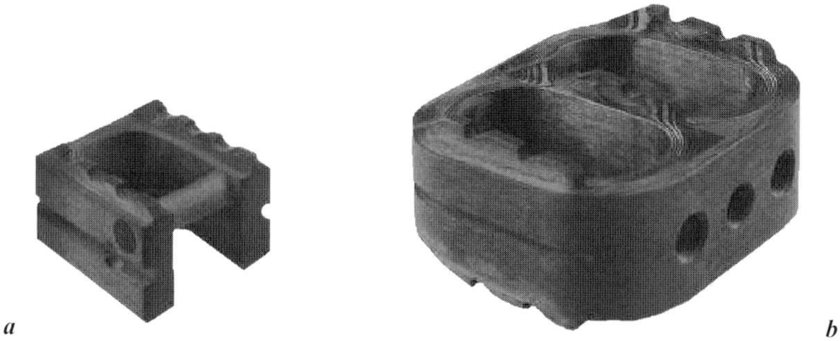

Fig. 2. CFRP implants: cervical interbody fusion cage (CORNERSTONE-SR C, ***a***) and anterior lumbar interbody fusion cage (UNION, ***b***).

Table 2. Primary diagnoses of all studies

Diagnosis	Retrospective study		Prospective study	
	cervical	lumbar	cervical	lumbar
Failed back disc surgery syndrome	2	40	–	18
Segmental instability	55	19	6	8
Disc herniation	77	2	28	10
Spondylolisthesis (grade 1–3)	–	25	–	–
Spinal stenosis	2	3	–	–
Osteochondrosis	2	–	–	–
Fracture	1	–	–	–

In a retrospective study preoperative, peroperative, and postoperative data were collected and entered in case report forms and a comparison was made between preoperative and postoperative clinical status (diagnoses see table 2).

In the cervical group 206 cages were used in 139 patients. There were 69 men and 70 women (36.2% smokers), with a mean age of 46.5 years (from 17 to 68), a mean weight of 75.4 kg (from 48 to 114 kg) and a mean height of 170.2 cm (from 151 to 196 cm). 25.2% of the patients had 1 previous spinal surgery and 4.2% had 2 previous spinal surgeries. In 91.4% of cases tibia was used as an autologous graft.

In the lumbar group 146 cages were used in 89 patients. There were 54 men and 35 women (36.8% smokers), with a mean age of 44.2 years (from 21 to 65), a mean weight of 76.3 kg (from 51 to 114 kg) and a mean height of 172.6 cm (from 155 to 197 cm). 64.0% of the patients had 1 previous spinal surgery and 6.7% had 2 previous spinal surgeries. In 94.4% of cases the pelvic bone was used as an autologous graft.

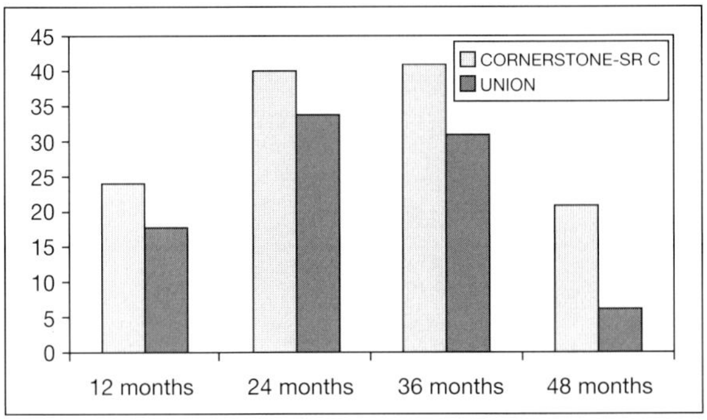

Fig. 3. Minimum follow-up of the CFRP cervical and lumbar fusion implants: CORNERSTONE-SR C (n = 126) and UNION (n = 89).

In 2% of the cervical cases there was a supplemental anterior fixation; in 97.8% an anterior-lateral approach was used. C3–C4 was operated on in 1.5%, C4–C5 in 11.7%, C5–C6 in 52.4%, C6–C7 in 34.0%, and C7–T1 in 0.5% of the cases. In 91% of the lumbar cases there was a supplemental posterior fixation; in 94.4% an anterior approach was used. L5–S1 was operated on in 50.7%, L4–L5 in 39.0%, L3–L4 in 8.9% and L2–L3 in 1.4% of the cases.

In addition a prospective study was performed on 34 cervical and 36 lumbar patients (diagnoses see table 2). The group of 34 cervical patients consisted of 19 males and 15 females with an average age of 47.1 years (range 26–77), an average weight of 76.5 kg and an average height of 169.6 cm. The group of lumbar patients consisted of 17 male and 19 female patients with an average age of 48 years (range 16–73), an average weight of 74.3 kg and an average height of 170.6 cm. In the cervical group 27 patients had no and 7 patients had 1 or 2 previous spinal operations in the affected areas; in the lumbar group 18 patients had no and 18 patients more than 1 operation.

In 7 cervical patients a supplemental screw and plate fixation was performed. The patients were treated with fusion surgery using the CFRP CORNERSTONE-SR C cages filled with the bone regeneration substance Colloss®, an osteoinductive natural protein complex. Monosegmental surgery was performed; in 10 patients a multisegmental procedure was carried out. There were 28 patients for the 3-month follow-up, 17 patients for the 6-month follow-up and 8 patients for the 12-month follow-up.

In the lumbar group, 34 patients were treated with the CFRP UNION cages and posterior pedicle fixation devices were used; the other 2 patients underwent stand-alone procedures. In 29 patients, one camber of the cage was filled with autologous cancellous bone and the other camber with Colloss. In 7 patients both cambers were filled exclusively with Colloss. In 26 of the patients, monosegmental surgery was performed; in 10 patients a multisegmental procedure was carried out.

The following radiographical criteria were used to detect fusion: bone in the fusion area is more dense and more mature than originally achieved in surgery, no interface between donor bone and vertebral bone; sclerotic line between graft and vertebral bone, mature bone trabeculae bridging the fusion area, resorption of anterior vertebral traction spurs, fusion of facet joints and 'ring' phenomenon on CT.

The neurological status was assessed postoperatively using a comprehensive neurological status scale ranging from 0 (worst) to 100 (best). Pre- and postoperatively each patient rated the frequency of their back/leg pain on a scale of 1–10. Patient satisfaction questions and success are defined as either a 'completely recovered', 'much improvement', or 'slightly improved' response.

For the prospective study the arm/neck score was used to evaluate and compare the pain intensity and frequency in the cervical groups (with 1 equal to 'no pain' or 'never' and 10 equal to 'extremely painful' or 'always'). The results of the lumbar group were evaluated and compared using the Oswestry score. In this scale patients can receive a maximum value of 5 points and a minimum value of 0 points on each of the 10 criteria being used.

Clinical examination and comparative measurements were performed on AP and lateral radiographs as well as on flexion/extension films in order to estimate the position of the cages, the degree of restoration of the disc height of the intervertebral discs and the density of the fusion area. MRIs were taken at defined times to verify possible edema that had been reported when using graft material. CTs and regular tomograms were also used to evaluate new bone formation inside the cages.

Results and Discussion

The standard mechanical tests showed the superior strength of the CFRP fusion devices. The cervical fusion device (CORNERSTONE-SR C) has a high compression and shear load (see fig. 7) which is more than 20 times above the normal load in the cervical spine [18]. Pull-out and torsion tests show significant differences between designs with and without the fins (see fig. 8) but even for the nonfin version the values reached are above the daily loads [18]. Figure 9 shows the compression and shear behavior of the CFRP lumbar fusion device UNION.

No significant differences could be detected between different sizes (small and medium) and different heights (10 up to 20 mm) of the implants. The compression load is more than 4 times higher than the load during daily activities [18]. The fatigue behavior due to compression and shear load is shown in figure 10. Run-out load is much higher than could be detected during daily activities. In the clinical studies no intraoperative or device-related complications were observed in either group. In all cervical and lumbar cases of the retrospective study, 100% fusion was determined.

In the cervical group the mean preoperative back/leg pain frequency score was 7.3 and the mean postoperative back/leg pain frequency score was 5.2 (28.8% improvement) (one clinical case, see fig. 4a–f). In the lumbar group the mean preoperative back/leg pain frequency score was 7.9 and the mean postoperative back/leg pain frequency score was 6.2 (21.5% improvement) (two clinical cases, see fig. 5a–c, 6a–d).

In the cervical group patients were satisfied with the results of surgery in 81.6%, surgery helped as much as patient thought it would in 79.0%, and

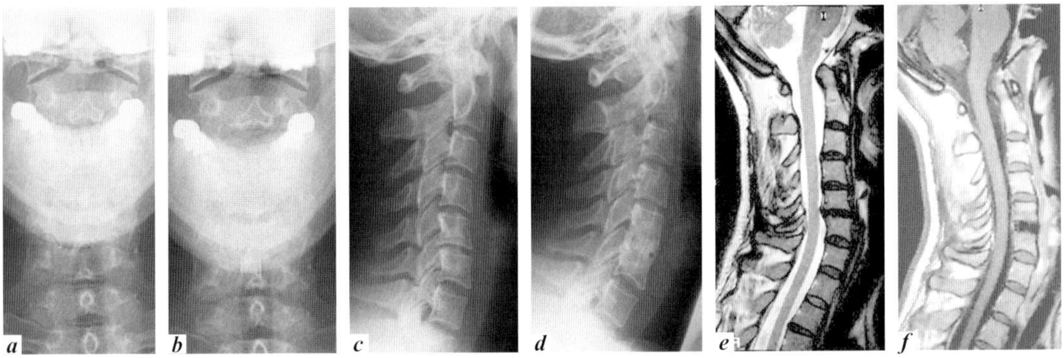

Fig. 4. a–f Radiography showing the CFRP fusion implant CORNERSTONE-SR C (visible due to a $BaSO_4$ layer in the implants): 40-year-old female, vertical segmental instability C5–C6, radicular pain with dysesthesia C5, severe neck pain, unsuccessful conservative treatment. Good realignment of cervical lordosis and secure fusion at the 6-month checkup.

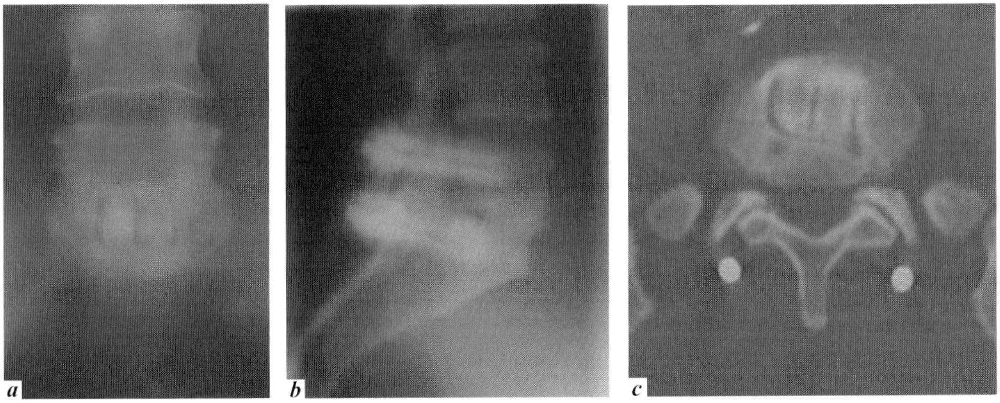

Fig. 5. a–c Conventional tomogram and CT scan show excellent visualization also inside the UNION cage. Secure determination of fusion showing the CFRP fusion implant UNION (visible due to a $BaSO_4$ layer in the implants); here at 6 months checkup is possible.

patients would have the same surgery again in 80.7% of the cases. In the lumbar group patients were satisfied with results of surgery in 71.4%, surgery helped as much as patient thought it would in 57.2%, and patient would have the same surgery again in 67.5% of the cases. The independent physician's assessment showed in 95.3% of the cervical and 97.7% of the lumbar cases excellent or good results (see table 3). 6% of the cervical and 13% of the lumbar patients in the retrospective study showed general and local complications.

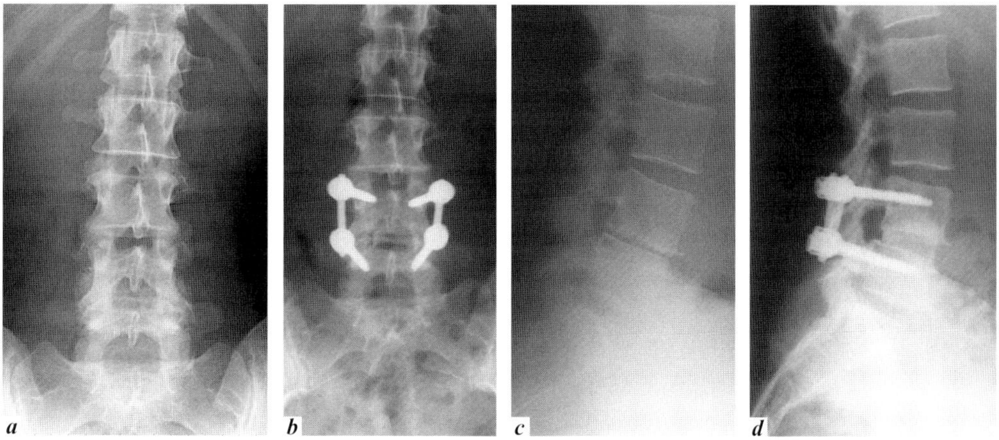

Fig. 6. ***a–d*** Radiography showing the CFRP fusion implant UNION-L (L4–L5, visible due to a $BaSO_4$ layer in the implants): 42-year-old female, failed back disc surgery in 1999, vertical segmental instability L4–L5, severe low back pain, minor radicular pain, unsuccessful conservative treatment. Posterior neurolysis L5 and stabilization L4–L5, ALPA approach. Good realignment of lumbar lordosis and secure fusion at the 12-month checkup.

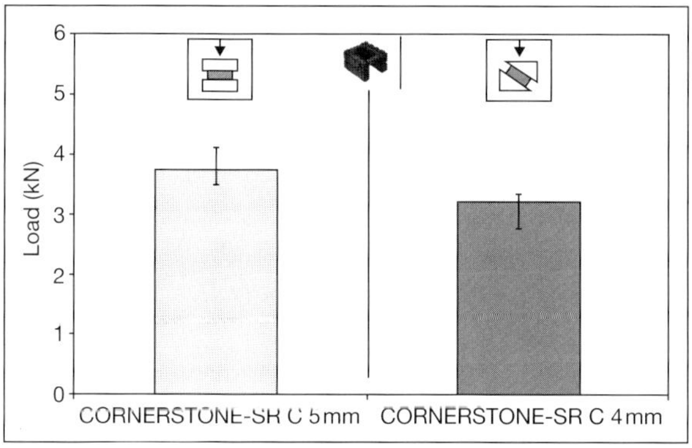

Fig. 7. Compression and shear strength of the CFRP cervical interbody fusion cage CORNERSTONE-SR C tested according to ASTM F2077-00.

In the cervical group of the prospective study 97% fusion could be detected radiographically; in 1 patient (3%) due to only one early check-up at 6 weeks after surgery fusion could not be evaluated. The mean arm/neck pain score improved significantly from 7.6 preoperatively to 4.2 after 12 months (45% improvement), the arm/neck pain frequency score from 8.8 to 5.4 after 12 months (39% improvement). 87.5% of the patients felt there was an improvement

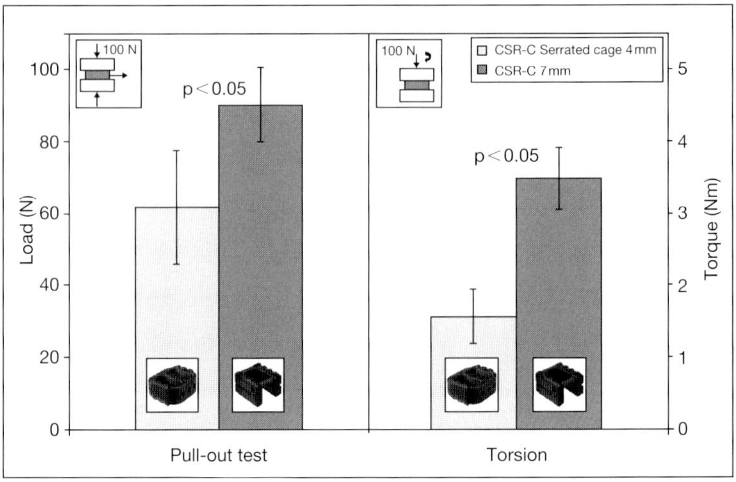

Fig. 8. Pull-out force and torsion behavior of CFRP cervical interbody fusion devices: comparison of implants with rails (CORNERSTONE-SR C) and without rails (CORNERSTONE-SR C serrated).

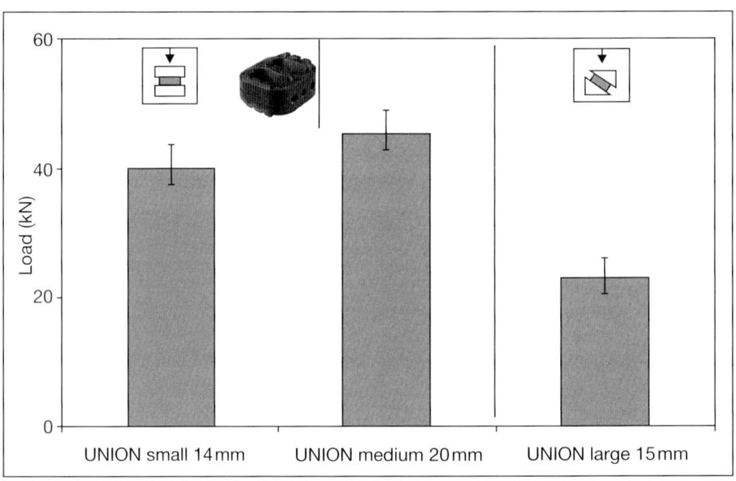

Fig. 9. Compression and shear strength of the CFRP anterior lumbar interbody fusion cage UNION tested according to ASTM F2077-00.

and were satisfied after 12 months, the results of surgery met the expectations of 75%, and 87.5% would have the same surgery again.

In the lumbar group 100% fusion could be detected radiographically; no pseudarthrosis was determined. The mean Oswestry score was 52.3 before surgery and improved after 6 months to 16.2 (69% improvement). 90.0% of the

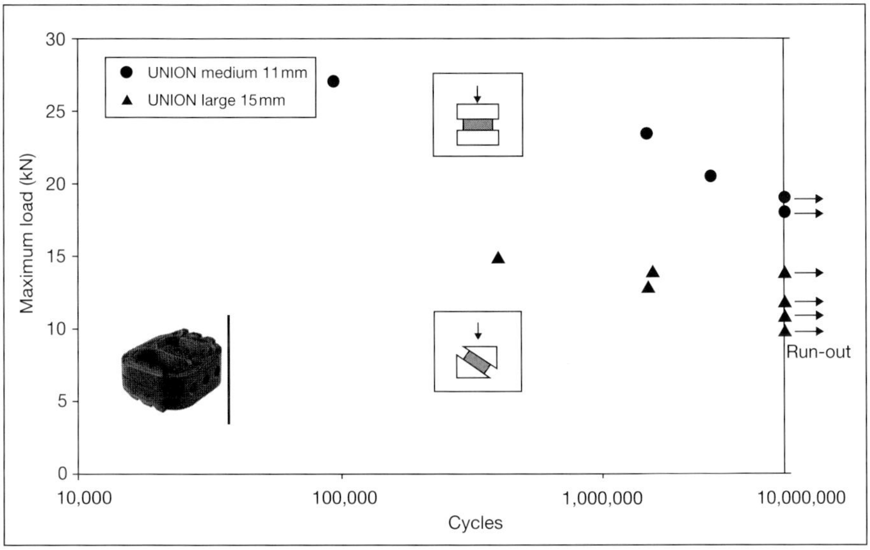

Fig. 10. S/N curve of compression and shear strength of the CFRP anterior lumbar interbody fusion cage UNION tested according to ASTM F2077-00.

Table 3. Independent physician's assessment of the retrospective study

	Cervical, %	Lumbar, %
Excellent	73.4	86.5
Good	21.9	11.2
Fair	4.7	2.3
Poor	0.0	0.0

patients felt there was an improvement and were satisfied after 6 months, the results of surgery met the expectations of 80%, and 60.0% would have the same surgery again. Only 1 patient was not satisfied with the result.

Conclusion

Spine stabilization is an important area of orthopedic surgery, especially due to an increasing number of patients with chronic low back pain and DDD. For interbody fusion, besides autologous or allograft bone grafts, fusion cages composed of metal or polymer as a space holder are increasingly used. Especially CFRP are used in the medical field when radiolucency, high mechanical strength and innovative design are required. During the manufacturing process of the material CFRP carbon fibers are embedded into a thermoset (e.g. epoxy resin EPN/DDS) or thermoplastic (e.g. PEAK) resin matrix. CFRP is biocompatible, radiolucent and has a higher mechanical potential compared to other implant materials and has clinically been used since 1993 for fusion implants of the cervical and lumbar spine. The clinical experience of cervical and lumbar fusion systems showed high fusion rates and no carbon fiber-related complications. In addition prospective studies have shown that the use of osteoinductive bone graft material in conjunction with CFRP cages is a safe and effective method with high fusion rates in the treatment of DDD.

References

1 Boenisch B, Ascherl R, Liebendörfer A, Geissdoerfer K, Schmeller ML, Kerschbaumer S, Scherer MA, Erhardt W, Scheer W, Bluemel G: Five-year functionality study of carbon fibre reinforced acetabular implants in dogs; in Heimke G, Soltész U, Lee AJC (eds): Clinical Implant Materials. Advances in Biomaterials. Amsterdam, Elsevier, 1990, vol 9, pp 391–396.

2 Bertagnoli R: Continuum of care in degenerative disc disease. Backup 2001;1:4–8.

3 Sandhu HS: Anterior lumbar interbody fusion with osteoinductive growth factors. Clin Orthop 2000;371:56–60.

4 Summers BN, Eisenstein SM: Donor site pain from the ilium. A complication of lumbar spine fusion. J Bone Joint Surg Br 1989;71:677–680.

5 Brantigan JW, McAfee PC, Cunningham BW, Wang H, Orbegoso CM: Interbody lumbar fusion using a carbon fiber cage implant versus allograft bone. An investigational study in the Spanish goat. Spine 1994;19:1436–1444.

6 Ciapetta P, Boriani S, Fava GP: A carbon fiber reinforced polymer cage for vertebral body replacement: Technical note. Neurosurgery 1997;41:1203–1206.

7 Jost B, Cripton PA, Lund T, Oxland TR, Lippuner K, Jaeger P, Nolte LP: Compressive strength of interbody cages in the lumbar spine: The effect of cage shape, posterior instrumentation and bone density. Eur Spine J 1998;7:132–141.

8 Kandziora F, Pflugmacher R, Schafer J, Born C, Duda G, Haas NP, Mittlmeier T: Biomechanical comparison of cervical spine interbody fusion cages. Spine 2001;26:1850–1857.

9 Shono Y, McAfee PC, Cunningham BW, Brantigan JW: A biomechanical analysis of decompression and reconstruction methods in the cervical spine. Emphasis on a carbon-fiber-composite cage. J Bone Joint Surg Am 1993;75:1674–1684.

10 Steinhauser E, Bader R, Rechl H, Bertagnoli R, Mittelmeier W, Gradinger R: Mechanical testing of spinal interbody implants – Characteristics and limitations of a standardized testing procedure. Biomed Tech 2001;46:325–332.

11 Agazzi S, Reverdin A, May D: Posterior lumbar interbody fusion with cages: An independent review of 71 cases. J Neurosurg 1999;91:186–192.

12 Diedrich O, Perlick L, Schmitt O, Kraft CN: Radiographic characteristics on conventional radiographs after posterior lumbar interbody fusion: Comparative study between radiotranslucent and radiopaque cages. J Spinal Disord 2001;14:522–532.

13 Brantigan JW, Steffee AD, Lewis ML, Quinn LM, Persenaire JM: Lumbar interbody fusion using the Brantigan I/F cage for posterior lumbar interbody fusion and the variable pedicle screw placement system: Two-year results from a Food and Drug Administration investigational device exemption clinical trial. Spine 2000;25:1437–1446.

14 Tullberg T, Brandt B, Rydberg J, Fritzell P: Fusion rate after posterior lumbar interbody fusion with carbon fiber implant: 1-year follow-up of 51 patients. Eur Spine J 1996;5:178–182.

15 Commarmond J: One-segment interbody lumbar arthrodesis using impacted cages: Posterior unilateral approach versus posterior bilateral approach. Rev Chir Orthop Reparatrice Appar Mot 2001;87:129–134.
16 Brooke NSR, Rorke AW, King AT, Gullan RW: Preliminary experience of carbon fibre cage prostheses for treatment of cervical spine disorders. Br J Neurosurg 1997;11:221–227.
17 Tullberg T: Failure of a carbon fiber implant. A case report. Spine 1998;23:1804–1806.
18 White AA, Panjabi MM: Clinical Biomechanics of the Spine, ed 2. Philadelphia, Lippincott, 1990.

Dr. med. Rudolf Bertagnoli
Kay 2a, D–94315 Straubing (Germany)
Tel. +49 171 4325300, Fax +49 9421 530475, E-Mail bertagnoli@ogp.de

Haid RW Jr, Subach BR, Rodts GE Jr (eds): Advances in Spinal Stabilization.
Prog Neurol Surg. Basel, Karger, 2003, vol 16, pp 188–203

Thoracic Pedicle Screw Placement

Lawrence G. Lenke

Orthopaedic Surgery, Pediatric and Adult Spinal, Scoliosis and Reconstructive Surgery, Washington University Medical Center, Shriners Hospital in St. Louis, St. Louis, Mo., USA

The use of thoracic pedicle screws in the treatment of various spinal disorders has shown a dramatic increase in the last decade [1–4]. The biomechanical stability afforded by transpedicular fixation, the ability to correct various sagittal and coronal plane spinal malalignments and deformities, and the available room for bone grafting around the implants provide an optimal environment for spinal fusion success [5–10]. This chapter will discuss the technique of free-hand thoracic pedicle screw placement using anatomic landmarks, and a special thoracic pedicle probe combined with appropriate surgical 3-dimensional orientation and 'feel' to access the vertebral body via the pedicle channel [11]. This free-hand technique can be adopted by any surgeon comfortable placing lumbar pedicle screws and experienced with thoracic spinal anatomy and surgical techniques, and does not require the use of continuous or intermittent intraoperative fluoroscopy, radiography or navigational systems.

Preoperative Assessment

One of the first assessments that needs to be made by the surgeon contemplating the use of thoracic pedicle screws for the treatment of various surgical spinal disorders is whether the thoracic pedicle is large enough to probe down with a pedicle probe and subsequently accept a screw of appropriate and available diameter and length. There is a wide spectrum of individual pedicle dimensions, with the limiting dimension always being the medial to lateral diameter at the isthmus in millimeters [12–15]. This can range from only 2–3 mm in the mid thoracic region up to >10 mm at the lower thoracic levels. Interestingly, the smallest pedicle dimensions are usually found at the T5–T7 levels. Pedicle isthmus dimensions increase both above and below these mid thoracic levels, being consistently larger in the lower thoracic region (T10–T12), and somewhat smaller in the proximal thoracic region (T1–T3). Because of the varied anatomy and pedicle sizes, it is extremely important to have a variety of choices for pedicle screw diameters available ranging from a 4.0-mm all the way through a 7.5-mm diameter in 0.5-mm increments. The goal should be to maximize fit into the pedicle cortex with the largest screw that will safely fit. The lengths of the screws will vary but range from 40–50 mm in length in the lower thoracic regions to 25–35 mm in length in the proximal thoracic levels. The lengths will depend on patient size, and orientation of the screw, and will be shorter if the trajectory is somewhat lateral. It is also helpful to have both fixed head and multiaxial screws available. I tend to use fixed head screws in the thoracic spine, for they are lower profile and allow more room for bone grafting. However, multiaxial screws can easily be used as well.

In most instances, standard AP and lateral radiographs will adequately demonstrate the pedicle dimensions required to confirm the size of the thoracic pedicles and the ability of the surgeon to navigate down them into the body. One must remember that in a true frontal plane radiograph of the thoracic spine, the pedicles that are perfectly perpendicular to the x-ray beam will have the most accurate representation of their overall dimensions. With increasing thoracic kyphosis, the ability to adequately assess the pedicles above and below the apex will be diminished and occasionally additional views may be helpful in assessing pedicle dimensions in these specific cases. As an alternative, a preoperative CT scan can be obtained with a single slice through each mid pedicle level to check on overall isthmus dimensions. In my experience, these CT dimensions somewhat underestimate the diameter of the screw that can be placed since there does appear that cortical expansion occurs with aggressive tapping and final screw placement. This will be discussed further in the techniques section of this report. I would caution against using a preoperative MRI to assess pedicle dimensions as it appears to underestimate the true cortical size due to artifacts that can occur during the acquisition process.

It is much more difficult to assess rotated pedicles, such as those located at the concave apex of scoliosis deformities. For scoliosis cases, we rely on the assessment of pedicle dimensions noted at proximal and distal levels away from the apex where the vertebrae become more neutral in orientation. Routinely, if the pedicle dimensions are adequate at these more neutral levels, the pedicles will be accessible at the concave apical levels. Also, analyzing the convex-sided pedicle dimensions can provide information on the corresponding concave pedicles. The major difference is that the concave pedicles will tend to be more cortical than the more cancellous centered convex pedicles, although they appear to be relatively the same size at least in adolescent idiopathic scoliosis patients [16].

Free-Hand Pedicle Screw Technique

The technique of 'free-hand' thoracic pedicle screw placement is identical to that utilized in the lumbar spine and includes eight specific steps: (1) exposure, (2) locating the appropriate starting point with burring of the dorsal cortex, (3) use of the thoracic pedicle probe to navigate down the pedicle into the vertebral body, (4) intraosseous palpation, (5) undertapping by 0.5 mm of the intended screw diameter, (6) repalpating to confirm intraosseous borders, (7) screw placement, and (8) confirmation of intraosseous screw placement (table 1, fig. 1–8).

It is extremely important to have a well-exposed posterior spine with minimal oozing of blood into the field. The free-hand technique requires the identification of specific posterior element landmarks to help confirm the appropriate starting point. In addition, the vertebral body can often bleed a fair amount through the pedicle and thus blood loss can be an issue if multilevel screws are placed throughout the thoracic spine. So the initial spinal dissection must be meticulous and the pedicle tract should be liberally plugged with bone wax to minimize oozing from the body through the pedicle. It is also recommended to perform a partial inferior facetectomy which serves several purposes including to remove the cartilage off the facet joint, to improve the fusion rate, and also to gain access to the base of the facet joint which will be utilized as the starting point for the mid thoracic pedicle levels (T7, T8, T9).

Next a specific starting point on the posterior elements must be located for the creation of a cortical defect which should be at the superficial base of the pedicle. We have discovered that there are specific starting points for each thoracic pedicle between T1 and T12 that are fairly consistent for patients with or without a coronal and/or sagittal spinal deformity present [11]. Beginning distal at T12, the starting point is the down slope of the medial portion of the bisected transverse process where it meets the lamina which should be just at or lateral to the lateral portion of the pars. And as one proceeds to the T11 and T10 spinal levels, the starting point moves slightly more proximal and more medial such that by T10 the starting point is the proximal edge of the transverse process where it meets the lamina and facet. The starting points for T7, T8 and T9 are fairly consistent being the proximal portion of the transverse process where it meets the facet joint, just lateral to the mid portion of the superior facet. Then as one proceeds proximal from T7, the starting point becomes more lateral and distal, based off the anatomic landmarks of the thoracic transverse process-lamina junction. Thus at T6, similar to T10, the starting point is the proximal edge of the transverse process base at the junction of the lamina. Then by T3, the starting point is the bisected transverse process where the transverse process meets the lamina. This also holds true for T1 and T2, which are slightly larger pedicles, but have a greater medial inclination in the transverse plane [13].

Table 1. 8 steps of the 'free-hand' technique of thoracic pedicle screw placement

Step	Description
Exposure (see fig. 1)	Thorough and meticulous exposure to the tips of all transverse processes to be included in the instrumentation/fusion.
Starting point and cortical burr (see fig. 2)	Visualize the starting point based upon as much anatomical information as possible. For noncontiguous levels, this may be limited to a review of the pre- and intraoperative radiographs and orientation of the posterior elements. However, with successive levels, much information is provided by making fine adjustments to the trajectory of the previous level's screw or contralateral screw. Use a 5.0-mm acorn-tipped burr (or smaller burr in smaller patients) to thin the posterior cortex and enter the pedicle. The pedicle 'blush' should be visualized suggesting entrance into the cancellous bone of the pedicle. In cases with smaller pedicles, especially in the apical concavity of scoliosis patients, there will be very limited intrapedicular cancellous bone and therefore a pedicle blush may not be observed.
Pedicle gearshift-lateral (see fig. 3)	Use a 2-mm blunt-tipped, slightly curved pedicle finder (thoracic gearshift) facing laterally to enter the pedicle. Often the endosteal diameter of the pedicle is quite small, so allowing the finder to 'fall' into the pedicle. The thoracic gearshift should be perpendicular to the plane of the superior facet and/or lamina. Aiming slightly laterally initially will help to avoid medial wall perforations. Rotate the pedicle finder to a medially faced orientation after a depth of approximately 15–20 mm is attained (the average length of a typical pedicle). Carefully place the tip to the base of the prior hole before advancing the pedicle finder. Advance the finder to approximately the length of the desired screw and then rotate the finder 180° to make room for the screw. Make sure you feel bone the entire length of the pedicle. Any sudden advancement of the gearshift suggests penetration into soft tissue and thus a pedicle wall violation or vertebral body violation. These should be investigated immediately in order to possibly salvage the pedicle and avoid complications.
Pedicle palpation (see fig. 4)	Use a flexible ball-tipped sounding device to palpate all 5 walls of the pedicle (cephalad, caudad, medial, lateral, and floor). Pay special attention to the junction of the middle and upper portions of the tract as this is the region of the pedicle where the spinal canal is located. If any wall besides the medial wall has been breached, the pedicle may be salvageable. In this circumstance, place bone wax in the pedicle hole to limit bleeding and reangle the pedicle finder with a more appropriate trajectory.
Pedicle tapping (see fig. 5)	Tap the pedicle with a tap that is 0.5 mm smaller than the proposed screw. If there is difficulty passing the tap, use the next smaller tap and then retap the pedicle. If there is no anterior wall violation, one can use a K wire to assist with guiding the path of the cannulated taps. If there is any question of whether the anterior wall is intact, do not use a K wire as cardiac tamponade due to K-wire-induced trauma to a coronary artery has been reported.

Table 1 (continued)

Step	Description
Repeat pedicle palpation (see fig. 6)	Use the palpating device a second time to assess the bony pedicle walls and remeasure the tract length with a hemostat. Compare this measurement directly adjacent to the screw to be placed to ensure appropriate screw length.
Screw placement (see fig. 7)	Place the screw slowly to confirm it is threaded properly and allow for viscoelastic expansion of the pedicle. Make sure the angle of screw insertion matches the tract previously palpated and tapped.
Confirmation of intraosseous screw placement (see fig. 8)	After all the screws have been placed, intraoperative radiographs are repeated prior to placing the rods in order to confirm accurate placement of the screws. Some surgeons prefer to use fluoroscopy in order to obtain a true AP of each level. The coronal plane should show harmonious screw positions from proximal to distal. The sagittal plane should demonstrate parallel orientation to the superior end-plate so that no screw tip is anterior to the anterior vertebral body line. Perform EMG assessment of the screws based upon rectus abdominis data. Frequently we use active EMGs via the same approach through the pedicle finder or cannulated tap to assess real-time monitoring of the thoracic nerve root. The screws with the lowest impedance are removed and rechecked with a ball-tipped sounder prior to replacement of the screw if intraosseous borders are confirmed.

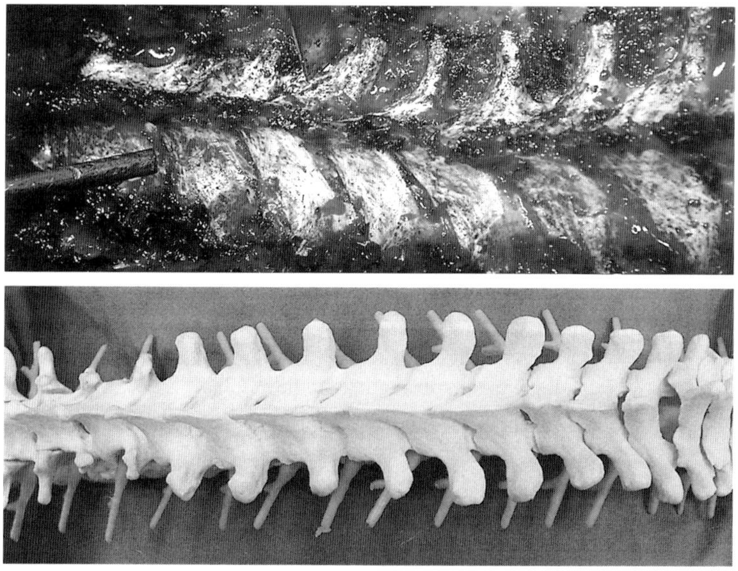

Fig. 1. Complete exposure of the bony anatomy.

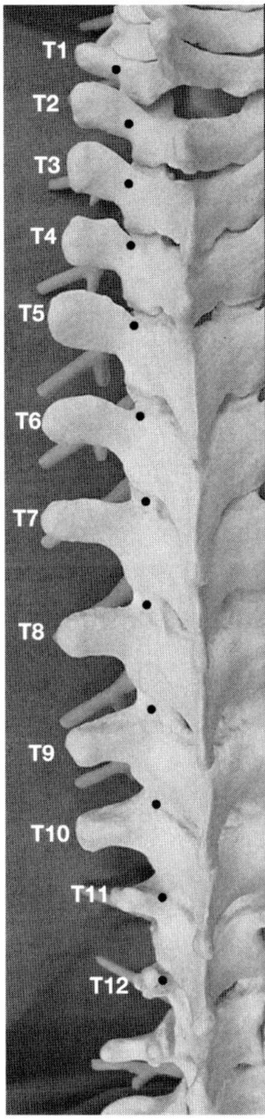

Thoracic Pedicle Screw Starting Points		
Level	Cephalad-Caudad Starting Point	Medial-Lateral Starting Point
T1	Midpoint TP	Junction: TP-Lamina
T2	Midpoint TP	Junction: TP-Lamina
T3	Midpoint TP	Junction: TP-Lamina
T4	Junction: Proximal third-Midpoint TP	Junction: TP-Lamina
T5	Proximal third TP	Junction: TP-Lamina
T6	Junction: Proximal edge-Proximal third TP	Junction: TP-Lamina-Facet
T7	Proximal TP	Midpoint Facet
T8	Proximal TP	Midpoint Facet
T9	Proximal TP	Midpoint Facet
T10	Junction: Proximal edge-Proximal third TP	Junction: TP-Lamina-Facet
T11	Proximal third TP	Just medial to lateral pars
T12	Midpoint TP	At the level of lateral pars

Fig. 2. Thoracic pedicle screw starting points.

A specially designed thoracic pedicle probe ('Lenke Probe', Medtronic Sofamor-Danek Memphis, Tenn., USA) helps probe down the small-sized pedicle channel into the vertebral body. The pedicle probe has a 2-mm tip, which will be required for navigating smaller pedicles versus a conventional 4- to 5-mm tip used as a lumbar pedicle probe. The probe tip becomes thicker as one proceeds away from the tip of the probe, which will make the probe somewhat snugger as one proceeds down into the body past the pedicle. It is also calibrated in 5-mm increments with a rectangular tip going to a round shaft at 35 mm in length. The probe is also shaped with a slight

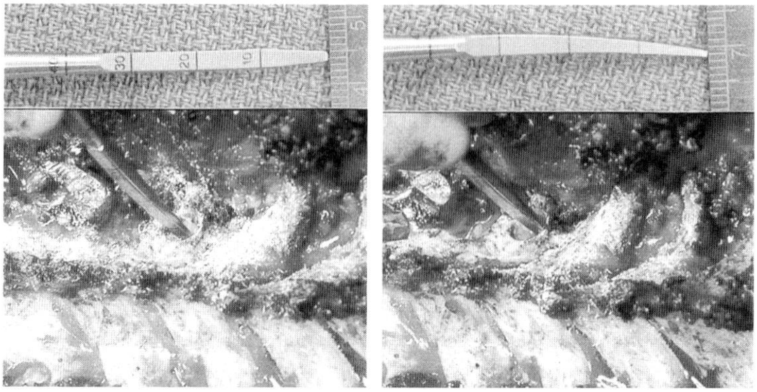

3

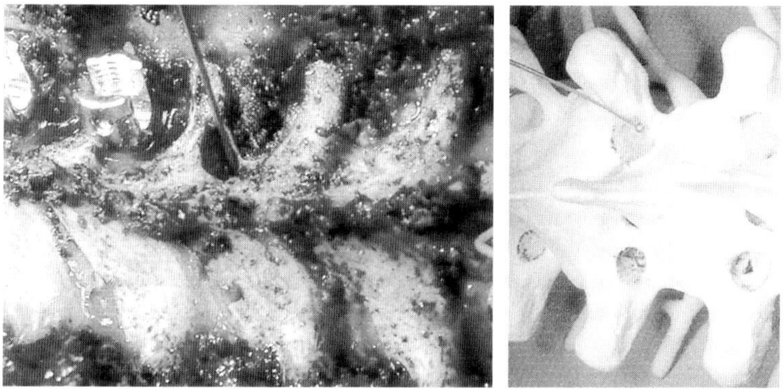

4

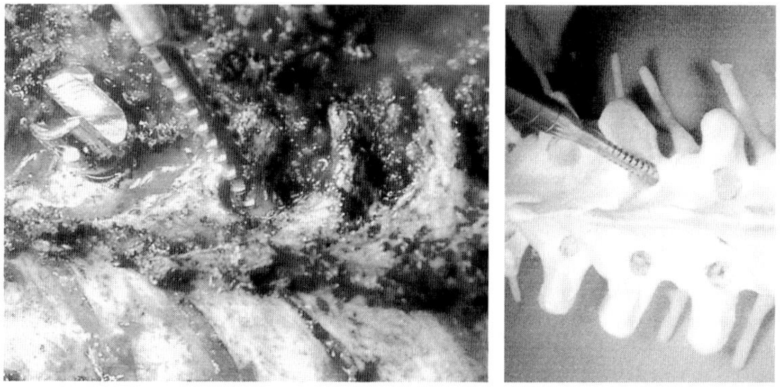

5

Fig. 3. Use a 2-mm blunt-tipped, slightly curved pedicle finder (thoracic gearshift) facing laterally to enter the pedicle.

Fig. 4. Sounding device to palpate all 5 walls of the pedicle (cephalad, caudad, medial, lateral, and floor).

Fig. 5. Tap the pedicle with a tap that is 0.5 mm smaller than the proposed screw.

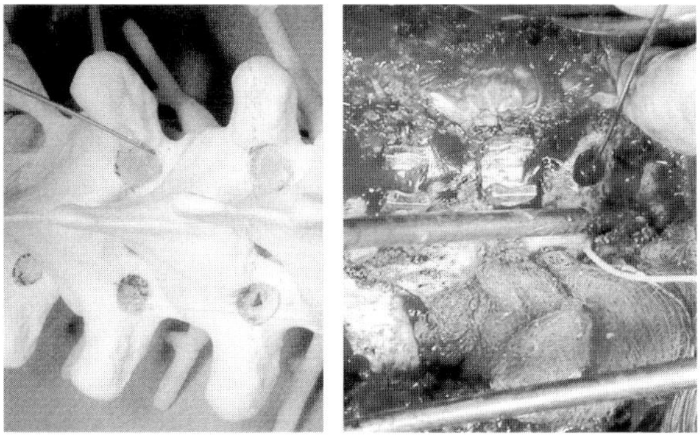

6

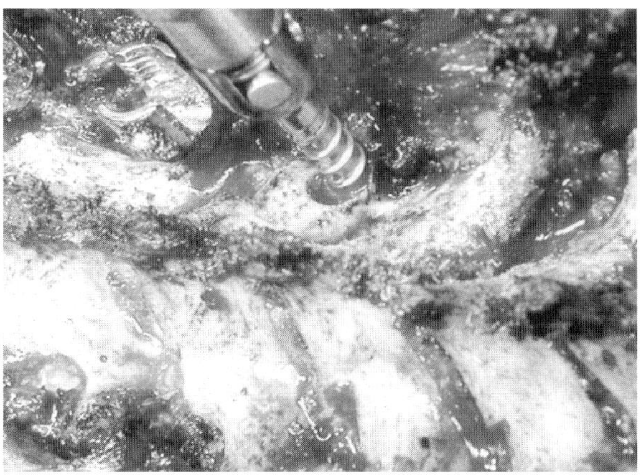

7

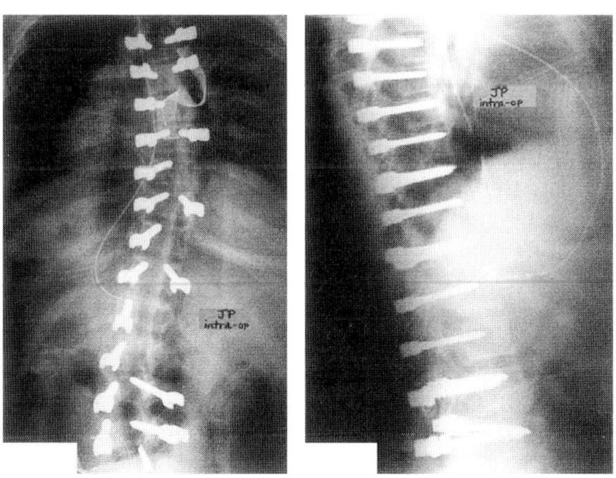

8

Fig. 6. Use the palpating device a second time to assess the bony pedicle walls.
Fig. 7. Place the screw slowly.
Fig. 8. Intraoperative x-rays.

curvature, which is utilized to avoid penetration of the spinal canal at all times [17]. We almost always start our probe with the curve facing lateral for this purpose.

After a cortical window is drilled with a 4.0-mm burr, the gearshift is taken and placed perpendicular to the plane of the lamina at the level being instrumented. This 'perpendicularity' is an extremely important feature for obtaining both correct sagittal plane and transverse plane angulation to allow placement of the screw parallel to the superior end-plate of the instrumented level. The pedicle probe tip starts out with the curve facing lateral in the pedicle tract. A 'soft spot' of the cancellous pedicle is identified with an initial light push of the probe tip into the burred surface. Once this 'soft spot' is acknowledged by 'feel', then the probe is advanced deeper into the pedicle past the spinal canal. Once the pedicle probe has been engaged down to 15–20 mm (i.e. past the spinal canal and into the posterior portion of the body), the probe is removed, and turned in a medially curved direction and the probe is then advanced medially into the vertebral body. If the probe was left continually in the lateral curved position, it would deflect out of the vertebra laterally, which is less than desirable. It is important as one is advancing the probe to rotate it slightly so as to allow the tip to fall into the soft portion of the pedicle and then into the body quite readily. If resistance is being met, then the probe tip is usually positioned either too medial or too lateral. One should make multiple small permutations of probe tip positioning and orientation to seek out the best fit of the pedicle probe down the shaft of the pedicle without breaking out of the pedicle. Certainly, this 'feel' is an extremely important component to the free-hand screw placement technique. Thus, one should ideally have mastered this in the lumbar spine before proceeding up to the thoracic spine where medial penetration may render the thoracic spinal cord at risk during probe placement and/or screw placement.

After the probe has been advanced to a depth between 30 and 35 mm (proximal thoracic region) or up to 40–45 mm (lower thoracic region), the probe is removed and the pedicle tract palpated with a fine ball-tipped palpation device. It is absolutely essential to feel the floor and four bony walls (medial, lateral, superior, and inferior) confirming intraosseous placement. One must carefully rule out a ledge that will be indicative of a medial wall breech that will be present in the proximal to mid third of the pedicle tract where the spinal canal is located. A tip-off of a medial breach is fairly aggressive bony oozing of venous blood from the pedicle tract out of proportion to other levels. Although this bleeding can be indicative of intraosseous bleeding, it may also signal epidural bleeding secondary to a medial pedicle wall defect. Liberal use of bone wax will plug the hole between the various maneuvers before the screw is placed, if intraosseous borders are confirmed.

Next, the pedicle tract is tapped with a tap undersized from the final pedicle screw by 0.5 mm. I use a variety of color-coded cannulated taps that range in diameter from 4.0 up to 6.5 mm with the threaded portion 35 mm in length (Medtronic Sofamor-Danek). If necessary, a short K wire can be placed into the pedicle tract as long as there is a floor for the K wire not to advance through while tapping is undertaken. The K wire can be especially helpful if more than one attempt is made to probe down the pedicle and a false passage has been created. A K wire leading down the correct pathway can guide the tap into the appropriate position. We have also found clinically, and confirmed biomechanically, that undertapping by 0.5 mm will improve the screw ultimate pullout strength. It is not necessary to tap the entire length of the pedicle screw tract, only the portion deep into the isthmus of the pedicle usually meaning approximately 20–25 mm.

Following tapping, the pedicle is palpated again with a fine ball-tipped sounding probe. Once again the floor and four walls (medial, lateral, superior and inferior) should be confirmed intact to be completely intraosseous. There is often a very nice cortical bony ridge that is palpated following the tapping that absolutely confirms an intraosseous screw tract. It is important at this time to confirm the appropriate length of the screw by measuring the length of the sounding device while it is held deep against the floor of the vertebral body. We will place a screw of a slightly smaller length so as not to penetrate anterior or lateral to the vertebral body with an inadvertently long screw. The screw is then placed in the same orientation as the pedicle tract was probed and tapped.

If the initial pedicle probe tract is found to be either medial or lateral, it often can be redirected with the probe down the appropriate pedicle shaft. Even with a medial wall defect, a new medial wall can be created with a pedicle probe placed correctly down the pathway of the pedicle. However, this is not always the case and in very tiny pedicles, often only one pass will be allowed to successfully navigate the pedicle. Almost always if the initial pedicle probe is lateral, the true pedicle pathway can be salvaged with a more medially directed probe. Similar to the lumbar spine, if one is having difficulty finding the start of the pedicle, it is best to err slightly more lateral. If one does exit lateral initially, virtually no structures are at risk from minor lateral wall penetrations, and the correct pedicle tract can almost always be salvaged in these circumstances.

Confirmation of Intraosseous Screw Placement

Following screw placement, it is imperative that the surgeon confirm accurate screw placement. This is done intraoperatively by several methods including previously mentioned tract palpation, visual orientation and line-up of the screws, intraoperative AP and lateral radiographs and/or fluoroscopy, and pedicle screw stimulation with EMG recordings [18]. The use of CT scans postoperatively to confirm appropriate screw position is strongly recommended to those beginning their experience [19].

Probably the more important intraoperative confirmation of an intraosseous screw is the palpation method. This is utilized twice: initially after the probe is in place and then following tapping of the pedicle. Once the screw is placed, intraoperative coronal and sagittal plane radiographs or fluoroscopy should be used to check all screws. In the frontal plane, the screws should be fairly harmonious with a lack of crossing of the screw tips in the midline. Although this does not absolutely predict medially directed screws, it certainly heightens one's suspicion. Also, lateral placement needs to be checked because this is fairly common in the thoracic spine especially since the vertebral bodies thin out laterally in mid and proximal thoracic vertebral levels. In the lateral view, I prefer to have the screw parallel to the superior end-plate. And also, the screw tips should not extend past the anterior border of the vertebral body so as to make sure the screws are not excessively long. It is important to confirm that the top and bottom screws are not penetrating the superior end-plate extending into the adjacent disc space. This is especially true for the most proximal level thoracic screw, as it is often difficult to angle one's pedicle probe, tap and screw in the appropriate kyphotic angulation of the proximal thoracic region, with resultant cephalad positioning.

We perform thoracic pedicle screw stimulation with EMGs recorded from the rectus abdominis muscles to confirm intraosseous screw placement [20]. An identical technique is used for screws placed between L1 and S1 with recording in the various lower extremity myotomes. Screws are stimulated with an ascending method of simulation to obtain a compound muscle action potential from the rectus abdominis muscles bilaterally. A recent study of 677 screws placed between T6 and T12 (innervation of the rectus) predicted a medially placed screw by a combination of threshold response less than 6 mA in absolute value and also a threshold intensity averaging 65% below the mean of all other thoracic screw responses in the same patient. Although this is not absolutely indicative for a medially misplaced screw, it is another method utilized to heighten one's suspicion of a pedicle wall defect intraoperatively.

It also is advisable for surgeons beginning with the technique of thoracic pedicle screw placement to obtain postoperative CT scans of their patients [19]. It can be quite enlightening to see exactly where the screws are placed, where the tips of the screws are located, and it can only help the surgeon improve his or her technique over time.

Results and Correlations of Thoracic Pedicle Screws Placed by the Free-Hand Technique

All thoracic pedicle screws placed by the free-hand placement technique have been reviewed by an independent spine surgeon performing a 2-year clinical research fellowship (Y.J. Kim, MD, Seoul, Korea) [21]. 2,199 thoracic pedicle screws have been placed by this technique in the last 9 years, the vast majority of which over the last 4 years. The majority of screws have been placed in the treatment of pediatric and adult spinal deformity, but also include use in nondeformity conditions such as spinal trauma, tumor and infection. Our results in spinal deformity treatment include increasing correction rates with a decreased use of preliminary anterior release and fusions in some circumstances, and the rare use of any postoperative external immobilization (fig. 9).

There were no screws removed for any type of neurologic, vascular or visceral complications [11, 21]. Specifically, there have been no screw-related neurologic deficits, unexplained thoracic chest wall pain or radicular lower extremity pain, or unexplained neurologic symptoms. There have been no cases of revision surgery needed up to this stage in the cases with thoracic pedicle

9a
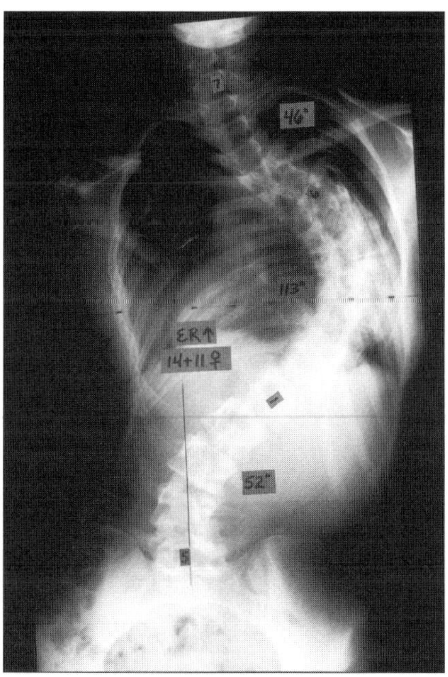

9b
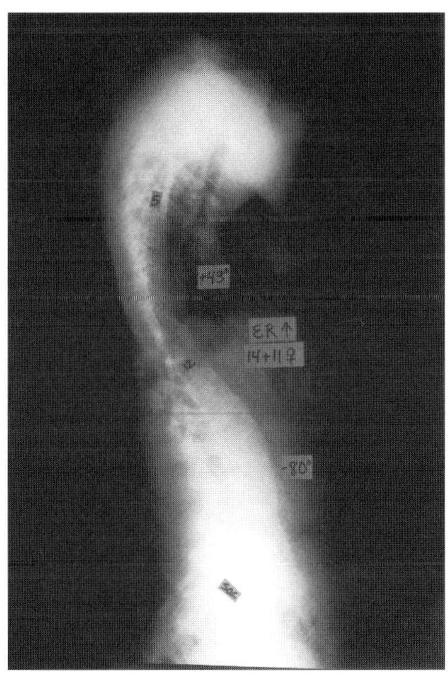

(For legend see p. 201.)

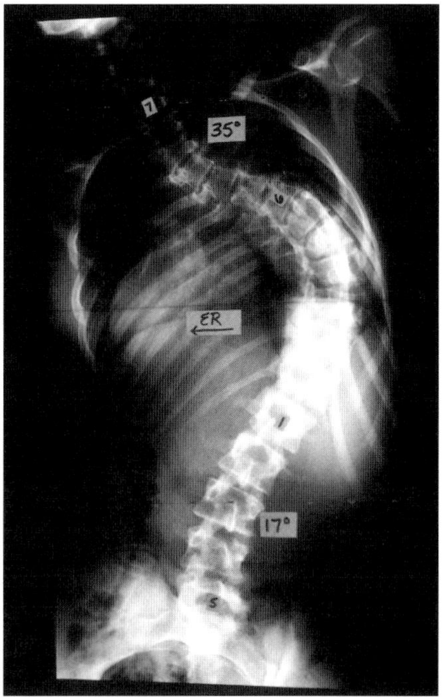

9c

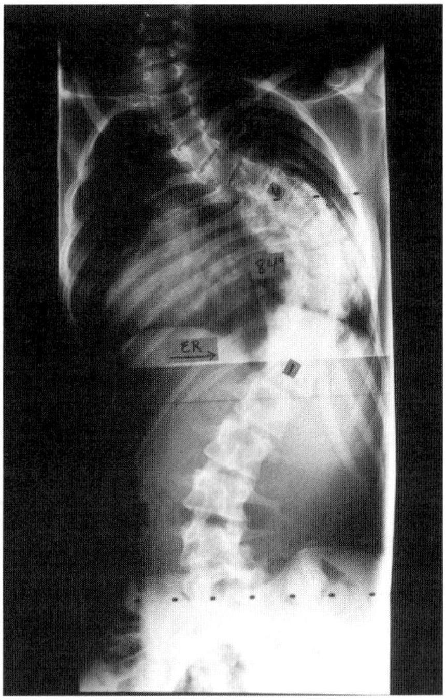

9d

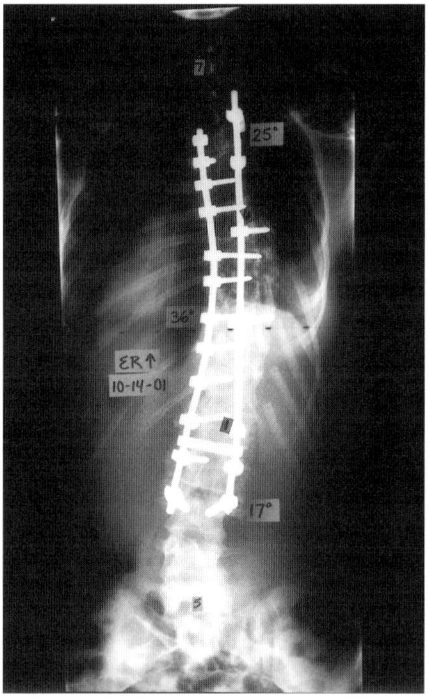

9e

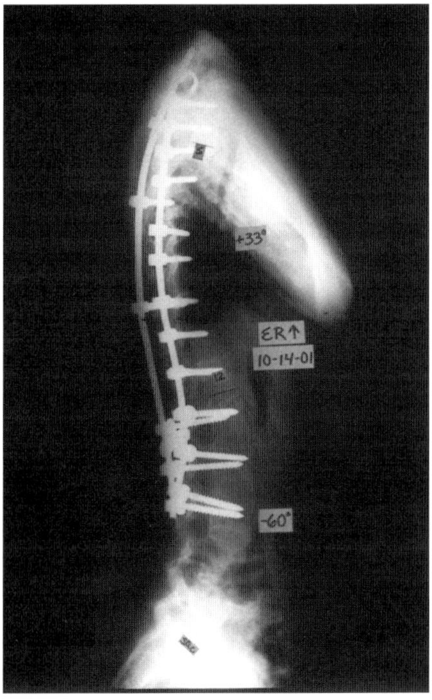

9f

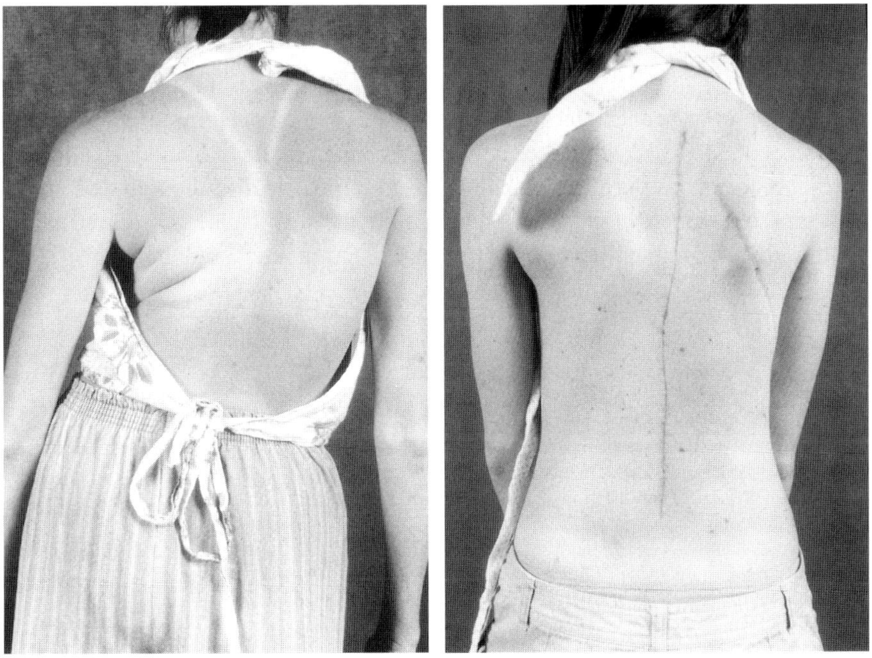

9g 9h

Fig. 9. ***a*** ER is a 14 + 11-year-old female who presented with a severe 113° right thoracic idiopathic scoliosis. Proximal thoracic curve measured 46° and lumbar compensatory curve 52°. ***b*** Her sagittal plane showed 43° of thoracic kyphosis between T5 and T12 and –80° of lumbar lordosis between T12 and the sacrum. ***c*** Her left side bender showed a structural proximal thoracic curve bending out to only 35°, with a flexible lumbar curve bending out to 17°. ***d*** Her right side bender showed a stiff main thoracic region as expected with correction to only 84°. ***e*** She underwent an open anterior release and fusion from T5 to T12 and a posterior segmental screw instrumentation and fusion from T3 to L3 and in a staged fashion. Her upright postoperative coronal radiograph demonstrates excellent correction of her main thoracic curve to 36°, with well balanced curves both above and below. Note the marked apical translation occurring with use of multisegmental screw instrumentation. ***f*** Her upright lateral x-ray shows normalized thoracic kyphosis of +33° and overall good sagittal balance. ***g*** Her preoperative upright photograph demonstrates her right thoracic trunk shift and rib prominence on the right side. ***h*** Her postoperative clinical photo demonstrates excellent balance of her trunk on her pelvis and level shoulders with a diminished rib prominence.

screw constructs, except for 1 patient 2 years postoperatively from an adolescent idiopathic scoliosis surgery with a chronic deep wound infection treated by implant removal. Because of these results, we have continued to utilize pedicle screws as our main anchor attachment to the thoracic and lumbar spine in all forms of pediatric and adult deformity and nondeformity conditions requiring spinal instrumentation and fusion.

Conclusions

The free-hand placement of thoracic pedicle screws in both pediatric and adult patients with or without spinal deformity can be performed in a safe and reliable manner. This technique should be mastered in the lumbar spine and thoracolumbar junction prior to extending it more proximal in the mid and proximal thoracic spine. Strict and meticulous attention to detail is required along with a precise surgical technique to safely place thoracic pedicle screws for a variety of spinal conditions.

References

1 Gaines RW: The use of pedicle-screw internal fixation for the operative treatment of spinal disorders. J Bone Joint Surg Am 2000;82:1458–1476.

2 Liljenqvist UR, Halm HF, Link TM: Pedicle screw instrumentation of the thoracic spine in idiopathic scoliosis. Spine 1997;22:2239–2245.

3 Suk SI, Kim WJ, Lee SM, Kim JH, Chung ER: Thoracic pedicle screw fixation in spinal deformities: Are they really safe? Spine 2001;26:2049–2057.

4 Suk SI, Lee CK, Kim WJ, Chung YJ, Park YB: Segmental pedicle screw fixation in the treatment of thoracic idiopathic scoliosis. Spine 1995;20:1399–1405.

5 Hamill CL, Lenke LG, Bridwell KH, Chapman MP: The use of pedicle screw fixation to improve correction in the lumbar spine of patients with idiopathic scoliosis. Is it warranted? Spine 1996; 21:1241–1249.

6 Hirano T, Hasegawa K, Takahashi HE, Uchiyama S, Hara T, Washio T, Surgiura T, Yokaichiya M, Ikeda M: Structural characteristics of the pedicle and its role in screw stability. Spine 1997;22: 2504–2510.

7 Krag MH, Weaver DL, Beynnon BD, Haugh LD: Morphometry of the thoracic and lumbar spine related to transpedicular screw placement for surgical spinal fixation. Spine 1998;13/1:27–32.

8 Liljenqvist UR, Link TM, Halm HF: Morphometric analysis of thoracic and lumbar vertebrae in idiopathic scoliosis. Spine 2000;25:1247–1253.

9 Lonstein JE, Denis F, Perra JH, Pinto MR, Smith MD, Winter RB: Complications associated with pedicle screws. J Bone Joint Surg Am 1999;81:1519–1528.

10 Vaccaro AR, Rizzolo SJ, Balderston RA, Allardyce TJ, Garfin SR, Dolinskas C, An HS: Placement of pedicle screws in the thoracic spine. II. An anatomical and radiographic assessment. J Bone Joint Surg Am 1995;77:1200–1206.

11 Kim Y, Lenke LG, Bridwell KH, Riew KD, Rhee JM, Hanson DS: Free hand pedicle screw placement in the thoracic spine (poster). Scoliosis Research Society 36th Annual Meeting, Cleveland, 2001.

12 Cinotti G, Gumina S, Ripani M, Postacchini F: Pedicle instrumentation in the thoracic spine. A morphometric and cadaveric study for placement of screws. Spine 1999;24/2:114–119.

13 Ebraheim NA, Xu R, Ahmad M, Yeasting RA: Projection of the thoracic pedicle and its morphometric analysis. Spine 1997;22/3:233–238.

14 Kothe R, O'Holleran JD, Liu W, Panjabi MM: Internal architecture of the thoracic pedicle. An anatomic study. Spine 1996;21/3:264–270.

15 Vaccaro AR, Rizzolo SJ, Allardyce TJ, Ramsey M, Salvo J, Balderston RA, Cotler JM: Placement of pedicle screws in the thoracic spine. I. Morphometric analysis of the thoracic vertebrae. J Bone Joint Surg Am 1995;77:1193–1199.

16 O'Brien MF, Lenke LG, Mardjetko S, Lowe TG, Kong Y, Eck K, Smith D: Pedicle morphology in thoracic adolescent idiopathic scoliosis: Is pedicle fixation an anatomically viable technique? Spine 2000;25:2285–2293.

17 Ebraheim NA, Jabaly G, Xu R, Yeasting RA: Anatomic relations of the thoracic pedicle to the adjacent neural structures. Spine 1997;22:1553–1557.

18 Brown CA, Lenke LG, Bridwell KH, Geideman WM, Hasan SA, Blanke K: Complications of pediatric thoracolumbar and lumbar pedicle screws. Spine 1998;23:1566–1571.

19 Kim YJ, Lenke LG, Bridwell KH, Riew KD, O'Brien M, Rhee JM, Hanson DS: CT scan accuracy of 'free hand' thoracic pedicle screw placement in pediatric spinal deformity (poster). Scoliosis Research Society Annual Meeting, Cleveland, 2001.

20 Raynor BL, Lenke LG, Kim Y, Bridwell KH, Hanson DS, Padberg AM: Can triggered EMG thresholds accurately predict thoracic pedicle screw placement? Spine, in press.

21 Kim Y, Lenke LG, Bridwell KH, Riew KD, Rhee JM, Hanson DS: Thoracic pedicle screw placement in deformity: Is it safe? (poster). Scoliosis Research Society 36th Annual Meeting, Cleveland, 2001.

Lawrence G. Lenke, MD
One Barnes-Jewish Hospital Plaza, Suite 11300, St. Louis, MO 63110 (USA)
Tel. +1 314 747 2509, Fax +1 314 747 2599, E-Mail lenkel@msnotes.wustl.edu

Haid RW Jr, Subach BR, Rodts GE Jr (eds): Advances in Spinal Stabilization.
Prog Neurol Surg. Basel, Karger, 2003, vol 16, pp 204–212

Percutaneous Lumbar Pedicle Screws: Indications, Technique, Results

Gerald E. Rodts, Jr.

Department of Neurosurgery, Emory University, Atlanta, Ga., USA

Lumbar pedicle fixation has proven to be a safe, effective means of lumbar stabilization. Prospective, randomized trials and community clinical experience using lumbar instrumentation have demonstrated an increased fusion rate. Lumbar instrumentation has also improved the ability to mobilize patients after surgery and perhaps brace them for shorter periods of time or not at all. To date, techniques of lumbar pedicle screw placement have involved a single midline or bilateral paramedian incision. Some degree of muscular tendon detachment from the bone and muscle retraction has been necessary. Without question, this is a source of postoperative pain and subsequent muscle atrophy and scar formation.

Until recently, techniques of percutaneous lumbar fixation have involved external instrumentation or epifascial techniques [1–3]. Described herein is a new technique to allow for direct subfascial lumbar pedicle fixation, rod insertion, distraction/compression, and final tightening, all with percutaneous entry points. Compared to open techniques, the presumed benefit of the percutaneous technique is avoidance of muscular tendon detachment, elimination of large-scale muscle retraction, diminished postoperative pain, less blood loss, and improved cosmetic result. In the future, improved minimally invasive fusion techniques and the use of bone morphogenetic protein may increase the applicability of percutaneous techniques.

Indications

The indications for percutaneous lumbar pedicle fixation initially are limited to a few specific clinical conditions. Currently, percutaneous lumbar pedicle fixation may be most useful when a surgeon wishes to create a posterior tension band. As posterior endoscopic or other minimally invasive techniques progress, percutaneous fixation may be combined with simultaneous laminectomy, discectomy, interbody or posterolateral fusion.

One indication for percutaneous posterior fixation is following a laparoscopic or open (retroperitoneal or transperitoneal) anterior lumbar interbody fusion (ALIF). Many surgeons do not rely on a stand-alone ALIF for the treatment of a mobile (unstable) lumbar spondylolisthesis. Whether threaded titanium cylinders, vertical carbon or titanium or ceramic cages, allograft femoral ring wedges or threaded allograft bone dowels are used for the ALIF, the placement of posterior instrumentation in the setting of a mobile spondylolisthesis provides greater biomechanical stability. Furthermore, studies have shown a higher rate of pseudoarthrosis following stand-alone ALIF using allograft bone. With posterior fixation, the rate of fusion following ALIF with bone-only is improved.

Another consideration for the use of posterior percutaneous fixation is in the case of a pseudoarthrosis following previous stand-alone ALIF. If a nonunion is present yet the surgeon is satisfied with the structural integrity of the previously implanted bone graft, posterior instrumentation ultimately can help to achieve a successful arthrodesis. An example would be a case of previous femoral ring ALIF with an intact graft, absence of subsidence or vertebral body lysis, but no evidence of bone union on plain radiographs or CT with reconstructions.

Percutaneous pedicle fixation is also a reasonable alternative to open placement of instrumentation in the setting of a pseudoarthrosis following previous posterolateral fusion. In this setting, decortication of the previous fusion mass and placement of bone graft can be done through the same portals used for percutaneous screw placement.

More recently, advances in less invasive techniques using tubular retractors and blunt dissection through muscle have allowed for lumbar bone decompression (laminectomy, laminotomy, medical facetectomy, discectomy), posterolateral fusion, and interbody fusion. Percutaneous pedicle screw fixation using the same or different stab incisions may be a beneficial adjunct to these newer approaches to decompression and arthrodesis.

Materials and Techniques

For percutaneous pedicle screw fixation, radiographic image guidance is essential. Several options may be considered. Placing the instrumentation using plain radiographs is not recommended. A single fluoroscopic C-arm can be alternated between anterior-posterior (AP), oblique or 'owl's eye', and straight lateral views. The owl's eye view allows a coaxial view down the barrel of the pedicle. Performing percutaneous screws with a single fluoroscopic

C-arm is possible; however, it is tedious and significant time must be devoted to changing sterile drapes and moving the C-arm into different positions.

Simultaneous biplanar fluoroscopy offers immediate feedback in two planes. Ergonomically, it is challenging to operate inside of and around two C-arms placed for lateral and AP or lateral and oblique views. Simultaneous dual views allow for instant feedback when an instrument trajectory is altered manually by the surgeon in one plane. One limitation of biplanar fluoroscopy in percutaneous procedures, however, is the difficulty in seeing the tip of an instrument at the level of the skin surface. This is particularly true in patients with a large body habitus where there is a great distance between skin surface and the spine.

Computer-assisted, virtual fluoroscopic systems offer a tremendous advantage. We have had extensive experience using the FluoroNav™ virtual fluoroscopic system (Medtronic Sofamor Danek, Memphis, Tenn., USA). With this technology, a stereotactic reference arc with light-emitting diodes is attached rigidly to the patient's spine through a small stab incision. The arc can also be attached to the ileum using a screw. Routine lateral, oblique or owl's eye, and AP images are obtained. The images are obtained with an overlying calibration array of 'fiducials' attached to the C-arm. Images are then transferred automatically from the C-arm monitor to the Stealth™ or ION™ (intraoperative navigation) computer monitor. The images are automatically 'registered' and ready for navigation. Left and right oblique images are recommended for each level to be instrumented. Up to four images can be displayed and monitored simultaneously on the same screen. Digitized instruments with light-emitting diodes are then recognized by the camera and their location in the room is thereby known by the computer. In short, a surgeon can navigate on two-dimensional images as if the C-arm were operating 'live' continuously. No further irradiation is necessary. Virtual cartoons or representations of the surgical instruments move real time on the monitor as the surgeon moves them in surgery.

Perhaps the most powerful component of the virtual fluoroscopic system is the ability to virtually 'extend' the tips of the various instruments from the skin surface down to the spine. Thus, when an instrument is held on the skin surface, the tip is extended down to recognizable radiographic landmarks that represent the entry point for pedicle fixation. This is not possible with conventional fluoroscopy or radiography unless a wire is actually passed through the skin and soft tissues to simulate a trajectory. The lateral view identifies the center of the pedicle and appropriate trajectory in the sagittal plane. The owl's eye or oblique view gives the surgeon feedback in the axial plane. Straight AP images represent the coronal plane. One helpful technique is to extend the tip of the virtual instrument on the computer screen to the point where the pedicle enters the posterior aspect of the vertebral body (fig. 1, 2). In the sagittal view, therefore, the instrument would have virtually probed the entire length of the pedicle in the AP direction. When one then looks simultaneously at the oblique view, the very tip of the extended instrument should be within the cortical confines (margins) of the pedicle. If the tip is medial, medial wall perforation may be possible. In short, the surgeon's brain is able to imagine three-dimensional trajectories based on multiple two-dimensional fluoroscopic images. Once the desired skin entry point is identified, a small stab incision is made (approximately 10–12 mm) (fig. 3).

In open placement of lumbar pedicle screws, slight variations of the same technique are used to identify the entry point for pedicle fixation. It is recommended that the proximal or medial-most aspect of the transverse process be considered for the entry point. This is as opposed to performing a partial inferior-medial facetectomy for a more medial entry point. For obvious reasons, one would favor a technique for percutaneous placement that does not

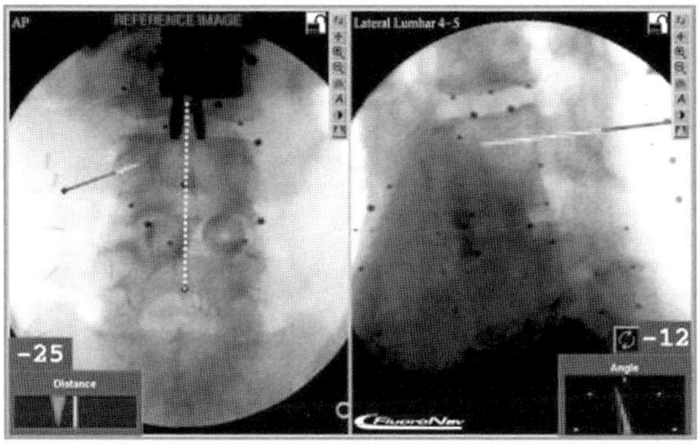

Fig. 1. Virtual representation of probe extending through skin down to the level of vertebral body (AP and lateral views) (photo courtesy of Kevin Foley, MD).

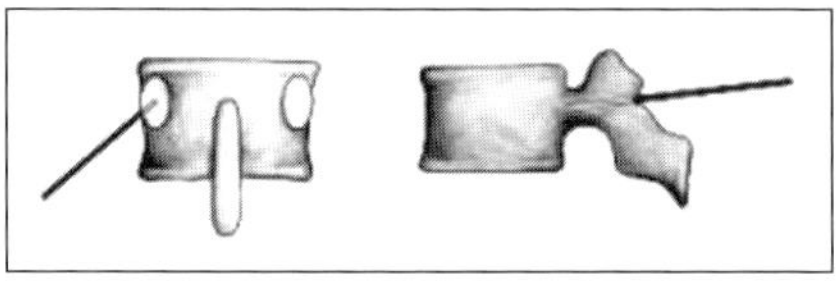

Fig. 2. Schematic drawing of extending virtual tip of probe beyond length of pedicle to help stay within confines of cortex.

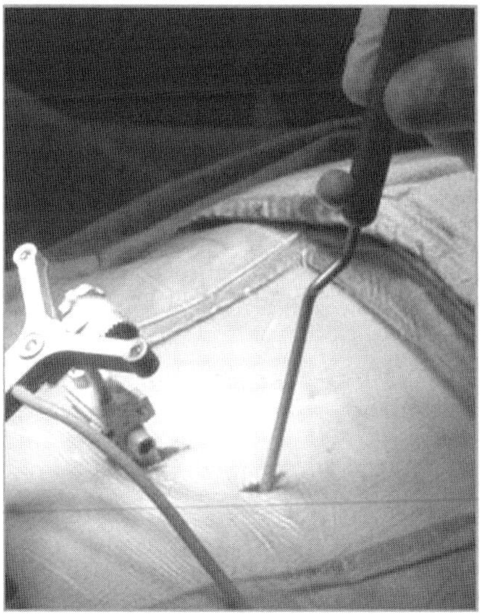

Fig. 3. Reference arc and digitized probe just beneath skin surface.

require bone removal. Another advantage of using the medial transverse process is that the surgeon can palpate with a wire or other image-guided probe the superior and inferior edges of the transverse process at the same time that visual feedback is given from the AP virtual fluoroscopic view. One can then feel the slight groove where the transverse process meets the superior facet process.

4 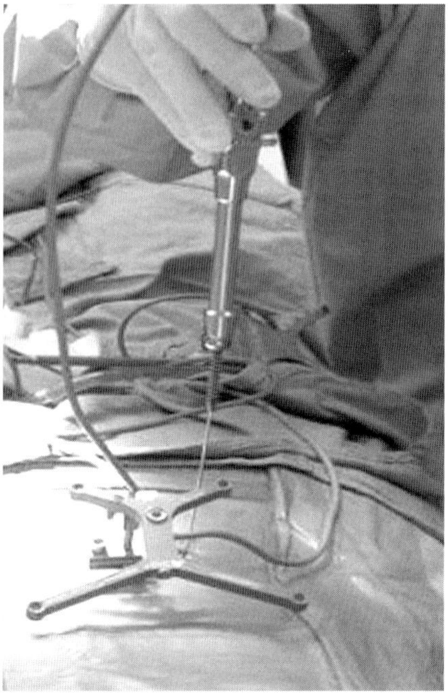 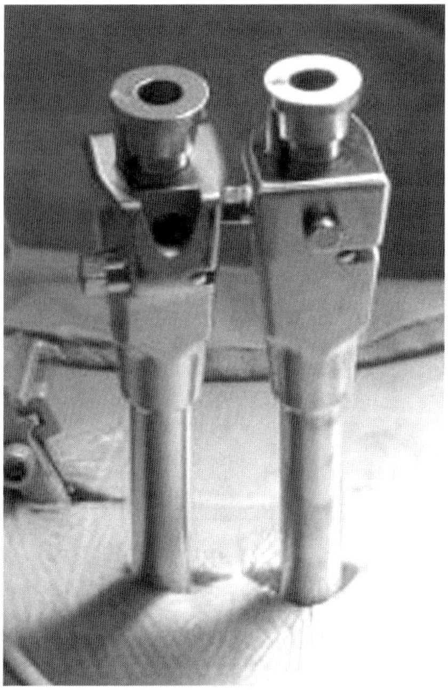 5

Fig. 4. Percutaneous placement of cannulated pedicle screw with screw extender (over K wire).

Fig. 5. Pedicle screw extenders.

Using an image-guided drill guide, a K wire is drilled into the pedicle approximately 20 mm, allowing for entry into the posterior vertebral body. A cannulated pedicle probe can then be passed or a cannulated drill bit can be used to drill the pedicle. A cannulated tap is passed (usually) to the depth of the posterior vertebral body (fig. 4). Patients with sclerotic or very firm bone may require tapping the full length of the intended screw. The pedicle is now ready for screw placement.

An important part of the percutaneous instrumentation is the screw extender. A multiaxial screw (M8, Medtronic Sofamor Danek) is attached to a long arm that will cross the distance between the posterior pedicle and the skin edge (fig. 5). A locking screw is preloaded into the chamber of the screw extender. The outer end of the screw extender will attach to the Sextant™ device.

For L5–S1 fixation, a single longer stab incision can be made to accommodate placement of both the L5 and S1 screws and screw extenders. For L4–L5 and higher levels, separate stab incisions will be necessary. Thus, once one screw has been placed, the sequence of steps is repeated for placement of the second screw. When both screws have been placed, the ends of the screw extenders are snapped together. The Sextant device with detachable trocar is then attached to the end of the screw extender complex (fig. 6). The arm of the Sextant is rotated down to the skin surface. This site is identified and a small stab incision is made. The trocar is passed through the adipose layer, fascia, and bluntly through the muscle to the heads of the multiaxial screws (fig. 7, 8). The arm is rotated back out. This step helps prepare for

6

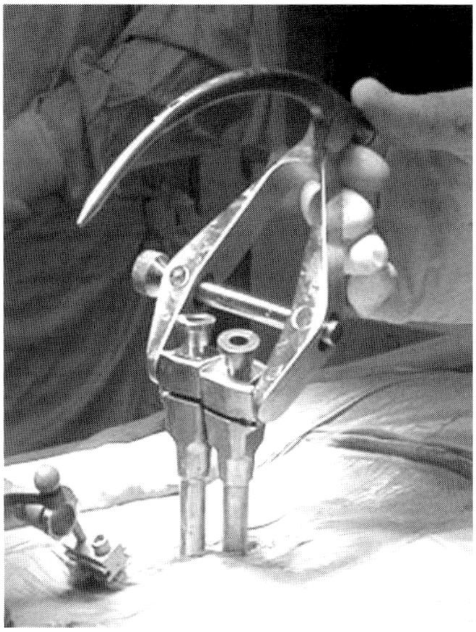

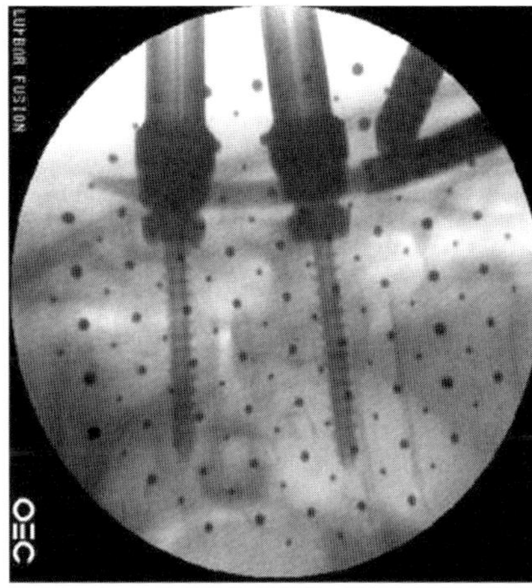

7

Fig. 6. Sextant device with rod attached and screw extenders prior to percutaneous delivery.

Fig. 7. Fluoroscopic view of rod inserted with tip of Sextant device visible inferiorly.

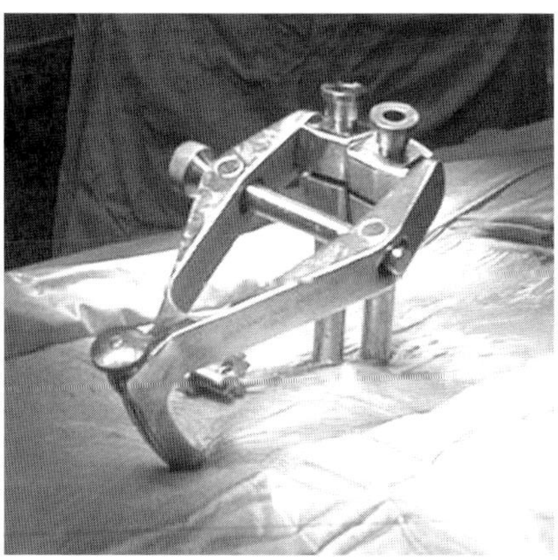

Fig. 8. Sextant device at moment of final rod engagement.

passage of the rod. The trocar is removed and a lordotic rod is attached to the arm of the Sextant. The rod is delivered through the same fixed arc into the side openings of the multi-axial screws. One additional real-time fluoroscopic image is recommended to ensure proper placement of the rod, though the fixed geometry of the screw extender Sextant system provides for consistent accurate placement. The rod is detached from the delivery arm, and the arm removed. The locking screws previously loaded into the screw extender chambers are tightened to the appropriate torque tension with a screwdriver. Then, the complete apparatus

9 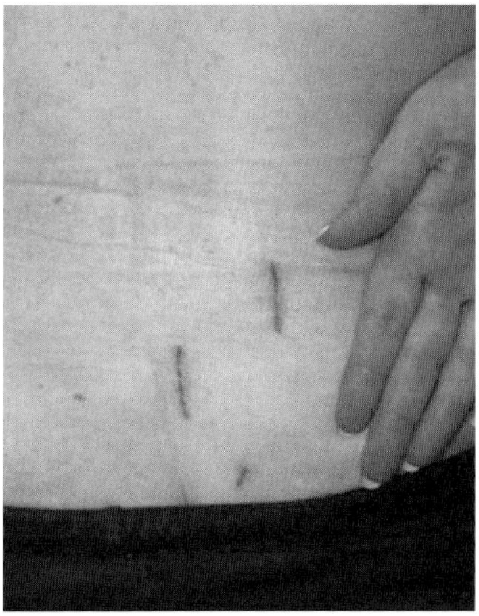

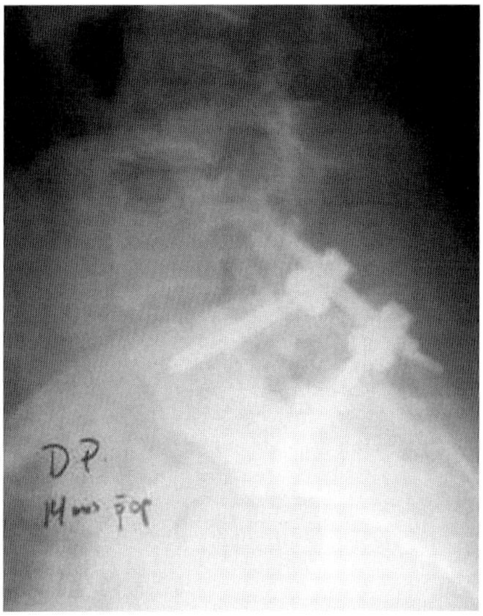 10

Fig. 9. Postoperative scars from unilateral percutaneous pedicle screw-rod fixation.

Fig. 10. L5–S1 ALIF with allograft femur wedge and unilateral percutaneous pedicle fixation, 14 months postoperatively.

is pulled out of the three (or if L5–S1, two) stab incisions. Subcuticular closure is then possible (fig. 9). The entire process can be repeated on the opposite side, though some surgeons may perform unilateral fixation when the biomechanical goal is to provide a posterior tension band following ALIF (fig. 10).

Results

The preliminary results of this technique confirm that it is a safe, effective way to place lumbar pedicle screws and rods. Lefkowitz and Foley [4] presented their results for 10 patients with spondylolisthesis. Patients underwent ALIF followed by posterior percutaneous pedicle screw/rod fixation. There were no complications related to the percutaneous technique. The average total operating time for both the ALIF and the percutaneous screw placement in this initial series was 7.3 h. Blood loss was markedly decreased compared to open techniques. The average hospital stay was 2.9 days.

Nockels et al. [5] presented their experience in 15 patients with a wide range of pathology. A total of 64 screws with rods were placed. Two cases of a two-level instrumentation were done. Patients were evaluated postoperatively with plain radiography and CT scan. Most cases were performed in combination with an ALIF. The average time for the percutaneous placement of lumbar screws with rods was 65 min. No complications were reported due to the percutaneous technique. There were no cases of implant failure during the initial follow-up.

Lefkowitz et al. [6] also reported on their experience using percutaneous pedicle screw fixation following minimally invasive posterior lumbar interbody fusion (PLIF). This latter technique was performed through endoscopic tubular retractors but with the use of the operating microscope or surgical loupes. Six patients underwent this technique. The indications were spondylolisthesis or degenerative disc disease. One dural tear was reported but was not related to the screw technique (it occurred during the PLIF technique). The average operating time for the entire procedure was 6 h 45 min. The average blood loss was 183 ml. The average duration of hospitalization was 2.3 days.

Rodts [7] presented preliminary data of 5 patients who underwent unilateral posterior percutaneous pedicle screw fixation following ALIF. The indication for surgery was spondylolisthesis in 4 patients and recurrent disc herniation in a fifth. All patients received unilateral instrumentation alone. Follow-up ranged from 10 to 22 months. Solid arthrodesis has been achieved in all patients. Postoperative CT scans were performed showing satisfactory screw placement in all screws except one. One S1 screw had 3 mm of lateral cortical perforation of no clinical significance.

Conclusion

Lumbar instrumentation has proven to be a useful component of current lumbar fusion surgery. The advantages include higher rates of arthrodesis, provision of immediate spinal stability, and the ability to more effectively reduce or correct deformity [8–11]. For patients who require extensive posterior decompression with fusion, open placement of pedicle instrumentation remains a useful technique.

In some patients, however, the goals of arthrodesis may be achieved with an ALIF, a minimally invasive PLIF, or a minimally invasive posterolateral fusion technique. In cases of mobile spondylolisthesis, previous surgery (and suboptimal fusion bed, vascular supply), metabolic bone disease, or smoking, a surgeon may wish to supplement the ALIF or PLIF arthrodesis with instrumentation. In this setting, the percutaneous technique may offer an advantage over open techniques. Several very small stab incisions may be cosmetically superior to one longer midline or paramedian incision. The paraspinal musculature is spared the ill-effects of midline tendinous release and wide retraction causing ischemia and subsequent atrophy and scar formation. Blood loss is markedly less compared to open techniques. In their initial experience, surgeons using the percutaneous pedicle screw technique have found that their patients have substantially less back pain in the postoperative period.

The key component to safe, effective passage of percutaneous instrumentation is image guidance. Whether a surgeon chooses to use a single or biplane live fluoroscopy or computer-assisted virtual fluoroscopy, the proper radiographic identification of important landmarks is critical. Virtual fluoroscopy offers several advantages, including the ability to view four images at once (e.g. right and left oblique, AP, lateral), and the ability to virtually extend various instruments from the surface of the skin down to the spine on the radiographic images.

Further experience with percutaneous and minimally invasive techniques will not only lead to less postoperative pain, smaller incisions and soft tissue trauma, shorter operating time, and less blood loss, but it will also enable the surgeon to achieve the same desired result as in open procedures: successful arthrodesis. With the advent of new biological products such as bone morphogenetic protein, and with the refinement of interbody fusion implants, the role of minimally invasive surgery may expand.

References

1 Wiesner L, Kothe R, Ruther W: Anatomic evaluation of two different techniques for the percutaneous insertion of pedicle screws in the lumbar spine. Spine 1999;24:1599–1603.

2 Lowery GL, Kulkarni SS: Posterior percutaneous spine instrumentation. Eur Spine J 2000;9: S126–S130.

3 Magerl F: External skeletal fixation of the lower thoracic and the lumbar spine; in Uhtoff HK, Stahl E (eds): Current Concepts of External Fixation of Fractures. Berlin, Springer, 1982, pp 353–366.

4 Lefkowitz M, Foley KT: Percutaneous pedicle fixation for spondylolisthesis. Annual Meeting of the AANS/CNS Joint Section on Disorders of the Spine and Peripheral Nerves, Orlando, 2002.

5 Nockels R, et al: Percutaneous pedicle screw fixation. Annual Meeting of the AANS/CNS Joint Section on Disorders of the Spine and Peripheral Nerves, Orlando, 2002.

6 Lefkowitz M, Palmer S, Foley KT: Percutaneous pedicle fixation following minimally-invasive PLIF. 2002 Annual Meeting of the AANS/CNS Joint Section on Disorders of the Spine and Peripheral Nerves, Orlando, 2002.

7 Rodts GE: Unilateral percutaneous lumbar pedicle screw/rod fixation following ALIF. Global Spine Meeting, Mexico, 2002.

8 Tribus CB, Belanger TA, Zdeblick TA: The effect of operative position and short-segment fusion on maintenance of sagittal alignment of the lumbar spine. Spine 1999;24/1:58–61.

9 Zuckerman JF, Zdeblick TA, Bailey SA, et al: Instrumented laparoscopic spinal fusion: Preliminary results. Spine 1995;20:2029–2034.

10 Yuan HA, Garfin SG, Dickman CA, Mardjetko SM: A historical cohort study of pedicle screw fixation in thoracic, lumbar and sacral spine fusions. Spine 1999;19(suppl 20):2279S–2296S.

11 Foley KT, Gupta SK: Percutaneous pedicle screw fixation of the lumbar spine: Preliminary results. J Neurosurg 2002;97:7–12.

Gerald E. Rodts, Jr., MD
Department of Neurosurgery, Emory University
550 Peachtree St., NE, Suite 806, Atlanta, GA 30308 (USA)
Tel. +1 404 686 8101, Fax +1 404 686 4805, E-Mail gerald_rodts@emoryhealthcare.org

Haid RW Jr, Subach BR, Rodts GE Jr (eds): Advances in Spinal Stabilization.
Prog Neurol Surg. Basel, Karger, 2003, vol 16, pp 213–224

Thoracolumbar Deformity Advances

1. Nonoperative Treatment of Thoracolumbar Deformity

Praveen V. Mummaneni[a], *Stephen L. Ondra*[b], *Rick C. Sasso*[c]

[a] Department of Neurosurgery, Emory University, Atlanta, Ga.,
[b] Department of Neurosurgery, Northwestern University, Chicago, Ill., and
[c] Department of Orthopaedic Surgery, Indiana University School of Medicine, Indiana Spine Group, Indianapolis, Ind., USA

The terms 'scoliosis, kyphosis, and lordosis' were first coined by the Greek physician Galen in the second century AD [1]. Since that time, significant advances have occurred in the classification and management of patients with spinal deformities.

Early physicians attempted to correct thoracolumbar deformities with non-operative treatments. Hippocrates, and later Galen, unsuccessfully used longitudinal traction to try to pull the deformed spine back into alignment [2]. Ambrose Pare was the first physician to use an orthosis to brace a scoliotic patient (approximately 1,500 AD). Pare soon realized that bracing was not useful once a patient had reached skeletal maturity [1].

During the past several centuries, more sophisticated and effective non-operative treatment modalities for spinal deformity have been developed.

Evaluation of Deformity

There are multiple causes of thoracolumbar deformity; a full discussion of all of these entities is beyond the scope of this chapter. We will limit our discussion to the most frequently encountered entities: adolescent idiopathic scoliosis, adult scoliosis, and thoracic hyperkyphosis. When the surgeon encounters any of these entities, the first step in the treatment paradigm is to evaluate the patient fully.

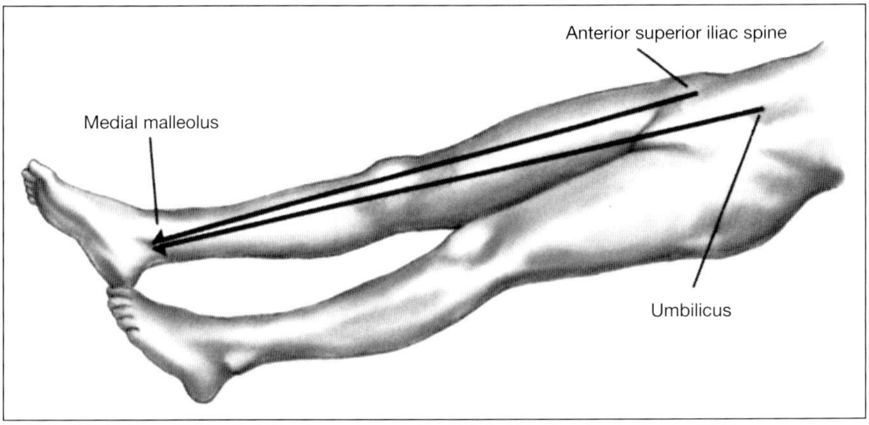

Fig. 1. Measurement of leg length from the umbilicus or the anterior superior iliac spine to the medial malleolus.

History

The patient's medical and family history should be documented. Documentation of the age of onset of the deformity and the rate of progression of the deformity are important factors that may influence treatment. Since the rate of curve progression often accelerates after puberty, the age of onset of menarche should also be noted. In addition, since spinal deformities can be inherited, it is important to identify all relatives with deformity and to attempt to classify the type of deformity and the rate of progression of the deformity in family members.

Physical Examination

Initially, a global survey is performed to evaluate overall spinal balance. Obvious curvatures are noted. Pelvic obliquities and abnormal skin folds are often seen with moderate to severe scoliotic curvatures. In the pediatric population, secondary sex characteristics are also noted. Additionally, in scoliotic patients, leg lengths are measured and discrepancies are noted. Leg lengths can be measured either from the umbilicus or the anterior superior iliac spine to the medial malleolus (fig. 1). In addition, overall coronal balance can be quantified in the upright position by dropping a plumb line from the C7 spinous process (fig. 2). Normally the line should extend down the intergluteal crease.

Patients with scoliotic curvatures may be in overall coronal balance if their secondary curves are of sufficient magnitude to recenter C7 over the intergluteal crease in the coronal plane. Patients are asked to perform side bends to assess if their curves are flexible or rigid.

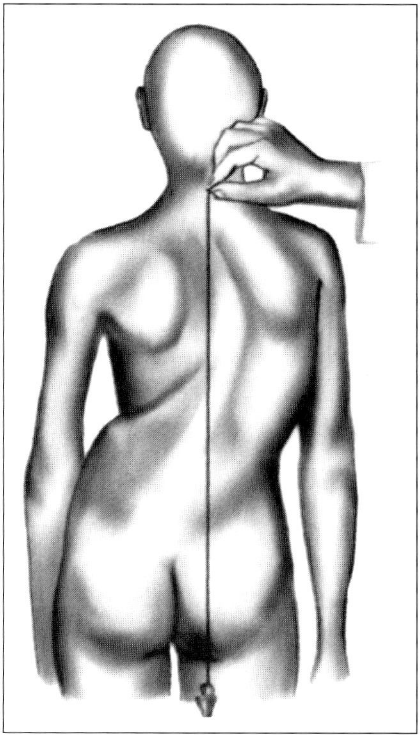

Fig. 2. C7 plumb line. Normally line should fall into intergluteal crease indicating coronal plane balance. The plumb line in this illustration falls to the right of the intergluteal crease indicating coronal plane imbalance.

In order to further evaluate scoliosis, the patient is asked to stand upright with their palms opposed in the 'praying position' and with their arms extended perpendicular to their torso. The patient is asked to bend forward at the waist until the shoulders and hips are in the same axial plane. The physician then views the patient from both the front and the back noting any spinal curvature or asymmetric rib/flank elevation. For lumbar curves, more forward flexion is required to bring out the maximal asymmetry; for thoracic curves, less forward flexion is required to bring out the maximal asymmetry. Some physicians elect to use an inclinometer to quantify their patient's scoliotic curvature. The patient is maneuvered to a flexed position where the asymmetry is most striking before the inclinometer is used.

Patients with kyphotic deformities are observed in the neutral position to see if they are able to look straight ahead when facing forward, and to assess for compensatory extension at the hips and flexion at the knees. In addition, these patients are asked to perform the forward bending test, which makes thoracolumbar apex kyphosis obvious. Finally, these patients are asked to extend and flex their spines at the apex of the curvature to check for curve flexibility.

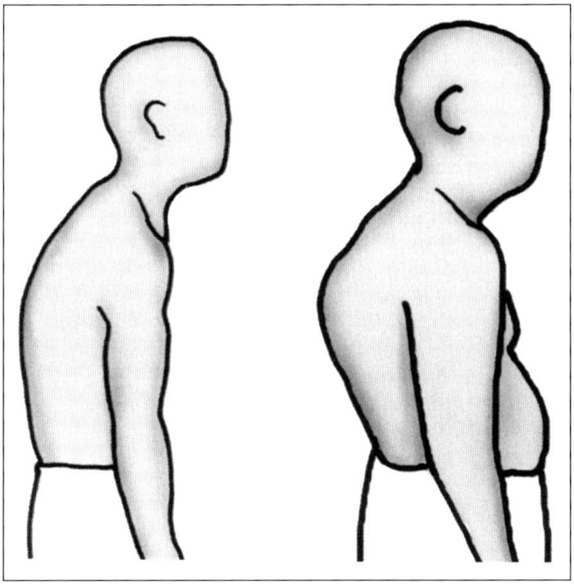

Fig. 3. Postural and structural thoracic kyphosis. The illustration on the left shows a patient with a postural kyphosis. Note the rounded, smooth curve. The illustration of the patient on the right has a structural kyphosis with a pronounced gibbus in the midthoracic spine.

Kyphotic curves are classified as either postural or structural. Kyphotic curves that correct in extension are classified as postural. Postural kyphotic curves are smooth curves and are usually due to poor posture and not to a pathological process. Structural kyphotic curves, on the other hand, do not correct in extension, often have a sharp, angular gibbus at the apex of the curve on forward flexion, and are due to a pathological process (fig. 3).

Radiographic Evaluation

Standard radiographic evaluation for deformity begins with standing full length (36 inch) posterior-anterior (P/A) and lateral spine x-rays. In patients who cannot stand, recumbent x-rays are acceptable. The flexibility of the patient's scoliotic curve is evaluated with recumbent side-bending x-rays. Side-bending x-rays are taken in the recumbent position in order to avoid locking the facet joints during the bending motion. In patients who do not have adequate muscle mass to perform side bends, a manual push may be administered during the x-ray.

Scoliosis x-rays differ from nonscoliosis x-rays in several ways. First of all, they are shot in the P/A direction in order to minimize the radiation dose to the

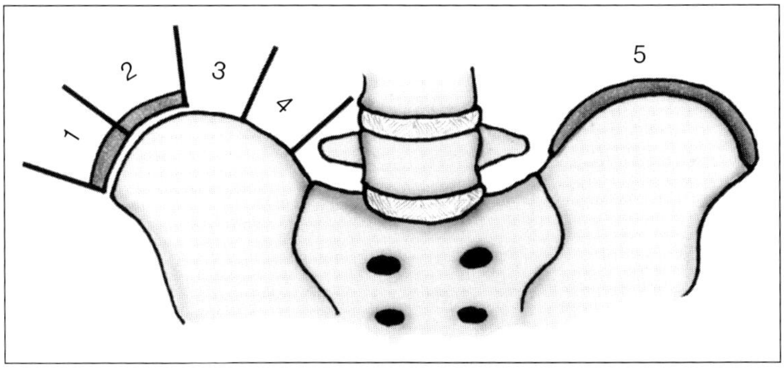

Fig. 4. The Risser classification (grades 0–5) is used to quantify skeletal maturity. Risser grade 1 patients have ossified only 25% of their iliac apophysis. Risser grade 4 patients have ossified 100% of their iliac apophysis, but have not fused their iliac wing to their ileum. Risser grade 5 patients are skeletally mature and have ossified their entire iliac apophysis and fused their iliac wing to the ileum.

breast tissue in adolescent girls. Secondly, scoliosis x-rays are placed on the x-ray viewer in the opposite orientation from other x-rays. The reader looks at scoliosis x-rays as if he is looking at the patient's back, i.e. the right side of the x-ray is on the right side of the viewer.

In younger patients, special attention is paid to the pelvis on the P/A x-ray to assess skeletal maturity. In 1958, Risser [3] noted that the growth of the vertebral body endplate parallels the ossification of the iliac apophysis. The Risser classification (grades 0–5) is used to quantify skeletal maturity. Risser grade 1 patients have ossified only 25% of their iliac apophysis. Risser grade 4 patients have ossified 100% of their iliac apophysis but have not fused their iliac wing to their ileum. Risser grade 5 patients are skeletally mature and have ossified their entire iliac apophysis and fused their iliac wing to the ileum (fig. 4). Furthermore, the pelvic x-ray is examined to see if the triradiate acetabular cartilage is still open (indicating skeletal immaturity).

The lateral x-rays are inspected to assess overall sagittal balance. Normally, a plumb line dropped from the posterior vertebral body of C7 should pass through a point within 2.5 cm of the posterosuperior corner of S1. If the plumb line passes more than 2.5 cm anterior to this point, then the patient is noted to have a 'positive sagittal imbalance'. Likewise, if the plumb line passes more than 2.5 cm posterior to this point, then the patient is noted have a 'negative sagittal imbalance'.

The P/A x-rays are evaluated to assess coronal balance and rotatory deformity. Overall coronal balance is assessed by dropping a plumb line from the C7 spinous process. Normally, this line should pass through the midline of the sacrum.

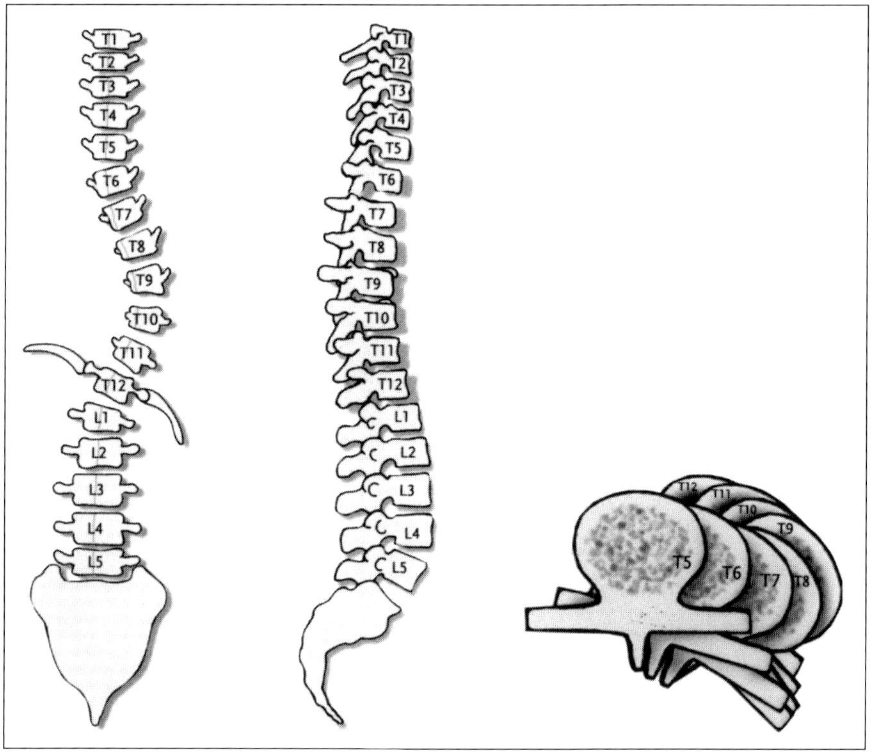

Fig. 5. Coronal, sagittal, and axial illustrations of a scoliotic deformity. Note that this single right thoracic curve has a significant rotatory component.

When there is a loss of coronal balance, as seen occasionally with scoliosis, the head and shoulders are no longer centered over the pelvis. In order to compensate, the patient often tries to bend the spine above or below the primary curve in the opposite direction. Over time, a fixed, secondary scoliotic curve can develop as a result of this bending. The apex of the secondary curve is opposite that of the primary curve, and the magnitude of the secondary curve is smaller than that of the primary curve.

Rotatory deformities result in loss of axial balance and often complicate scoliotic curvatures. They transmit loads unevenly between successive vertebral segments (fig. 5). Rotatory deformity can be evaluated on the P/A x-rays by assessing the symmetry in the pedicle positions at each level. Nash and Moe [4] classified the rotatory deformity by grading it from zero (no rotation) to grade IV (only one pedicle shadow is visible and it is rotated past the center of the vertebral body).

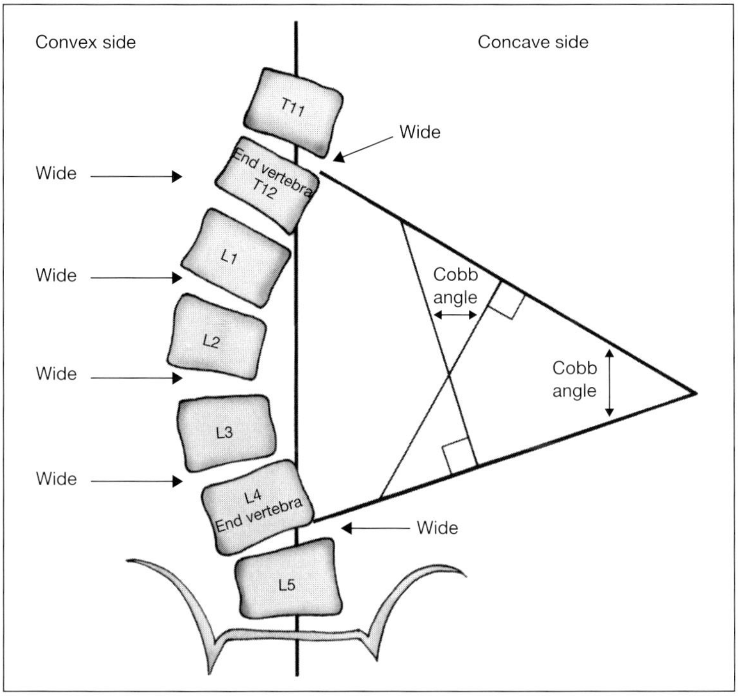

Fig. 6. Measurement of the Cobb angle. End vertebrae are the last levels that are tilted into the curve concavity. A line is drawn from the superior endplate of the superior end vertebral body, and another line is drawn from the inferior endplate of the inferior vertebral body. The angle of the intersection of these lines is the Cobb angle.

Curve Measurement

Scoliosis x-rays are evaluated to establish the number of curves, the location of the curve(s), the direction of the curve(s), and the magnitude of the curve(s). When multiple scoliotic curves are present, the major curve is defined as the largest, rigid curve. Minor curves are compensatory curves that are created to try to return to overall spinal balance. Minor curves are smaller than the major curve and usually are flexible on side-bending x-rays.

The magnitude of each coronal plane curve is quantified through the Cobb angle measurement. To measure the Cobb angle, the physician identifies the end vertebrae of the curve on the P/A x-ray. End vertebrae are the last levels that are tilted into the curve concavity. A line is drawn from the superior endplate of the superior end vertebral body, and another line is drawn from the inferior endplate of the inferior vertebral body. The angle of the intersection of these lines is the Cobb angle (fig. 6).

Indications for Treatment and Nonoperative Treatment Modalities

Adolescent Idiopathic Scoliosis

Adolescent idiopathic scoliosis is the most common form of scoliosis seen in the United States. School screening programs are effectively screening for this disorder, and the prevalence of scoliosis in the school age population is estimated to be 1–3% [5, 6]. Most patients with adolescent idiopathic scoliosis are female with a right thoracic curve. Patients with atypical thoracic curve patterns (i.e. left thoracic curve) also should be evaluated with spinal axis MRI to rule out other causes of adolescent scoliosis (i.e. tumor).

Indications for treatment are dependent on the initial Cobb angle, the skeletal maturity of the patient, and the progression of the curve. Skeletally immature patients (Risser score of 0–3) with curves less than 25° usually are not treated and are followed with serial x-rays at 4- to 6-month intervals to check for curve progression.

If the curve progresses to greater than 30° (but less than 40°), then nonoperative treatment with bracing is initiated [7]. For curves with their apex above T6, a cervical extension may be needed. Otherwise, underarm, rigid, thoracolumbar braces are satisfactory. Bracing requires cooperation and compliance from the patient and the family. Braces should be worn daily for over 18 h per day until skeletal maturity.

For braced patients, follow-up radiographs are obtained at 4- to 6-month intervals until skeletal maturity is reached. If the curve remains under 40° and the patient reaches the end of growth (Risser 4 status and at least 18 months since menarche), then the brace is discontinued. If the curve progresses beyond 40°, then surgical treatment is indicated [8, 9].

Adult Scoliosis

Adult scoliosis has two primary etiologies: adolescent idiopathic scoliosis (which has progressed after skeletal maturity) and degenerative adult-onset (de novo) scoliosis.

Adult Patients with Progressive Adolescent Idiopathic Scoliosis

Studies have shown that adolescent idiopathic scoliosis can progress after skeletal maturity, especially if the magnitude of the curve is greater than 30° [8, 10]. Consequently, it is important to continue to periodically follow patients with adolescent idiopathic scoliosis with curves greater than 30° at skeletal maturity. Patients with adolescent idiopathic scoliosis suspected of progressing during adulthood should be evaluated with serial scoliosis x-rays at 6-month intervals to document progression.

Adult patients with progressive adolescent idiopathic scoliosis typically become symptomatic in the fourth and fifth decades of life. These patients are usually female with thoracic or thoracolumbar junction curves. The most frequent presenting complaint in this patient population is back pain (lumbar more common than thoracic), and the etiology of the back pain may be multifactorial. Causes of back pain in this population include muscle fatigue, facet arthropathy, radiculopathy from foraminal compression, and lumbar degenerative disc disease. Other presenting complaints in this population include cosmetic deformity or, rarely, cardiopulmonary dysfunction.

For patients presenting with pain, the surgeon must deduce the cause of the pain via the patient's history, exam, and/or diagnostic testing. Fatigue-related back pain, for example, usually occurs on the convex side of the curve, is absent in the morning, worsens as the day progresses, and resolves with rest. It is often alleviated with physical therapy (strengthening of the back and abdominal muscles). If patients fail physical therapy, then bracing may be tried to reduce the workload on the muscles (bracing in the adult does not prevent curve progression).

Patients with facet arthropathy, on the other hand, often have pain on the concave side of their curve or in the lower lumbar spine. This pain is also activity related. Facet arthropathy can be confirmed by, and effectively treated by, facet joint injections.

Patients with thoracic or lumbar radiculopathy can be diagnosed by their history of radiating pain. The diagnosis can be confirmed by selective nerve root sleeve injection. The selective nerve root sleeve injections can be periodically repeated to give long-term pain relief.

Patients with degenerative disc disease causing mechanical low back pain should undergo a trial of physical therapy to strengthen their low back and abdominal muscles. This often alleviates their pain because these muscle groups can then function to decrease the workload of the lumbar discs. If physical therapy is ineffective, then further evaluation can be done with discography. If the discogram correlates with their pain and with disc degeneration seen on MRI, then lumbar fusion may be considered (if the patient is not osteoporotic).

For scoliotic patients presenting with pulmonary limitations, one key treatment option is cessation of smoking.

In general, initial management of adults with progressive idiopathic scoliosis should be nonoperative. Most patients will respond to the measures above in combination with oral nonsteroidal anti-inflammatory medications.

Degenerative Adult-Onset Scoliosis

Patients with degenerative adult-onset scoliosis typically present during the sixth or seventh decade of life. These patients have primarily lumbar deformities, and the male to female ratio is equal. The presenting complaints are usually related to lumbar stenosis or extraforaminal stenosis with radicular pain and neurogenic claudication. Extraforaminal stenosis usually occurs at the apex of the scoliosis on the concave side as a result of the transverse processes abutting each other.

Low back pain may be due to facet arthropathy or degenerative disc disease. Discogenic pain commonly occurs below the scoliotic deformity in the 'normal' region of the lumbar spine because this region is compensating for the scoliotic curvature. Loss of lumbar lordosis (flat back) is common. The etiology of the low back pain must be ascertained. On physical exam, the facet joints can be loaded by asking the patient to extend the lumbar spine posteriorly and laterally; pain caused with this maneuver is indicative of ipsilateral lumbar facet arthropathy. Facet arthropathy can be confirmed by and treated with facet joint injections.

The workup and treatment for degenerative disc disease has been previously mentioned and will not be repeated here.

For symptoms of stenosis and radiculopathy, epidural steroid injections and selective nerve root sleeve injections may assist with the diagnosis and provide temporary relief from symptoms.

Kyphosis

Normal thoracic kyphosis ranges from 20 to 40°. Hyperkyphosis is a sagittal plane deformity with excessive flexion of the thoracic spine. Hyperkyphosis is subclassified as either postural or structural (fig. 3).

Postural kyphosis is due to poor posture, and the patient can consciously correct the curve by 'standing up straight'. Postural kyphosis is characterized by a smooth, rounding pattern in the thoracic spine. There is no gibbus on forward flexion. For patients with cosmetic issues related to their postural kyphosis, we recommend physical therapy with back strengthening exercises to improve posture. No operative intervention is indicated.

Structural kyphosis, on the other hand, cannot be consciously corrected by the patient. Often, a gibbus is seen when the patient is asked to flex forward, and there is often a sharp angular pattern to the kyphosis on x-ray. Structural kyphosis can either be primary or secondary. The most common cause of primary structural kyphosis is Scheuermann's disease (juvenile kyphosis). Scheuermann's disease is defined as three consecutive levels of at least 5° of segmental kyphosis (anterior wedging) at each level [11]. The etiology of Scheuermann's disease is unknown; however, there does appear to be a familial occurrence. Nonoperative treatment for Scheuermann's disease is indicated for progression of the kyphosis beyond 40° (but under 70°) in a skeletally immature patient (Risser 1–4). For these patients, an underarm, hyperextension, thoracolumbar orthosis is often satisfactory to halt progression of the kyphosis [12, 13].

Secondary structural kyphosis, on the other hand, has an underlying pathological process. The most common etiologies include multiple level degenerative disc disease, vertebral body fracture or tumor, or prior multilevel laminectomy. Multilevel thoracic degenerative disc disease can result in thoracic hyperkyphosis, whereas multilevel lumbar degenerative disc disease is the most common cause of lumbar flat backs. Normally, lumbar discs are taller anteriorly than posteriorly and thus create lumbar lordosis. As the lumbar discs dehydrate, the lumbar spine loses this normal lordosis and becomes straight. The patient often loses overall spinal sagittal balance as a result and tries to compensate by flexing at the hips and knees. Patients with secondary structural kyphosis are often older adults, and the typical presenting complaint is back pain. The physician must, once again, determine the cause of the pain. The pain may be due to muscle fatigue, which typically worsens as the day progresses. Pain related to muscle fatigue can often be effectively treated by back strengthening physical therapy. Another treatment modality is daytime bracing with an underarm thoracolumbar orthosis in those unable to perform back strengthening exercises. The orthosis can share the load with the posterior spinal musculature and reduce muscle fatigue and pain. However, in the skeletally mature patient, an orthosis will not prevent progression of the kyphosis. In addition, the orthosis can contribute to further weakening and atrophy of the lumbar musculature by shielding these muscles from spinal loads.

Pain may be due to degenerative disc disease (the workup and treatment have been previously mentioned and will not be repeated here). Pain may be due to facet arthropathy. This pain also tends to worsen as the day progresses. Facet joint injections can be both diagnostic and therapeutic for this problem.

Conclusion

For the majority of patients with mild or moderate spinal deformities, initial evaluation and a course (or several courses) of the appropriate nonsurgical treatment are often satisfactory to alleviate symptoms.

For those patients who fail to have relief of their symptoms with conservative treatment, and for those patients who have severe deformities, surgical intervention is often necessary. Part 2 will focus on the indications for surgical treatment and the options for surgical treatment of spinal deformity [14].

Acknowledgments

We are grateful to Drew Imhulse and Tom Fletcher for assistance with the radiographic images in the figures. We are grateful to Sherry Ballenger for editorial assistance.

Disclosure Statement

The following authors are consultants for Medtronic Sofamor Danek: Stephen L. Ondra, MD and Rick C. Sasso, MD.

References

1 Ogilvie JW: Historical aspects of scoliosis; in Lonstein JE, Bradford DS, Winter RB, Ogilvie JW (eds): Moe's Textbook of Scoliosis and Other Spinal Deformities. Philadelphia, Saunders, 1995, pp 1–3.
2 Huebert HT: Scoliosis. A brief history. Manit Med Rev 1967;47:452–456.
3 Risser JC: The iliac apophysis: An invaluable sign in the management of scoliosis. Clin Orthop 1958;11:111.
4 Nash CL Jr, Moe JH: A study of vertebral rotation. J Bone Joint Surg Am 1969;51:223–229.
5 Lonstein JE, Carlson JM: The prediction of curve progression in untreated idiopathic scoliosis during growth. J Bone Joint Surg Am 1984;66:1061–1071.
6 Lonstein JE, Bjorklund S, Wanninger MH, Nelson RP: Voluntary school screening for scoliosis in Minnesota. J Bone Joint Surg Am 1982;64:481–488.
7 Nachemson A, Peterson L: Effectiveness of treatment with a brace in girls who have adolescent idiopathic scoliosis. J Bone Joint Surg Am 1995;177:815–822.
8 Weinstein SL, Ponseti IV: Curve progression in idiopathic scoliosis: Long-term follow-up. J Bone Joint Surg Am 1983;65:447.
9 Weinstein SL: Natural history. Spine 1999;24:2592.
10 Ascani E, Bartolozzi P, Logroscino CA, Marchetti PG, Ponte A, Savini R, Travaglini F, Binazzi R, Di Silvestre M: Natural history of untreated idiopathic scoliosis after skeletal maturity. Spine 1986;11:784–789.
11 Sorensen KH: Scheuermann's Juvenile Kyphosis. Copenhagen, Munksgaard, 1964.
12 Sachs BL, Bradford DS, Winter RB, Lonstein J, Moe J, Willson S: Scheuermann kyphosis. Follow-up of Milwaukee-brace treatment. J Bone Joint Surg Am 1987;69/1:50–57.
13 Murray PM, Weinstein SL, Spratt KF: The natural history and long-term follow-up of Scheuermann's kyphosis. J Bone Joint Surg Am 1993;75/2:236.
14 Mummaneni PV, Ondra SL, Sasso RC: Thoracolumbar deformity advances. 2. Operative treatment of thoracolumbar deformity. Prog Neurol Surg. Basel, Karger, 2003, pp 225–239.

Praveen V. Mummaneni, MD
Assistant Professor, Department of Neurosurgery, The Emory Clinic
550 Peachtree St., Suite 806, Atlanta, GA 30308 (USA)
Tel. +1 404 686 8101, Fax +1 404 686 4805, E-Mail praveen_mummaneni@emoryhealthcare.org

Haid RW Jr, Subach BR, Rodts GE Jr (eds): Advances in Spinal Stabilization.
Prog Neurol Surg. Basel, Karger, 2003, vol 16, pp 225–239

Thoracolumbar Deformity Advances

2. Operative Treatment of Thoracolumbar Deformity

Praveen V. Mummaneni[a], *Stephen L. Ondra*[b], *Rick C. Sasso*[c]

[a] Department of Neurosurgery, Emory University, Atlanta, Ga.,
[b] Department of Neurosurgery, Northwestern University, Chicago, Ill., and
[c] Department of Orthopaedic Surgery, Indiana University School of Medicine, Indiana Spine Group, Indianapolis, Ind., USA

Surgical fusions to treat spinal deformity were first developed in the 1900s. In 1911, Hibbs [1] performed a noninstrumented, posterior spinal fusion for deformity related to tuberculous spondylitis. In 1962, Harrington [2] revolutionized spinal fusion for deformity with the use of his distraction rod instrumentation system.

In the past 50 years, there has been a revolution in the use of instrumentation for the treatment of deformity, and new techniques and new constructs have improved the surgical outcomes for deformity patients.

Indications for Surgery and Surgical Techniques

Adolescent Idiopathic Scoliosis

Surgical treatment is indicated for adolescent idiopathic scoliosis (AIS) that progresses beyond 40–50° in the growing child. Typically, curves over 40° in a growing child will continue to progress if not treated surgically. The primary reasons to perform surgical correction of these curves is to halt and reverse curve progression as well as to improve cosmesis. Curves between 40 and 90° usually do not cause cardiopulmonary difficulties. However, curves greater than 90° may cause cardiopulmonary compromise, and this is an additional indication to surgically correct these curves. Preoperative planning for these patients should include a radiographic assessment (with 36-inch standing x-rays) of curve magnitude, pedicle rotation, location of curve apex, vertebral levels marking the ends of the curve, and overall sagittal and coronal alignment.

The ends of the curve are defined as the vertebrae that are both stable and neutral. The stable vertebra is the end vertebra that is most closely bisected by the center sacral line. The neutral vertebra is the end vertebra that is the least rotated. Usually the stable vertebra is also the neutral vertebra, but if they do not correspond then fusion to the stable vertebra (not the neutral vertebra) is recommended [3].

This will give the surgeon a good idea of the amount of correction needed to reestablish spinal balance. Lateral bending films are useful to identify structural (usually rigid thoracic curves) and compensatory curves (usually flexible, lower magnitude, lumbar curves without pedicle rotation). In addition, the size of the rib hump should also be measured, and the surgeon can consider thoracoplasty for significant rib hump deformity.

Curve Classification

Classification of AIS curves is important because the selection of fusion levels is dependent on the classification. Over the past few decades, the King classification system has been the most commonly used system to classify AIS curves. Recently, however, Lenke et al. [4] described a more comprehensive and descriptive classification system for AIS.

We prefer to use the Lenke classification system for several reasons. The King system only describes curves in the coronal plane and does not take sagittal balance into account. In addition, interobserver variability in classification with the King system is high. The Lenke system, on the other hand, takes into account sagittal alignment with a sagittal modifier. In addition, the Lenke system is highly descriptive and uses a three-tiered classification scheme (6 curve types, lumbar spine modifier, and sagittal thoracic modifier) (fig. 1) [4]. The most frequent curve types with the Lenke system were found to be type 1 (main thoracic curve) and type 2 (double thoracic curve) with the most frequent curve classifications found to be types 1AN, 1BN, and 2AN [4].

Surgical Correction

The Lenke classification system can be used to predict which levels should be instrumented to correct AIS [5]. For type 1 curves, only the main thoracic curve should be instrumented. For type 2 curves, both the proximal and main thoracic curves should be fused. For type 3 curves (double major), both the main thoracic and the thoracolumbar/lumbar curves should be fused. For type 4 curves (triple major), all three curves should be instrumented.

Surgical treatment for AIS is usually reserved until the patient is close to skeletal maturity. If the patient is not near skeletal maturity, then the patient may be at risk for a crankshaft phenomenon in the years following surgery. The crankshaft is due to continued growth from the vertebral endplates while

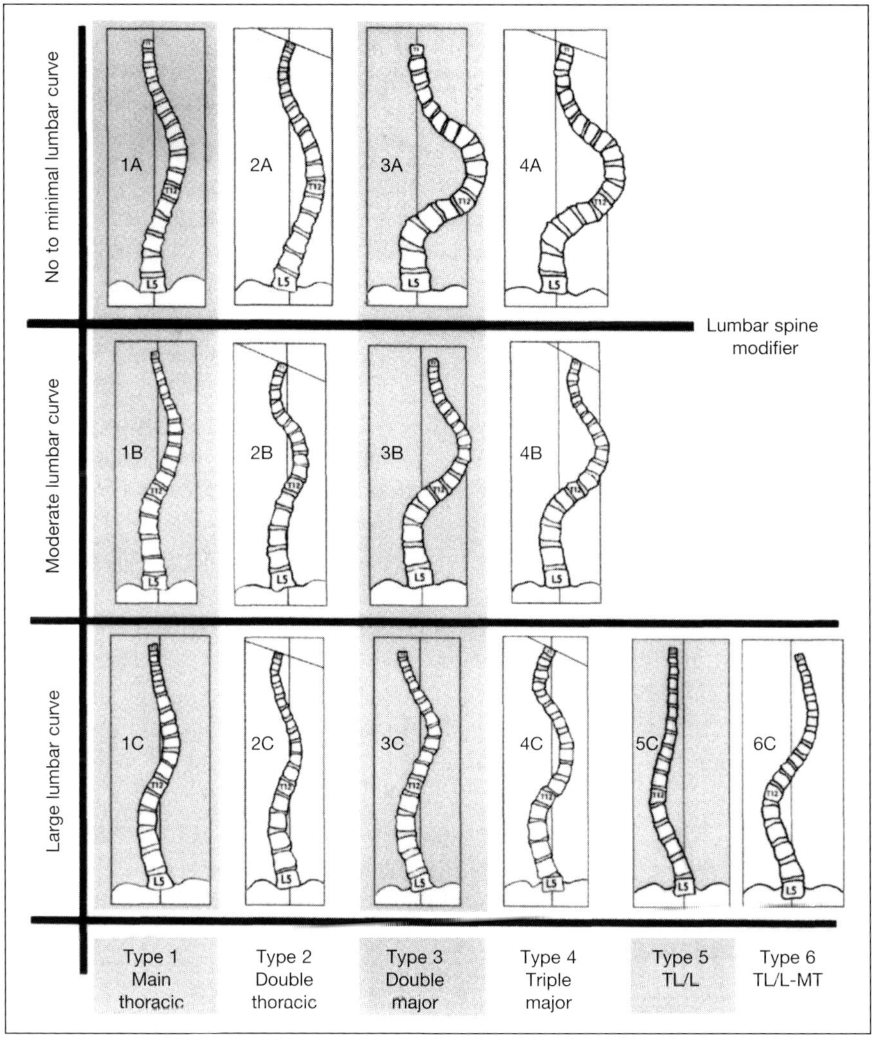

Fig. 1. Artist's illustration of the Lenke classification system for scoliosis. The Lenke system is highly descriptive and uses a three-tiered classification scheme (6 curve types, a lumbar spine modifier, and a sagittal thoracic modifier). TL = Thoracolumbar; L = lumbar; MT = main thoracic.

the posterior tension band is secured by instrumentation; the spine then crankshafts from side to side to accommodate the vertebral body growth.

In the past few decades, hook-rod instrumentation has been used successfully for the correction of AIS. In the 1990s, however, pedicle screw-rod instrumentation has gained in popularity. Pedicle screws are stronger anchors than hooks. In addition, unlike laminar hooks, pedicle screws do not occupy the spinal canal nor do they disrupt the ligamentum flavum.

Structural Right Thoracic Curve (Lenke Type 1)

The structural right main thoracic curve with a compensatory (flexible, low-magnitude, nonrotated) lumbar curve is classified as a King type II or a Lenke type 1 curve. It is the most common curve type in AIS, and we will discuss its treatment further.

Posterior Approach

The classic operation performed for a structural right thoracic curve in an adolescent is a selective thoracic fusion. Classically, a selective thoracic fusion is maintained by distraction with hook-rod instrumentation on the concave side of the curve and compression with instrumentation on the convex side of the curve [6, 7].

Initially, the thoracic curve is instrumented with hooks on the concave side; a rod is attached to the concave hooks and a rod rotation maneuver is performed to correct the curve (i.e. attach a concave rod to the hooks and then rotate the rod until it is straight in the sagittal plane). On the concave side, up-going pedicle hooks are typically placed at the superior end of the curve, and down-going laminar hooks are typically placed at the inferior end of the curve. This hook pattern allows for distraction on the rod, which serves to maintain the correction after a rod rotation maneuver. On the convex side, a claw is placed at the superior end of the curve (the claw consists of down-going hooks above and up-going hooks at the next level below), an up-going hook is placed at the apex of the curve, and down-going hooks are placed inferiorly. This hook pattern allows for compression on the rod in order to maintain curve correction on the convex side of the curve. The compensatory lumbar curve is not instrumented and will typically correct to normal when the structural thoracic curve is straightened [8].

Alternative posterior fusion options include hybrid hook-screw-rod systems, hook-endplate screw systems, or pure pedicle screw-rod systems. In the hybrid system, hooks are placed superiorly (where the pedicle diameters are smaller) and screws are placed inferiorly (where the pedicle diameters are larger). In the pedicle hook-endplate screw system, a pedicle hook is placed and then anchored to an endplate screw; this rigid fixation technique is similar to pedicle screws in pullout strength. In pure pedicle screw systems, no hooks are used; instead, pedicle screws are placed in lieu of the hooks. In all three systems, a rod rotation maneuver is initially done on the concave side of the curve to correct the curve.

When we place thoracic pedicle screws, we have found the following surgical nuances to be helpful. We locate the entry point for thoracic pedicle screws by using a high-speed burr to decorticate the surface of the thoracic facet overlying the area of the pedicle. Once this mild decortication has been done, a blush of blood is usually noticeable, and this blush marks the entry to the pedicle. This blush of red arises from the cancellous bone at the center of the pedicle, which tends to bleed when uncovered. The surrounding facet area does not tend to 'blush' with this maneuver. The surgeon can reliably establish the pedicle entry point through this technique.

The typical location of the pedicle with respect to the thoracic transverse process and facet has been elucidated by Lenke et al. [9].

One word of caution is in order, however. If the central portion of the pedicle is corticated, then this 'blush' technique cannot be used, as there is no cancellous bleeding bone. In this case, we recommend the surgeon perform a laminoforaminotomy to feel the medial, superior, and inferior walls of the pedicle to guide the screw placement [10].

Once the entry point has been established, there are three options we use to establish a pathway through the pedicle for the pedicle screw. The first method we use entails tapping the pedicle from the entry point with a 3.5-mm tap from the VERTEX posterior cervical set (Medtronic Sofamor Danek, Memphis, Tenn., USA). This tap has fine cutting flutes and with minimal downward pressure, the tap has a tendency to find the appropriate trajectory for screw placement by cutting through the cancellous portion of the pedicle without violating the cortical pedicle walls. The screw can then be placed through this trajectory.

The second option is to use the thoracic pedicle probe recently created by Lenke et al. [9]. This small tap is ideal for the thoracic pedicles. It has a small angled end, and this end is initially placed through the pedicle entry point facing laterally (in order to avoid medial cortical wall violation and spinal canal penetration). After a depth of 15 mm (marked on the tap itself), the probe is then turned medially to enter into the vertebral body and to avoid lateral wall breakout from the vertebral body. It is important to note that after the first 15 mm, the probe is beyond the spinal canal in most patients, and the risk of spinal cord injury is minimized during the first 15 mm by the laterally directed angle of the probe [9].

We avoid drilling down the pedicle as cortical breakthrough can occur with the drill. However, when the pedicle is corticated, then drilling becomes a necessity (the third option). We guide our drill trajectory by feeling the outer walls of the pedicle after performing a laminoforaminotomy. When the pedicles are too small to accommodate 4.5-mm screws, several options should be considered. First, by using a 3.5-mm tap (we prefer to use the one available on the VERTEX posterior cervical system), we establish a pathway through the pedicle into the vertebral body. Then we use a 4.5-mm tap to 'dilate' the pedicle.

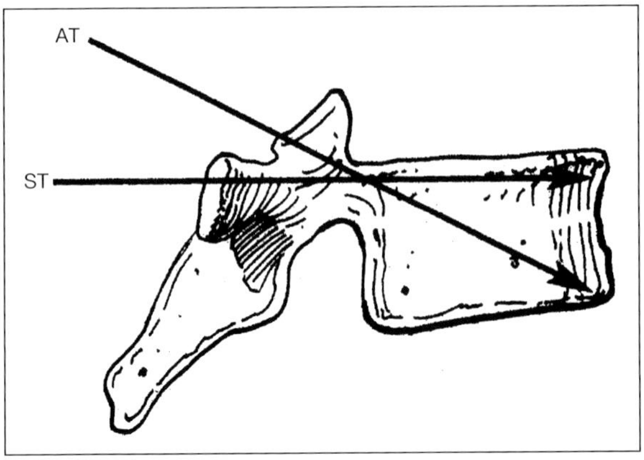

Fig. 2. Artist's illustration of the difference between the anatomic (AT) and the straightforward (ST) trajectories for thoracic pedicle screw placement. The thoracic pedicle screws can either be placed parallel to the endplates (straightforward trajectory), or they can be placed parallel to the axis of the pedicle itself (anatomic trajectory).

In adolescents, the pedicle often dilates with this successive tapping, and this allows for placement of a 4.5-mm screw.

Another option for dealing with a small pedicle is to use the 'in-out-in' technique for screw placement [11]. In this technique, the screw enters the pedicle and then is purposely placed through the lateral wall of the pedicle and engages the bone of the transverse process and rib head. The screw subsequently reenters the pedicle more anteriorly and ends in the vertebral body [12, 13].

The surgeon should keep in mind that the pedicle on the concave side of the curve may be smaller than the pedicle on the convex side. Consequently, different screw widths may be needed for the contralateral pedicles of the same level in scoliotic patients [14].

Use of fluoroscopy can be helpful in establishing the appropriate sagittal plane angulation of the pedicle screw. Thoracic pedicle screws can either be placed parallel to the endplates (straightforward trajectory), or they can be placed parallel to the axis of the pedicle itself (anatomic trajectory) (fig. 2). When placed parallel to the axis of the pedicle (anatomic trajectory), a longer screw can be used, and the tip of the screw is directed at the anterior, inferior vertebral endplate [15–17].

Anterior Approach

Another alternative is to perform the correction through an anterior approach by releasing the anterior longitudinal ligament, debriding the discs anteriorly, packing the disc spaces with bone graft harvested from a rib, placing vertebral body screws, and derotating the spine with a connected rod. This can be done either through a video-assisted thoracoscopic surgery (VATS), via an open thoracotomy, or via a 'mini-open' thoracotomy, which is a hybrid technique utilizing a small thoracotomy inferiorly and VATS superiorly [18, 19].

In patients who are not near skeletal maturity, an anterior operation may be required to release the spine anteriorly and remove the growing vertebral endplates. The surgeon can choose to perform only an anterior release and epiphysiodesis with a subsequent posterior instrumented procedure, or he can perform an anterior release, derotation, and fusion through a single anterior approach.

The anterior approach for derotation and fusion has advantages and disadvantages. VATS offers the advantages of decreased blood loss, sparing of the posterior muscular tension band, and a smaller surgical scar. However, VATS requires a lung takedown (with subsequent chest tube placement) and entails a longer operative time (often double the time of a posterior operation).

Anterior derotation and fusion procedures typically do not achieve the same degree of curve correction that posterior procedures do; this is likely due to the limitations in the number of segments that can be accessed via an anterior approach. When patients are hyperkyphotic the anterior approach is not possible, as access to the anterior vertebral bodies is limited. In addition, long-term follow-up of anterior derotation and fusion procedures is currently lacking. Consequently, a posterior derotation and fusion operation is still the gold-standard operation for correction of AIS.

Double Thoracic Curves (Lenke Type 2)

In progressive double thoracic curves, both curves are structural. Consequently, the fusion will need to extend to the stable vertebrae above and below both the curves. The preferred approach for the correction of double thoracic curves is the posterior approach.

An anterior approach for these curves may be necessary as an adjunct to a posterior correction and fusion (for an anterior release and epiphysiodesis), but instrumentation and curve correction via an anterior approach are very difficult, if not impossible due to the difficulty of accessing and instrumenting numerous thoracic levels.

Double Major Curves (Lenke Type 3)

Double major curves have a structural thoracic and a structural thoracolumbar or lumbar curve. In general, the instrumentation should extend to the stable vertebra above the thoracic curve and the stable vertebra below the thoracolumbar (or lumbar) structural curve.

An area of controversy in treating progressive structural curves that extend to the low lumbar spine is whether or not to extend the fusion to the sacrum. In general, in the treatment of AIS, the instrumentation should extend to the stable vertebra at the inferior end of the lowest structural curve (which is rarely at L4 or below) and fusion to the sacrum should be avoided unless the low lumbar discs are severely degenerated.

Extension of fusion to the sacrum has several disadvantages. First of all, the risk of pseudoarthrosis increases when a long construct is taken down to the sacrum [20]. Also, long constructs can fail due to screw pullout from the sacrum. In addition, extension of the fusion to the sacrum increases the risk of not completely correcting a patient's spinal imbalance. Patients often rebalance themselves following scoliosis corrections by accommodating any offset from the balanced state through alterations in the position of the lower lumbar spine. When the lumbosacral junction is fused, this accommodation potential is lost. Finally, extension to the sacrum runs the risk of creating flat-back syndrome if an appropriate amount of thoracic kyphosis and lumbar lordosis is not placed in the rods.

Adult Scoliosis

Adult Patients with Progressive AIS

The indications for surgery in this patient population are curve progression greater than 5° in a single year, back pain that is not relieved by conservative measures, pulmonary compromise from severe curvature, and unacceptable cosmetic deformity. Of these, the two most common indications are unrelenting back pain and cosmetic deformity.

Surgical Correction

The principles for surgical correction of adult patients with AIS are similar to those for adolescents with AIS. The curve can be evaluated and classified by the Lenke system. The instrumentation pattern is dependent upon the curve classification.

There are, however, two main differences between treating AIS in adults versus adolescents. First, the rate of pseudoarthrosis is higher for adults than for adolescents. Consequently, adults may need both anterior and posterior surgery to achieve a solid fusion. The anterior approach is often required in long curves to release the anterior longitudinal ligament and incise disc spaces to allow for a rigid curve to be corrected. The disc spaces can then be packed with structural graft to promote fusion, and a subsequent posterior procedure can be performed to instrument and correct the curvature.

The second major difference between adults and adolescents with AIS is that adults often have significant disc degeneration and spondylosis in the lumbar spine. Stopping a long segment fusion at a stable and neutral vertebra in the mid lumbar spine may not be appropriate in the face of significant lumbar spondylosis and degenerative disc disease (DDD). Patients with significant lumbar spondylosis and DDD may have progression of the spondylosis or significant low back pain from accelerated disc degeneration due to the greater loads on these segments following a long segment fusion above. Consequently, the need for extension of the fusion to the sacrum is greater in adults than it is in adolescents. However, if there is no significant lumbar spondylosis or disc degeneration, then stopping the fusion in the mid lumbar spine is appropriate.

Degenerative Adult-Onset Scoliosis

Degenerative adult-onset scoliotic curves are often rigid, lumbar curves. The indications for operative intervention are curve progression and unrelenting low back and radicular pain (not responsive to the conservative measures previously discussed). Often patients have significant radicular pain on the concave side of the curve due to severe foraminal compromise. Patients with these curves may be in overall spinal balance as many of them compensate at the thoracolumbar and lumbosacral junctions. Consequently, evaluation of overall spinal balance with 36-inch scoliosis x-rays is important. If a patient is a surgical candidate but is in overall spinal balance, then correction of the curve is not necessary.

Surgical Correction

In the subgroup of patients who are in overall spinal balance, there are two surgical treatment options. First, if the patient suffers from primarily radicular symptoms, then a unilateral Wiltse approach and decompression (posterolateral approach between the multifidus and longissimus muscles to perform an extraforaminal nerve root decompression) on the concave side of the curve are often sufficient to provide relief from radicular pain [21]. The advantage of this option is that the posterior ligamentous tension band is left intact and bony removal of the posterior column is kept to a minimum. Only the lateral portion of the facet joints is removed and the roof of the neural foramen is opened from lateral to medial.

If the patient, who is in overall spinal balance, is suffering from both low back and radicular pain, then another surgical treatment option is needed. For these patients, we recommend foraminal decompression on the concave side of the curve with an in situ instrumented fusion with pedicle screw-rod instrumentation. The foraminal decompression from a standard midline posterior approach will address the radicular symptoms. The fusion will relieve the low back pain (which is likely secondary to DDD and lumbar spondylosis). We always use autograft bone harvested from the iliac crest to establish the fusion.

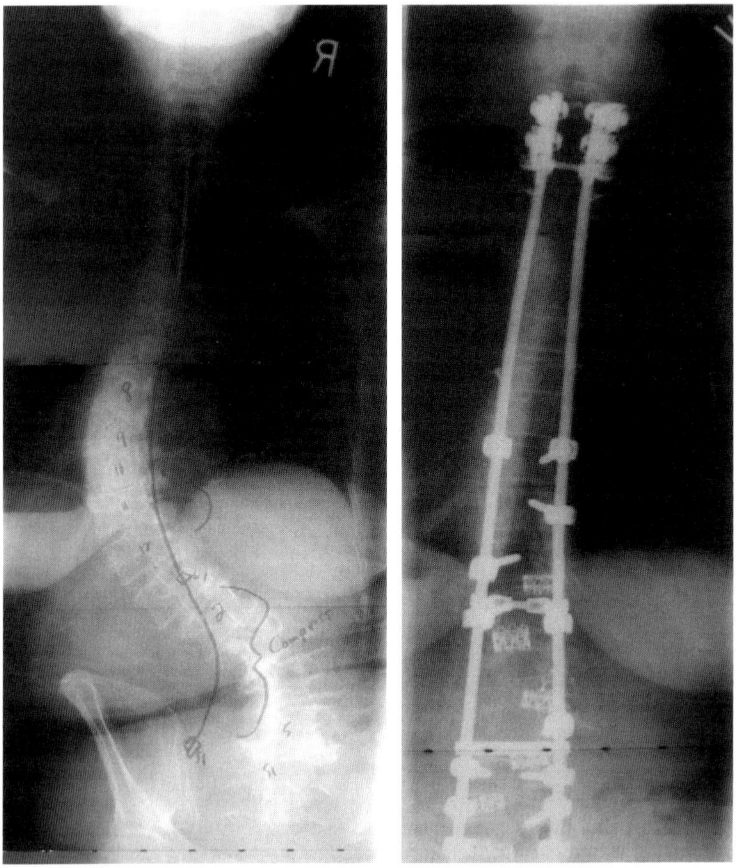

a *b*

Fig. 3. ***a*** Preoperative 36-inch x-ray of a fixed thoracolumbar scoliotic deformity in an adult. ***b*** Postoperative 36-inch anterior-posterior x-ray of the same patient following an anterior lumbar release with interbody fusion (Pyramesh, Medtronic Sofamor Danek) and a subsequent posterior multisegmental instrumented correction with thoracic hooks superiorly and thoracic and lumbar pedicle screws inferiorly (M-10 system, Medtronic Sofamor Danek).

When patients with degenerative adult-onset scoliosis are not in overall spinal balance and when their symptoms cannot be controlled by conservative measures, then correction of the scoliotic curvature is needed (fig. 3a). This is best accomplished by a combined anterior and posterior approach. An anterior approach is often helpful to release the rigid curve by incising the anterior longitudinal ligament and the anterior disc spaces. Autograft-filled Pyramesh cages (Medtronic Sofamor Danek) can be placed in the anterior interbody space to promote fusion (fig. 3b). If no anterior column support with autograft is performed, then the risk of pseudoarthrosis is high in this elderly patient population.

A subsequent posterior approach with a coronal plane wedge osteotomy of the convex facets is performed (i.e. the convex facets are removed from the pedicle above the neural foramen to the pedicle below the neural foramen). The wedge-shaped osteotomy of the convex side of the curve prevents compression of the exiting nerve roots on the convex side. This osteotomy is extended beyond the midline and includes the convex side of the laminae in order to avoid thecal sac compression when the convex side is compressed. Pedicle screws are then placed at all levels from the superior to the inferior stable vertebrae of the lumbar scoliotic curve. Rods are connected to the screws and the convex side of the curve is compressed while the concave side is distracted, and the curve is straightened.

If the surgeon wishes to perform the entire operation from a posterior approach, then multilevel transforaminal lumbar interbody fusions can be performed and Pyramesh cages filled with autograft can be placed into the interbody space through this approach. Fusion to the sacrum is avoided if the inferior stable vertebra is at L4 or above and if the L4/5 and L5/S1 discs are in good condition. If the lumbosacral junction is not fused, then additional curve compensation is possible for the patient. However, if the curve extends to L5 or if the low lumbar discs are significantly degenerated, then fusion to the sacrum is often needed. There are several options for extension of the fusion to the sacrum. First of all, S1 (and S2) pedicle screws can be placed. However, the sacral pedicles have large cancellous centers, and they often do not allow for solid screw purchase. Sacral pedicle screws have greater pullout strengths if they are bicortical, and lateral fluoroscopy can assist with bicortical placement.

Long segment fusions to the sacrum are subject to large cantilever loads, which can lead to pullout of sacral pedicle screws, sacral fractures, and lumbosacral pseudoarthrosis. Consequently, some surgeons elect to supplement sacral pedicle screws with intrasacral rods, transacral rods, and/or iliac screw fixation [22, 23]. Iliac screw fixation can be hindered by harvesting posterior iliac crest bone graft. However, the harvest of posterior iliac crest bone graft does not completely preclude the placement of iliac crest screws [24].

Kyphosis

Surgical treatment of kyphosis can be considered if there is a rigid thoracic or thoracolumbar kyphotic curve greater than 60–70° in either the adolescent or the adult. Curves of 60–70° are often cosmetically deforming, but they usually do not cause significant cardiopulmonary symptoms. However, these curves can cause intractable back pain that is not responsive to conservative treatment measures. Curves over 80–90°, on the other hand, can cause cardiopulmonary compromise and surgical correction is definitely indicated.

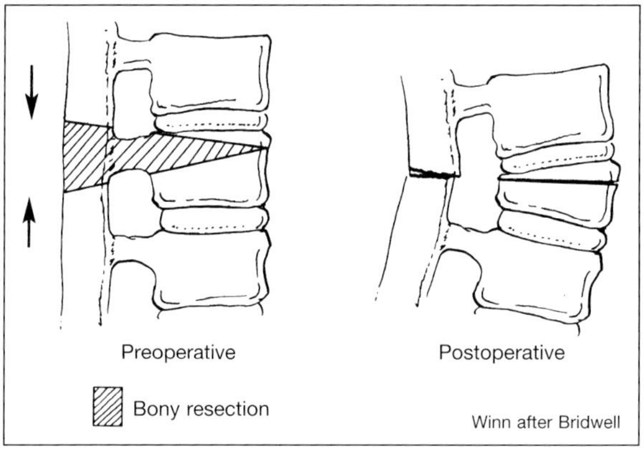

Fig. 4. Artist's illustration of a three-column PSO. The technique involves removing a large wedge of the posterior and middle columns (including the pedicle) of the vertebral body. The remainder of the posterior and middle columns is then approximated by pulling together pedicle screws above and below the osteotomy level. The anterior column of the PSO level acts as the fulcrum for this correction.

Surgical Correction

Surgical correction of large, structural thoracic or thoracolumbar curves can be performed through a posterior approach or a combined anterior and posterior approach. Correction through an anterior only approach is difficult because the severe thoracic kyphosis limits the surgeon's access to the anterior thoracic spine.

Curves of 60–70° can be treated via a posterior only approach, especially if the curves are flexible. The treatment strategy for these curves is to expose the ends of the curve, and then to either perform a pedicle subtraction osteotomy (PSO) or multilevel posterior closing wedge osteotomies (multiple Smith–Petersen osteotomies). PSO is useful for a focal thoracic kyphosis (i.e. thoracic wedge compression fracture) because with PSO, the majority of the correction is performed over a single segment. The technique involves removing a large wedge of the posterior and middle columns (including the pedicle) of the vertebral body. The remainder of the posterior and middle columns is then approximated by pulling together pedicle screws above and below the osteotomy level. The anterior column of the PSO level acts as the fulcrum for this correction (fig. 4), and up to 30° of correction can be achieved with a single level of PSO [25].

Prior to approximating the remainder of the posterior and middle columns in PSO, a Z-plasty of the underlying dura may be needed to avoid buckling of the dura into the spinal canal. We prefer to perform PSO below the conus to avoid injury to the spinal cord.

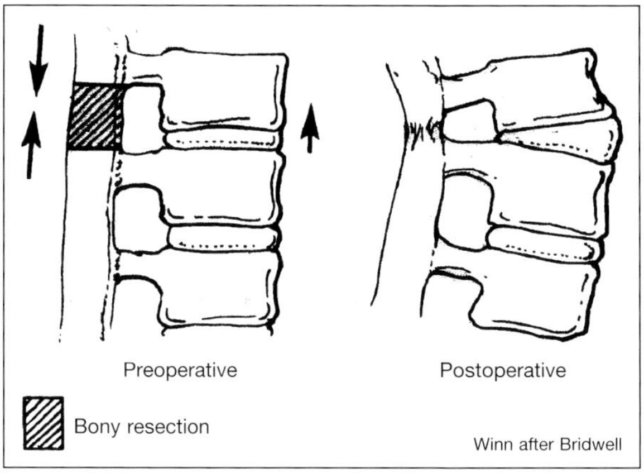

Fig. 5. Artist's illustration of a Smith–Petersen osteotomy. The technique involves removing multiple wedges of the facets bilaterally over several levels. The remaining posterior columns are then pulled together (by pedicle screw-rod instrumentation) while the neural foramina are monitored closely to ensure that excessive foraminal narrowing does not occur. The fulcrum of the correction is the anterior disc space, and, consequently, in rigid curves, an anterior procedure may be needed to first incise the anterior longitudinal ligament.

Multiple Smith–Petersen osteotomies, on the other hand, are much safer because the correction is spread out over multiple levels. Only 1° of correction can be expected for every 1 mm of bone removed with this technique. Consequently, multiple Smith–Petersen osteotomies are needed to correct a significant kyphosis. The technique involves removing multiple wedges of the facets bilaterally over several levels (fig. 5) [26]. The remaining posterior columns are then pulled together (by pedicle screw-rod instrumentation) while the neural foramina are monitored closely to ensure that excessive foraminal narrowing does not occur. The fulcrum of the correction is the anterior disc space, and, consequently, in rigid curves, an anterior procedure may be needed to first incise the anterior longitudinal ligament and the anterior disc space [27].

Conclusion

Surgical correction of spinal deformity has advanced rapidly over the past decade. Correction of severe scoliotic and kyphotic deformities can now be performed with low mortality rates. However, the morbidity rates for major deformity corrections remain very high. New advances will likely blend more minimally invasive techniques with the current instrumentation systems in an attempt to reduce the surgical morbidity associated with multisegmental correction and instrumented fusion.

Acknowledgments

We are grateful to Drew Imhulse and Tom Fletcher for assistance with the radiographic images in the figures, to Sherry Ballenger for editorial assistance, and to Bill Winn for assistance with the illustrations. We thank Medtronic Sofamor Danek for permission to use several of the illustrations.

Disclosure Statement

The following authors are consultants for Medtronic Sofamor Danek: Stephen L. Ondra, MD and Rick C. Sasso, MD.

References

1 Hibbs RA: An operation for progressive spinal deformities. NY Med J 1911;93:1013–1016.
2 Harrington PR: Treatment of scoliosis: Correction and internal fixation by spine instrumentation. J Bone Joint Surg Am 1962;44:591–610.
3 King HA, Moe JH, Bradford DS, Winter RB: The selection of fusion levels in thoracic idiopathic scoliosis. J Bone Joint Surg Am 1983;65:1302–1313.
4 Lenke LG, Betz R, Harms J, Bridwell KH, Clements DH, Lowe TG, Blanke KM: Adolescent idiopathic scoliosis: A new classification to determine extent of spinal arthrodesis. J Bone Joint Surg Am 2001;83:1169–1181.
5 Lenke LG, Betz RR, Clements D, Merola A, Haher T, Lowe T, Newton P, Bridwell KH, Blanke K: Curve prevalence of a new classification of operative adolescent idiopathic scoliosis: Does classification correlate with treatment? Spine 2002;27:604–611.
6 Cotrel Y, Dubousset J: New segmental posterior instrumentation of the spine. Orthop Trans 1985;9:118.
7 Lenke LG, Bridwell KH, Baldus C, Blanke K, Schoenecker PL: Cotrel-Dubousset instrumentation for adolescent idiopathic scoliosis. J Bone Joint Surg 1992;74:1056–1067.
8 Lenke LG, Betz R, Bridwell KH, Harms J, Clements D, Lowe T: Spontaneous lumbar curve coronal correction after selective anterior or posterior thoracic fusion in adolescent idiopathic scoliosis. Spine 1999;24:1663–1672.
9 Lenke LG, Rinella A, Kim YJ: Free hand thoracic pedicle screw placement. Semin Spine Surg 2002;14/1:48–57.
10 Mummaneni PV, Traynelis VC, Sasso RC: Cervical lateral mass advances. Prog Neurol Surg. Basel, Karger, 2003, pp 165–175.
11 Belmont PJ Jr, Klemme WR, Dhawan A, Polly DW Jr: In vivo accuracy of thoracic pedicle screws. Spine 2002;26:2340–2346.
12 Dvorak M, MacDonald S, Gurr KR, Bailey SI, Haddad RG: An anatomic, radiographic, and biomechanical assessment of extrapedicular screw fixation in the thoracic spine. Spine 1993;18:1689–1694.
13 Youkilis AS, Quint DJ, McGillicuddy JE, Papadopoulos SM: Stereotactic navigation for placement of pedicle screws in the thoracic spine. Neurosurgery 2001;48:771–778.

14 Liljenqvist UR, Link TM, Halm HFH: Morphometric analysis of thoracic and lumbar vertebrae in idiopathic scoliosis. Spine 2000;22:1247–1253.
15 Klemme WR, Belmont PJ, Polly DW: Transpedicular thoracic screws: General concepts and insertion technique using fluoroscopic guidance. Semin Spine Surg 2002;14/1:43–47.
16 McCormack BM, Benzel EC, Adams MS, Baldwin NG, Rupp FW, Maher DJ: Anatomy of the thoracic pedicle. Neurosurgery 1995;37:303–308.
17 Kuklo TR, Polly DW: Surgical anatomy of the thoracic pedicle. Semin Spine Surg 2002;14/1:3–7.
18 Newton PO, Wenger DR, Mubarak SJ, Meyer RS: Anterior release and fusion in pediatric spinal deformity: A comparison of early outcome and cost of thoracoscopic and open thoracotomy approaches. Spine 1997;22:1398–1406.
19 Lenke LG, Rhee J: Adolescent scoliosis: Anterior surgical techniques for adolescent idiopathic scoliosis. Curr Opin Orthop 2001;12/3:199–205.
20 Eck KR, Bridwell KH, Ungacta FF, Riew KD, Lapp MA, Lenke LG, Baldus C, Blanke K: Complications and results of long adult deformity fusions down to L4, L5, and the sacrum. Spine 2001;26:E182–E192.
21 Wiltse LL: The paraspinal sacrospinalis-splitting approach to the lumbar spine. Clin Orthop 1973; 91:48–57.
22 Mazda K, Khairouni A, Pennecot GF, Bloch J: The ideal position of sacral transpedicular endplate screws in Jackson's intrasacral fixation. An anatomic study of 50 sacral specimens. Spine 1998; 23:2123–2126.
23 Emami A, Deviren V, Berven S, Smith JA, Hu SS, Bradford DS: Outcome and complications of long fusions to the sacrum in adult spine deformity: Luque-Galveston, combined iliac and sacral screws, and sacral fixation. Spine 2002;27:776–786.
24 Kuklo TR, Bridwell KH, Lewis SJ, Baldus C, Blanke K, Iffrig TM, Lenke LG: Minimum 2-year analysis of sacropelvic fixation and L5–S1 fusion using S1 and iliac screws. Spine 2001;26: 1976–1983.
25 Kim KT, Suk KS, Cho YJ, Hong GP, Park BJ: Clinical outcome results of pedicle subtraction osteotomy in ankylosing spondylitis with kyphotic deformity. Spine 2002;27:612–618.
26 Smith-Petersen MN, Larson CB, Aufranc OE: Osteotomy of the spine for correction of flexion deformity in rheumatoid arthritis. Clin Orthop 1969;66:6–9.
27 Booth KC, Bridwell KH, Lenke LG, Baldus CR, Blanke KM: Complications and predictive factors for the successful treatment of flatback deformity (fixed sagittal imbalance). Spine 1999; 24:1712–1720.

Praveen V. Mummaneni, MD
Assistant Professor, Department of Neurosurgery, The Emory Clinic
550 Peachtree St., Suite 806, Atlanta, GA 30308 (USA)
Tel. +1 404 686 8101, Fax +1 404 686 4805, E-Mail praveen_mummaneni@emoryhealthcare.org

Haid RW Jr, Subach BR, Rodts GE Jr (eds): Advances in Spinal Stabilization.
Prog Neurol Surg. Basel, Karger, 2003, vol 16, pp 240–250

Vertebral Augmentation for Osteoporotic and Osteolytic Vertebral Compression Fractures: Vertebroplasty and Kyphoplasty

Isador Lieberman

The Cleveland Clinic Foundation, Cleveland, Ohio, USA

Osteoporosis is a systemic disease currently afflicting more than 40 million Americans; this figure is likely to rise further as the population ages. It results in progressive bone mineral loss and concurrent changes in bony architecture that leave bone vulnerable to fracture, often after minimal or no trauma. Osteolysis secondary to metastatic disease or multiple myeloma affects up to 70% of patients on initial presentation. The spine is the most common site of osteoporotic or osteolytic fracture, with vertebral compression fracture (VCF) occurring in up to 50% of women 80 years and older and 25% of women 70 years and older [1, 2]. Overall, 700,000 people per year in the US suffer a VCF secondary to osteoporosis, exceeding even the frequency of hip fractures [11]. Osteoporotic VCFs have been shown to be associated with up to a 30% age-adjusted increase in mortality [3]. The cost to society of managing osteoporotic VCF patients in the United States in 1995 was USD 746 million [4]. Possible acute complications of either osteoporotic or osteolytic vertebral fracture include cord compression, urinary retention, and ileus [10]. Long-term consequences include considerable pain (reported in 35% of detectable VCFs) [12], as well as pulmonary compromise (a 9% loss in predicted forced vital capacity with each vertebral fracture) [13]. Other chronic sequelae include deconditioning, deformity, insomnia, and depression, resulting in substantial physical, functional, and psychosocial impairment [13, 14].

Nonoperative Management of VCFs

Two thirds of patients with acute, painful osteoporotic VCFs improve regardless of the treatment applied. Traditional, nonoperative management includes bed rest, analgesics, and bracing. This type of medical management, however, fails to restore spinal alignment, and the lack of mobility itself can result in secondary complications, including worsening osteoporosis, atelectasis, pneumonia, deep vein thrombosis, decubitus ulcer, and pulmonary embolism. An alternative approach is supervised ambulatory mobility by a physiotherapist plus hydrotherapy [15]. In one third of patients, severe pain, limited mobility, and poor quality of life persist despite appropriate nonoperative management. No patient spontaneously achieves a realigned spine, corrected sagittal contour, or restoration of vertebral height.

Half the patients with metastases to the spine report pain relief after external beam radiation [31]. Patients with radiosensitive tumors (breast, prostate, myeloma) typically do well, however radiotherapy does not protect the spine from progressive osteolytic collapse and presents the treating surgeon with major concerns regarding postoperative wound healing and bone fusion should surgery be indicated [32]. Similar concerns exist when considering the use of chemotherapy to treat various metastases to the spine, although there are new investigational bisphosphonates which are promising reversal of bone loss [33].

Operative Management of VCFs

Historically, the only alternative to nonoperative management for symptomatic osteoporotic or osteolytic vertebral fractures was open surgical decompression (anterior or posterior decompression and stabilization via internal fixation hardware and bone grafting), and this was usually reserved for those patients with gross spinal deformity or neurologic impairment (<0.5%) [10, 32]. The reason for this surgical caution was due to the adverse risk/benefit ratio in this elderly or cancer population with poor bone quality and multiple comorbid conditions.

Percutaneous vertebroplasty (PVP) is a minimally invasive method that involves the percutaneous injection of polymethyl methacrylate (PMMA) into a collapsed vertebral body to stabilize the vertebra. Originally developed for osteolytic metastasis, myeloma, and hemangioma, the procedure resulted in quick, effective pain relief and a low complication rate [5–7]. PVP is now also increasingly used for the treatment of osteoporotic vertebral fractures [8]. However, PVP does not expand the collapsed vertebra, potentially locking the spine in a kyphotic posture. In addition, the PMMA bone filler has associated problems (epidural leakage, thermal necrosis, inability to integrate with bone, handling difficulties, toxicity to patient and operator) [2, 9].

Kyphoplasty is a newer minimally invasive technique with a number of potential advantages over PVP, including lower risk of cement extravasation and better restoration of vertebral body height [29]. A cannula is introduced into the vertebral body, followed by insertion of an inflatable bone tamp (IBT), which when deployed, reduces the compression fracture and restores the vertebral body toward its original height, while creating a cavity to be filled with bone cement. The cement augmentation is therefore done with more control into the low-pressure environment of the preformed cavity with viscous, partially cured cement.

Percutaneous Vertebroplasty

Background

Percutaneous vertebral augmentation (vertebroplasty, PVP) was first devised by Galibert et al. [16] in 1987, and initially involved the augmentation of the vertebral body with PMMA during open procedures to allow stable fixation of internal hardware. PVP was first described in the French literature in 1987 [16] but was not performed in the United States until 1994. Originally targeted for osteolytic metastasis, myeloma, and hemangioma, PVP resulted in early appreciable pain relief and a low complication rate [7, 16]. Its indications now include osteoporotic vertebral collapse with chronic pain, expanding further to include treatment of asymptomatic vertebral collapse and even prophylactic intervention for at risk vertebral bodies [17]. Nevertheless, the treatment of acute fractures in ambulatory patients and prophylactic treatment remains controversial [18]. In fact, vertebral augmentation itself is somewhat controversial, with questions concerning a lack of defined indications, expected complications, outcome measures, and the need for long-term follow-up data [2].

An open question in PVP is the mechanism of pain relief. The most intuitive explanation involves simple mechanical stabilization of the fracture; the cement stabilizes vertebral bodies and offloads the facet joints. However, another possibility is that analgesia results from local chemical, vascular, or thermal effects of PMMA on nerve endings in surrounding tissue [8, 19]. Supporting this concept is the lack of correlation between cement volume and pain relief [20, 21]. Further evidence against an effect resulting solely from mechanical stabilization is the fact that PVP typically does not restore lost vertebral body height and therefore does not correct altered biomechanics [1, 18].

Technique

Injection of opacified PMMA is performed via a transpedicular or paravertebral approach under continuous fluoroscopic guidance to obtain adequate filling and to avoid PMMA leakage. For complex or high-risk cases, CT and fluoroscopic guidance are sometimes combined [5, 18]. In routine cases, PVP can be performed under local anesthesia with slight sedation in less than an hour [1], although general anesthesia is sometimes required because pain may intensify during cement injection [8]. Preceding PMMA injection, intraosseous venography is often used to determine the filling pattern and identify sites of potential PMMA leakage (outline the venous drainage pattern, confirm needle placement within the bony trabeculae, and delineate fractures in the bony cortex). However, others have dispensed with routine venography [1].

Contraindications to vertebroplasty include coagulopathy, absence of facilities to perform emergency decompressive surgery in the event of a complication, and extreme vertebral collapse (>65–70% reduction in vertebral height) [8]. However, this last contraindication has been questioned recently [18, 22].

Results

The available clinical studies, mostly European, report pain relief in about 90% of cases treated for osteoporotic fracture, with only infrequent clinically significant complications (0–10%), most of them minor [7, 18]. In a series of 80 patients treated with PVP for osteoporotic vertebral collapse, 90% gained immediate pain relief [5]. During a follow-up of 1 month to 10 years, only one complication was reported: intercostal neuralgia treated by local anesthetic infiltration. In another prospective study of 45 vertebral body augmentations in 17 osteoporotic patients led to significant and lasting pain reduction during the 1-year follow-up [1]. Although cement leakage occurred in 20% of vertebral bodies, none had clinical sequelae. In a retrospective review of 70 augmented vertebrae in 38 consecutive patients with osteoporosis, treatment resulted in pain relief within 48 h in 36 patients (95%). The pain relief was durable in 34 of the patients (89%) during a follow-up averaging 18 months. Twenty-four patients (63%) experienced marked to complete pain relief, 12 (32%) moderate relief, and 2 (5%) no significant change [18]. Of 8 patients suffering malignant neoplasm of the spinal column and treated with vertebroplasty, 4 (50%) found pain relief in this series [18]. Cortet et al. [23] studied 16 patients with 20 osteoporotic vertebral compression fractures who underwent PVP. This study found a statistically significant decrease in pain with several standardized scoring systems at all observed time points during the 6-month follow-up, along with concurrent, significant improvement in overall health status. No adverse events and no vertebral fractures occurred during the follow-up period. Another study of 29 patients with 47 painful osteoporotic vertebral fractures reported a 90% success rate in terms of significant pain relief immediately after treatment [7]. Two patients sustained rib fractures during the procedure resulting in pain that subsequently resolved; otherwise, no clinically significant complications were noted.

Complications

The principal risk of PVP, which involves the forced injection of low-viscosity PMMA cement into the closed space of the collapsed vertebral body, is cement extravasation. Extravasation rates are as high as 40% when used to treat osteoporotic fractures [7]. The likelihood is greater when using cement with a liquid rather than paste consistency or with higher PMMA volume [24]. However, in most settings, the majority of extravasations have no clinical relevance, at least in the short term [1].

The consequence of an extravasation depends on its location. In epidural or foraminal extravasation, nerve root compression and radiculopathy are the major risk, occurring in 11 of 274 patients (4%) treated by Deramond et al. [5]. Three patients required surgical nerve root decompression, as has been described by others as well [10, 20]. Extravasation into perivertebral veins can cause cement embolism to the lungs; deaths attributed to cement embolism have been documented. However, the 2 deaths attributed to pulmonary embolism were reported to be unrelated to the procedure; no cement material was detected by chest x-ray of the first patient [8, 25], and the second pulmonary embolism arose from deep venous lower extremity thrombosis [5]. On the other hand, extravasation into adjacent disks or paravertebral tissue, although common, generally produces no patient symptoms and carries little clinical significance; many such extravasations can be avoided by careful needle positioning [5].

Other operative and long-term complications of PVP are specific to PMMA as a filler [1, 17, 26]. The physician may work with PMMA in large batches in order to keep it liquid and to extend the working time for vertebroplasty. However, its high polymerization temperature (86–107°C within cement core) [27] can damage adjacent tissue, including the spinal cord and nerve roots [9], leading to an inflammatory reaction and transitory exacerbation of pain [8]. When injecting PMMA monomer, vigilance and caution of the physician are required. Absorption of PMMA during the injection can induce hypotension by virtue of its cardiotoxic and arrhythmogenic properties [28]. Keeping in mind that placing a material in the spine affords proximity and access to the chest and the heart, vertebral augmentation with PMMA demands meticulous attention to technique.

Overall, the risk of complications that carry clinical significance following PVP for osteoporotic vertebral fracture is 1–3%, and most potential complications can be avoided with a good technique [5].

Kyphoplasty

Background

Kyphoplasty is a new technique evolved from a marriage of vertebroplasty with balloon angioplasty. It has a number of potential advantages, including lower risk of cement extravasation and better restoration of vertebral body height. A cannula is introduced into the vertebral body, via a transpedicular or

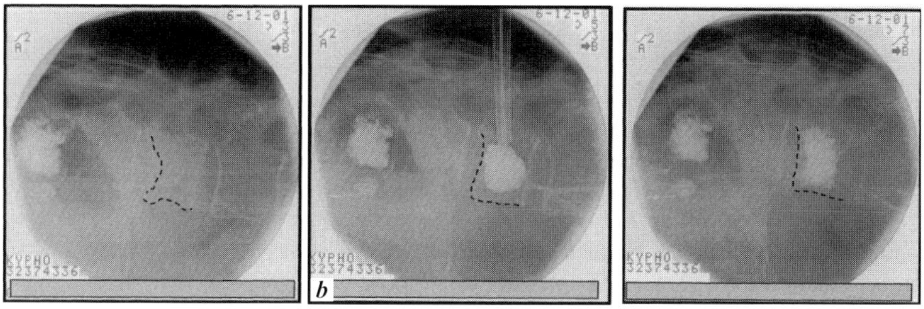

Fig. 1. ***a–c*** Kyphoplasty example, IBT inflation and PMMA augmentation.

extrapedicular route, followed by insertion of an IBT, which when deployed, reduces the compression fracture and restores the vertebral body toward its original height. This then creates a cavity to be filled with bone cement. The cement augmentation can now be completed with more control into the low-pressure environment of the preformed cavity with viscous, partially cured cement. Using a cannula for bone filler with a steel stylet as a plunger enables the operator to apply cement at considerably higher viscosity than is possible with injection through a 5-ml syringe and 11-gauge needle. Both the higher cement viscosity and lower-pressure injection reduce the risk of cement extravasation. Filling is performed under continuous lateral fluoroscopic guidance similar to vertebroplasty. The procedure can be performed under general anesthesia or local anesthesia with intravenous sedation; some patients are able to return home the same day of procedure.

Technique

With the patient under general or local anesthesia in prone position on a radiolucent spinal frame, two C-arms are positioned for anteroposterior and lateral fluoroscopic images. Once positioned the C arms or patient are not moved to ensure repeatable images throughout the case. Two 3-mm incisions are made at the vertebral level, parallel to the pedicles in both planes. Then a guide wire or biopsy needle is advanced into the vertebral body via a transpedicular or extrapedicular approach, depending on fracture configuration and patient's anatomy. The guide wire is then exchanged for the working cannula using a series of obturators. Once the working cannula is positioned the surgeon reams out a corridor to accommodate the IBT and positions IBT under the collapsed endplate. To deploy the IBT, inflation proceeds slowly under fluoroscopy until maximum fracture reduction is achieved or the balloon reaches a cortical wall (see fig. 1). At this point the surgeon deflates and removes the IBT, mixes the cement, prefills the cement cannulae and allows the cement to partially cure in the cement cannulae. Once partially cured PMMA is slowly extruded into the vertebral body through each pedicle under continuous lateral fluoroscopic guidance. This technique permits a low-pressure fill. In most instances, the volume of cement can slightly exceed that of the bone cavity to interdigitate filler from the central bolus with the surrounding bone. Once filling is complete and the cement has hardened the surgeon removes the cannula and closes the 3-mm incisions.

Results

Kyphoplasty has been slowly advanced through a few surgical centers participating in a multicenter study begun in 1999. A phase I efficacy study of 70 consecutive kyphoplasty procedures in 30 patients with painful, progressive osteoporotic/osteolytic VCFs was recently completed [29]. Mean duration of symptoms was 5.9 months. Symptomatic levels were identified by correlating the clinical data with MRI findings. Preoperative and postoperative x-rays were compared to calculate the percentage height restored. Outcome was further assessed by comparing the preoperative and latest postoperative survey of patient's self-reported health status using the 36-item Short Form Health Survey (SF-36) [30]. In 70% of the vertebral bodies, kyphoplasty restored on average 47% of the lost vertebral height ($p = 0.001$). SF-36 scores for bodily pain ($p = 0.0001$), physical function ($p = 0.002$), and vitality ($p = 0.001$) were among the subscales that showed substantial and significant improvement. Complications were infrequent. One patient experienced perioperative pulmonary edema and a myocardial infarction secondary to intraoperative fluid overload; 2 patients suffered rib fractures due to positioning during the procedure. Cement leakage occurred at 6 of 70 treated levels (8.6%); however, there were no complications that related directly to selection of this technique or to use of the IBT. In an ongoing evaluation the results of this initial series have been maintained in the most recent follow-up of over 70 consecutive patients up to 14 months.

In a second prospective evaluation the safety and efficacy of kyphoplasty in the treatment of osteolytic vertebral compression fractures due to multiple myeloma found similar satisfying results [34]. Fifty-five consecutive kyphoplasty procedures were performed in over 27 sessions in 18 patients. The mean age of patients was 63.5 years (48–79), the mean duration of symptoms was 11 months, and the mean follow-up 7.4 months. The range of levels treated were from T6 to L5 (T11 = 9, T12 = 7, L1 = 8, L2 = 7). There were no major complications related directly to the use of this technique. On average, 34% of height lost at the time of fracture was restored. After stratifying for those where height was not restored the remaining vertebral bodies showed an average of 56% height restoration. Asymptomatic cement leakage occurred at 2/55 levels (4%).

Significant improvement in SF-36 scores occurred for bodily pain: 23.2 to 55.4 ($p = 0.0008$) and physical function: 21.3 to 50.6 ($p = 0.0010$), vitality: 31.3 to 47.5 ($p = 0.010$), and social functioning: 40.6 to 64.8 ($p = 0.014$). The authors concluded that the kyphoplasty technique was efficacious in the treatment of osteolytic vertebral compression fractures due to multiple myeloma and associated with early clinical improvement of pain and function as well as some restoration of vertebral body height in these patients.

Vertebroplasty versus Kyphoplasty

Although both vertebroplasty and kyphoplasty provide excellent pain relief, kyphoplasty has the potential to improve spine biomechanics and decrease the risk of cement extravasation. PVP usually will not expand the vertebral body or regain normal spine alignment. Preliminary data indicate that kyphoplasty may restore near-normal height, preventing kyphosis that leads to respiratory and digestive problems. Restoration of height and sagittal alignment may also work to protect vulnerable vertebral levels above or below the site(s) treated by minimizing force transfer.

PVP is much more prone to cement leaks since the PMMA is injected in a liquid state and will take the path of least resistance through any cracks in surrounding bone. In administering vertebroplasty the operator injects the liquid cement, typically pausing or stopping once a leak becomes evident. On the other hand, in kyphoplasty, the expanded balloon creates a cavity and pushes bone to the edges of the cavity, thus sealing off potential fissures and cracks. Greater placement control is possible in a kyphoplasty, in which the operator can fill the cavity with a more viscous cement to the point at which the cement bolus reaches and interdigitates with the bony margins. The initial kyphoplasty findings show lower rates of cement extravasation compared with published vertebroplasty series, supporting the hypothesis that injection of high-viscosity cement into a previously formed cavity may be an improvement over the injection of low-viscosity liquid cement into the unreduced vertebral body.

Conclusion

Osteoporotic and osteolytic VCFs pose a significant clinical problem including spinal deformity, pain, reduced pulmonary function and mobility, as well as an overall increase in mortality in the elderly. Traditional medical and surgical options in many cases prove inadequate.

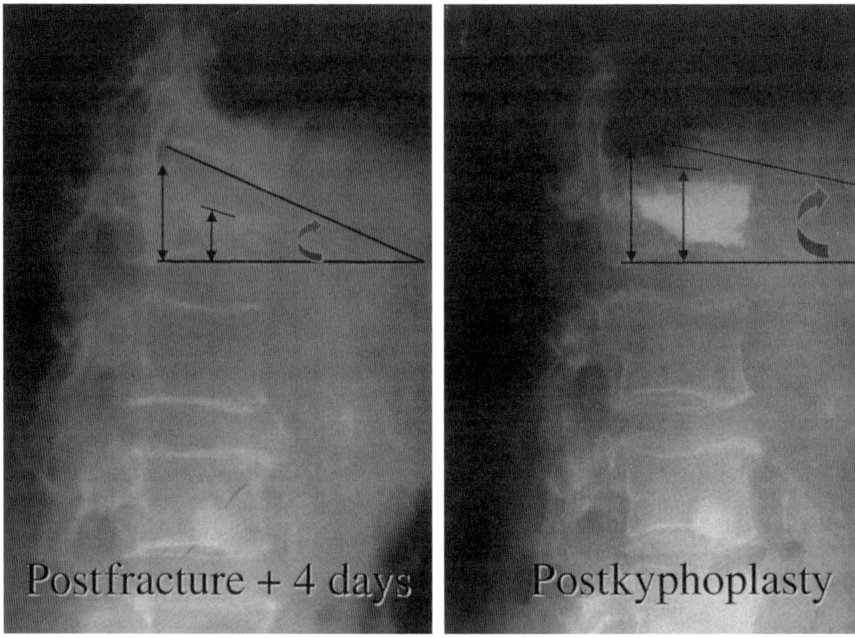

a *b*

Fig. 2. Kyphoplasty example, height and kyphosis restoration. ***a*** Postheight = 37 mm, midheight = 12 mm, kyphosis = 25°. ***b*** Postheight = 37 mm, midheight = 28 mm, kyphosis = 10°.

PVP is a relatively noninvasive technique that has gained increased acceptance over the last decade in the treatment of symptomatic osteoporotic vertebral fractures. The available clinical studies describe pain relief achieved in greater than 90% of symptomatic osteoporotic fractures, with only infrequent, mostly minor, complications. Some of the drawbacks of PVP stem from the use of PMMA, because of its toxicity and poor handling characteristics, rather than from the procedure itself.

Kyphoplasty is a modification of PVP that is still in evolution. It may add a margin of safety by virtue of a lower observed incidence of cement leakage. Kyphoplasty may be shown to be worthwhile in acute vertebral fracture, in high-risk patients to predictably restore vertebral height (see fig. 2) and to facilitate a low-pressure fill procedure. Favorable outcomes in early trials appear to permit early mobilization, which has the potential to decrease mortality. Considering the greater mortality that is associated with osteoporotic compression fractures, early mobilization in these patients is of prime importance.

The next logical step beyond treatment of evident vertebral fractures is prophylactic augmentation. Prevention of osteoporotic vertebral fractures with a combination of pharmacologics and timely reinforcement of at risk osteoporotic vertebrae is the ultimate goal aside from prevention of osteoporosis itself. It is here that new osteoconductive synthetic composites will figure more prominently as an emerging alternative to cement. Advances in minimally invasive surgical techniques, imaging, and synthetic engineering are rapidly changing the treatment protocols available for osteoporotic compression fracture.

References

1 Heini PF, Walchli B, Berlemann U: Percutaneous transpedicular vertebroplasty with PMMA: Operative technique and early results. A prospective study for the treatment of osteoporotic compression fractures. Eur Spine J 2000;9:445–450.

2 Einhorn TA: Vertebroplasty: An opportunity to do something really good for patients. Spine 2000; 25:1051–1052.

3 Kado DM, Browner WS, Palermo L, et al: Vertebral fractures and mortality in older women: A prospective study. Study of Osteoporotic Fractures Research Group. Arch Intern Med 1999;159: 1215–1220.

4 Ray NF, Chan JK, Thamer M, Melton LJ 3rd: Medical expenditures for the treatment of osteoporotic fractures in the United States in 1995: Report from the National Osteoporosis Foundation. J Bone Miner Res 1997;12:24–35.

5 Deramond H, Depriester C, Galibert P, Le Gars D: Percutaneous vertebroplasty with polymethylmethacrylate. Technique, indications, and results. Radiol Clin North Am 1998;36:533–546.

6 Chiras J, Depriester C, Weill A, Sola-Martinez MT, Deramond H: Percutaneous vertebral surgery. Techniques and indications. J Neuroradiol 1997;24:45–59.

7 Jensen ME, Evans AJ, Mathis JM, Kallmes DF, Cloft HJ, Dion JE: Percutaneous polymethylmethacrylate vertebroplasty in the treatment of osteoporotic vertebral body compression fractures: Technical aspects. Am J Neuroradiol 1997;18:1897–1904.

8 Cotten A, Boutry N, Cortet B, et al: Percutaneous vertebroplasty: State of the art. Radiographics 1998;18:311–320.

9 Deramond H, Wright NT, Belkoff SM: Temperature elevation caused by bone cement polymerization during vertebroplasty. Bone 1999;25(suppl 2):17S–21S.

10 Bostrom MP, Lane JM: Future directions. Augmentation of osteoporotic vertebral bodies. Spine 1997;15(suppl 24):38S–42S.

11 Riggs BL, Melton LJ 3rd: The worldwide problem of osteoporosis: Insights afforded by epidemiology. Bone 1995;17(suppl 5):505S–511S.

12 Cooper C, Atkinson EJ, O'Fallon WM, Melton LJ 3rd: Incidence of clinically diagnosed vertebral fractures: A population-based study in Rochester, Minnesota, 1985–1989. J Bone Miner Res 1992;7:221–227.

13 Leech JA, Dulberg C, Kellie S, Pattee L, Gay J: Relationship of lung function to severity of osteoporosis in women. Am Rev Respir Dis 1990;141:68–71.

14 Lyles KW, Gold DT, Shipp KM, Pieper CF, Martinez S, Mulhausen PL: Association of osteoporotic vertebral compression fractures with impaired functional status. Am J Med 1993;94: 595–601.

15 Patel U, Skingle S, Campbell GA, Crisp AJ, Boyle IT: Clinical profile of acute vertebral compression fractures in osteoporosis. Br J Rheumatol 1991;30.418–421.

16 Galibert P, Deramond H, Rosat P, Le Gars D: Preliminary note on the treatment of vertebral angioma by percutaneous acrylic vertebroplasty. Neurochirurgie 1987;33:166–168.

17 Bai B, Jazrawi LM, Kummer FJ, Spivak JM: The use of an injectable, biodegradable calcium phosphate bone substitute for the prophylactic augmentation of osteoporotic vertebrae and the management of vertebral compression fractures. Spine 1999;24:1521–1526.

18 Barr JD, Barr MS, Lemley TJ, McCann RM: Percutaneous vertebroplasty for pain relief and spinal stabilization. Spine 2000;25:923–928.
19 Mathis JM, Petri M, Naff N: Percutaneous vertebroplasty treatment of steroid-induced osteoporotic compression fractures. Arthritis Rheum 1998;41:171–175.
20 Cotten A, Dewatre F, Cortet B, et al: Percutaneous vertebroplasty for osteolytic metastases and myeloma: Effects of the percentage of lesion filling and the leakage of methyl methacrylate at clinical follow-up. Radiology 1996;200:525–530.
21 Dean JR, Ison KT, Gishen P: The strengthening effect of percutaneous vertebroplasty. Clin Radiol 2000;55:471–476.
22 O'Brien JP, Sims JT, Evans AJ: Vertebroplasty in patients with severe vertebral compression fractures: A technical report. Am J Neuroradiol 2000;21:1555–1558.
23 Cortet B, Cotten A, Boutry N, et al: Percutaneous vertebroplasty in the treatment of osteoporotic vertebral compression fractures: An open prospective study. J Rheumatol 1999;26:2222–2228.
24 Martin JB, Jean B, Sugiu K, et al: Vertebroplasty: Clinical experience and follow-up results. Bone 1999;25(suppl 2):11S–15S.
25 Padovani B, Kasriel O, Brunner P, Peretti-Viton P: Pulmonary embolism caused by acrylic cement: A rare complication of percutaneous vertebroplasty. Am J Neuroradiol 1999;20:375–377.
26 Cunin G, Boissonnet H, Petite H, Blanchat C, Guillemin G: Experimental vertebroplasty using osteoconductive granular material. Spine 2000;25:1070–1076.
27 Leeson MC, Lippitt SB: Thermal aspects of the use of polymethylmethacrylate in large metaphyseal defects in bone: A clinical review and laboratory study. Clin Orthop 1993;295:239–245.
28 Phillips H, Cole PV, Lettin AW: Cardiovascular effects of implanted acrylic bone cement. Br Med J 1971;iii:460–461.
29 Lieberman IH, Dudeney S, Reinhardt M-K, Bell G: Initial outcome and efficacy of 'kyphoplasty' in the treatment of painful osteoporotic vertebral compression fractures. Spine 2001;26: 1631–1638.
30 Ware JE Jr, Gandek B: Overview of the SF-36 Health Survey and the International Quality of Life Assessment (IQOLA) Project. J Clin Epidemiol 1998;51:903–912.
31 Sundaresan N, Krol G, Digiacinto G, Hughes J: Metastatic tumors of the spine; in Sundaresan N, Schmidek HH, Schiller AL, Rosenthal D (eds): Tumors of the Spine; Diagnosis and Clinical Management. London, Saunders, 1990, chap 29, pp 279–304.
32 McLain RF, Weinstein JN: Tumors of the spine; in Herkowitz HN, Garfin SR, Balderston RA, Eismont FJ, Bell GR, Wiesel SW (eds): Rothman-Simeone, the Spine. London, Saunders, 1999, chap 38, pp 1171–1206.
33 Rosen LS, Gordon D, Kaminski M, et al: Zoledronic acid versus pamidronate in the treatment of skeletal metastases in patients with breast cancer or osteolytic lesions of multiple myeloma: A phase III, double-blind, comparative trial. Cancer J, in press.
34 Dudeney S, Lieberman IH, Reinhardt MK, Hussein M: Kyphoplasty in the treatment of osteolytic vertebral compression fractures as a result of multiple myeloma. J Clin Oncol 2002;20: 2382–2387.

Isador H. Lieberman, B.Sc. MD, FRCS(C)
Department of Orthopaedic Surgery, A-41
The Cleveland Clinic Foundation, 9500 Euclid Ave., Desk A-41
Cleveland, OH 44195 (USA)
Tel. +1 216 445 2743, Fax +1 216 444 3328, E-Mail lieberi@ccf.org

Haid RW Jr, Subach BR, Rodts GE Jr (eds): Advances in Spinal Stabilization.
Prog Neurol Surg. Basel, Karger, 2003, vol 16, pp 251–265

Endoscopic Posterior Cervical Foraminotomy and Microdiscectomy

Mick J. Perez-Cruet, Richard G. Fessler

Institute for Spine Care, Chicago Institute of Neurosurgery and Neuroresearch, Rush-Presbyterian-St. Luke's Medical Center, Chicago, Ill., USA

Recently microendoscopic discectomy (MED) techniques have been applied to perform laminoforaminotomy and discectomy for unilateral cervical radiculopathy [1, 11] utilizing the MED technique and instrumentation (fig. 1) developed by Smith and Foley in 1997 for lumbar disc disease [4, 6]. The muscle-splitting approach used in this technique is effective in limiting postoperative pain and muscle spasms while maintaining the integrity of midline posterior muscular and ligamentous attachments to the spine. Minimally invasive posterior cervical microendoscopic discectomy and laminoforaminotomy (CMED) can provide a number of advantages including reduced approach-related morbidity, preservation of the motion segment, reduced patient postoperative pain and discomfort, and quicker patient recovery. In avoiding an anterior approach to the spine and maintaining segmental motion the incidence of hastened adjacent level disc degeneration may be reduced [3, 9, 10]. The muscle splitting approach used in this technique as apposed to the muscle stripping approach used in traditional posterior cervical discectomy and laminoforaminotomy may help to reduce paraspinal muscle denervation. Despite these many benefits there is a steep learning curve to mastering this technique, which may require additional training under the guidance of an experienced minimally invasive spine surgeon. Once trained in these techniques the results can be very satisfying for both clinician and patient. This chapter will focus on the technical considerations used in performing CMED effectively and safely.

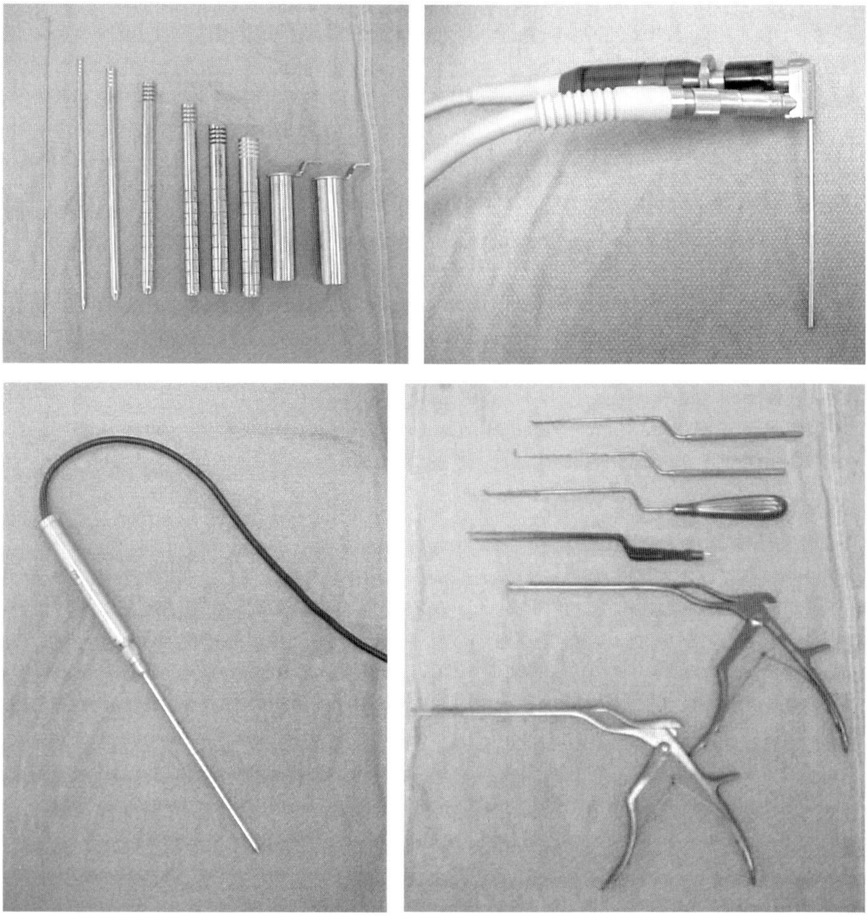

Fig. 1. METRx instrumentation used for performing CMED with figures showing K-wire, sequential dilators and tubular retractor (***a***), endoscopic assembly (***b***), long tapered Drill (***c***), and specialized instruments (***d***).

Background

Posterior cervical foraminotomy and microdiscectomy is a proven effective technique for the management of lateralized herniated disc and foraminal stenosis [2, 5, 7, 8, 12, 17–19]. The endoscopic approach is a further evolution of this technique with a primary benefit of reduction in approach-related morbidity. This is accomplished with a number of tubular dilators that allows for muscle splitting of the longitudinal muscular fibers to reach the facet complex as opposed to striping the muscle from the spinous process and lamina and aggressively retracting the muscles laterally to gain access to the facet complex. The instrumentations used to perform this technique were originally designed for the treatment of lumbar disc herniation (fig. 1). The ability to perform CMED was first determined in cadaveric studies [16]. These studies determined that the METRx system could be used effectively to treat degenerative cervical disease and then was applied safely in a clinical setting [1, 11].

Evaluation

Patient workups routinely include plain anteroposterior, lateral and oblique x-ray views to determine spine alignment, disc space height and foraminal encroachment. Additional radiographic evaluation of the cervical spine will include either a magnetic resonance image (MRI) or myelogram, and/or computed tomographic myelogram (CTM) to visualize the area of neural compression. CTM is particularly helpful in multilevel degenerative cervical disc disease to determine the level of maximal neural compression since this study clearly shows bone pathology, as well as foraminal stenosis and nerve root compression. In conjunction with thorough clinical history and physical examination, radiographic evaluation will help to determine the operative level. Further assessment can include selective nerve root blocks and or electromyelographic studies. Ultimately, it is critical to correctly identify the anatomic level from which the patient's radiculopathy originates in order to achieve surgical success.

Indications

Endoscopic posterior cervical foraminotomy is indicated for cases of lateralized disc herniation (fig. 2), osteophyte compression, and foraminal stenosis. Ideally, patients should present with painful cervical radiculopathy, which correlates with neural compression seen on MRI, myelogram, and/or CTM. This procedure is not recommended for cases of cervical myelopathy from spondylosis or central disc herniation. Whereas traditional surgical teaching guides us to address pathology from an anterior approach when there is straightening or kyphosis of the spine, the endoscopic posterior approach can be used for cases of posterolateral disc herniation or foraminal stenosis with mild to moderate kyphosis so long as there is no evidence of instability. For these patients, particular caution must be taken to avoid resecting too much of the medial facet complex during the decompression. Studies have shown that

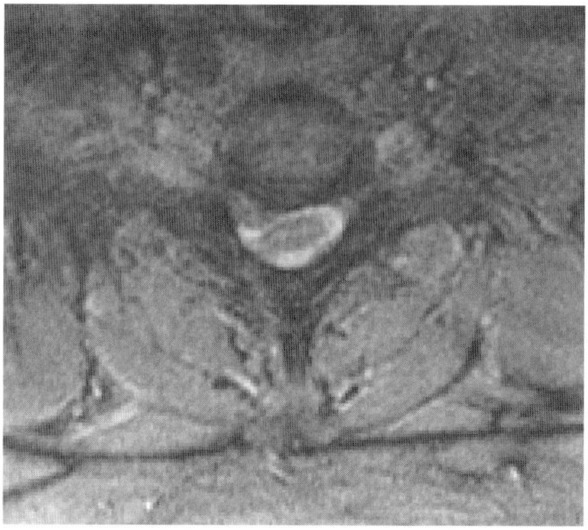

Fig. 2. Lateralized left C6,7 disc herniation ideal for treatment using the CMED approach.

up to 50% of the facet complex can be resected unilaterally without inducing iatrogenic instability [15]. Since the 30° angled endoscope allows for more extensive facet resection, care is taken during this procedure to avoid taking too much facet [16].

It is important to realize that even with a good clinical history of radiculopathy and a seemingly appropriate radiographic finding, a potential for misdiagnosis can exist. As the incidence of multilevel disc degeneration is high on MRI and CTM for elderly patients, it is statistically not uncommon that some degree of pathological change will be seen at any given level on imaging studies. For such patients, a careful search to exclude other causes of nerve root pain should be completed prior to operative intervention. The differential for nerve root pain includes spinal canal tumors, trauma, inflammatory diseases, demyelinating conditions, toxic and allergic conditions, hemorrhage, congenital defects, metabolic diseases, neuropathies, thoracic outlet syndrome, rotator cuff pathology, impingement syndromes, bursitis, arthritis of the shoulder, and bicipital tendonitis. It is important for spinal surgeons to be familiar with these disorders in order to properly exclude them from the list of possible etiologies before subjecting the patient to unneeded surgery. Electromyographic (EMG) and nerve conduction velocity studies done by a competent neurologist or physiatrist may be particularly helpful in this regard. Lastly, it is prudent to perform a psychological screening of all patients prior to performing this

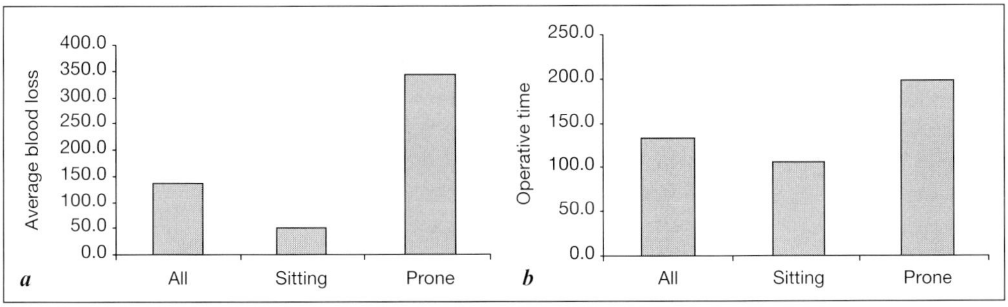

Fig. 3. Operative blood loss (***a***) and time (***b***) when performing the CMED procedure in all patients combined, in the semisitting position, and in the prone position.

procedure and to rule out secondary gain or psychological issues that may result in a poor surgical outcome.

Anesthesia and Operative Setup

After appropriate preoperative evaluation and medical clearance, patients were brought to the operative suite. Following the induction of general endotracheal anesthesia, adequate intravenous access was secured. An arterial line is placed to enable continuous blood pressure monitoring and control. Adequate blood pressure is maintained to assure spinal cord perfusion during this procedure. During the initial experience with the CMED technique, patients were placed in the prone position. However, this led to bleeding that often obscured the endoscopic image during the operative procedure and resulted in increased operative times and blood loss (fig. 3). A change to the semisitting position using a Mayfield head holder (fig. 4) has resulted in significantly improved operative visualization, relieved epidural venous congestion, and decreased operative blood loss and operative times (fig. 3). The advantage of this position is that blood does not accumulate at the bottom of the tubular retractor. Blood loss was found to be substantially less and the procedure can be preformed with the tubular retractor positioned at a comfortable height for the surgeon (fig. 5). Because of the slightly increased risk of air embolism, precordial Doppler as well as end tidal pCO_2 are measures. We do not routinely place a central venous line. Adequate intraoperative measures taken in the event of an air embolism should be familiar to the operative team prior to undertaking this procedure.

Before final patient positioning, utmost care is directed at ensuring that the cervical spine and neck musculature are not kinked or held in an unfavorable

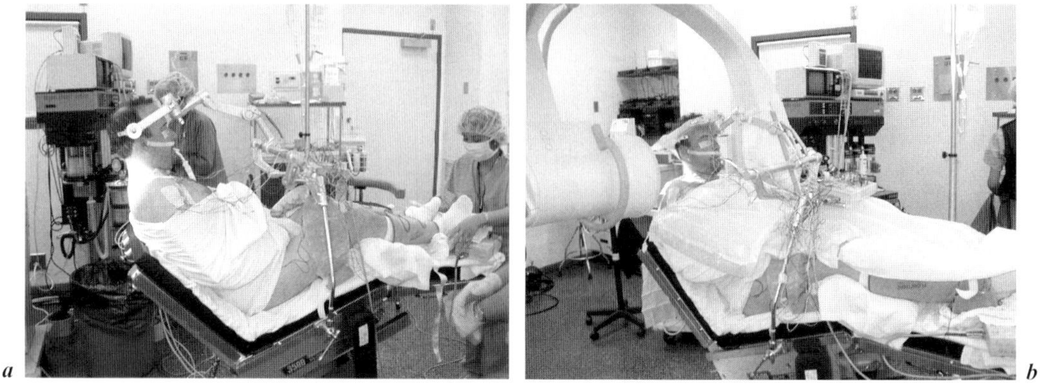

Fig. 4. Patient positioned in a semisitting position with head affixed in a Mayfield head holder (***a***) with lateral C-arm in place (***b***).

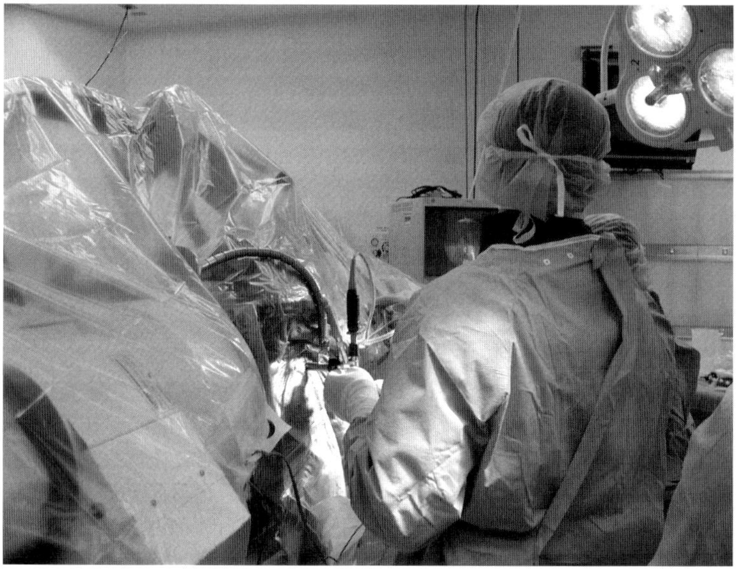

Fig. 5. The position of the surgeon, while standing behind the patient, viewing the endoscopic image on the operative monitor. Note the ergonomically favorable position of the surgeon's hands and body posture.

position. The neck is placed in a neutral or slightly flexed position to ensure adequate jugular venous drainage and the head is secured in the Mayfield holder to assure direct midline positioning. In most instances a Foley catheter is not placed except in instances where more than one level is performed.

Somatosensory evoked potentials, as well as EMG recordings, are measured to further ensure the safety of the procedure. After the initial induction of anesthesia, we have refrained from the use of neuromuscular paralytics to allow for improved feedback from the nerve root(s) during the operation. A single preoperative dose of either Ancef or vancomycin is used. We do not routinely employ Solumedrol or other glucocorticoids for neural protection.

The fluoroscopic C-arm is brought into the surgical field and positioned with the arc over the patient so that real-time lateral fluoroscopic images can easily be obtained (fig. 6). Although we have not typically use anteroposterior images, they can also be utilized to facilitate docking of the initial K-wire and tubular retractors on the facet complex. The surgeon generally stands directly behind the neck of the patient with the video and fluoroscopic monitors placed within direct view of the surgeon to allow optimal ergonomic flow during the procedure (fig. 5).

Surgical Technique

We employed the METRx system (Medtronic Sofamor-Danek, Memphis, Tenn., USA) of endoscopic retractors, camera, and instruments for the procedures (fig. 1). As this system was initially designed for lumbar discectomy, several modifications have been made to better optimize its use in the CMED procedure. These include lengthening of the table-mounted retractor as well as a better selection of smaller profile curettes and Kerrison punches for use in the more delicate cervical spine. An initial stab incision was made approximately 1–2 cm off midline ipsilateral to and at the level of the pathology. Under fluoroscopic guidance, a K-wire was inserted through the posterior cervical musculature and fascia down to the facet complex or lateral mass of the operative level. Particular caution was taken at this point to insure that the guidewire was docked on bone to avoid inadvertent dural penetration medially or slipping off the facet complex laterally (fig. 6). Once the guidewire is docked on the facet complex in question, the skin incision was extended above and below the K-wire for a total length of approximately 2.0 cm. The skin edges are retracted with a small retractor and the cervical fascia incised using either a Metzenbaum scissors or Bovey cautery. Care should be taken not to cut muscle fibers during this procedure as this can cause unnecessary blood loss. Due to the relative thickness of the posterior cervical fascia, this sharp opening of the fascia is required to allow for easier and safe passage of the sequential dilating cannulas with a minimum use of force. If a skin-covering barrier such as ioband was placed, it should be circumferentially removed from around the skin incision to prevent plastic sequestra that can occur during placement of the percutaneous

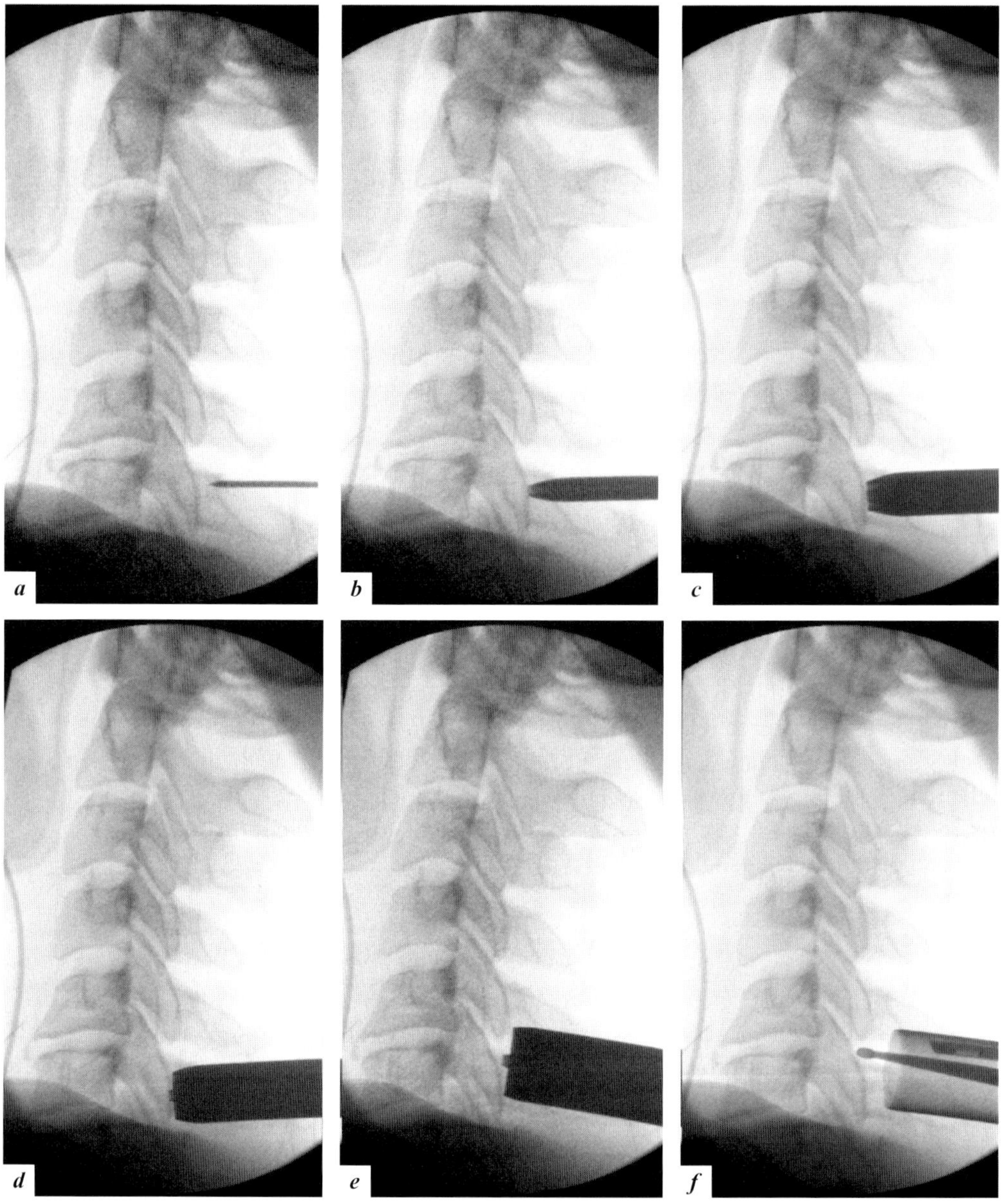

Fig. 6. Lateral fluoroscopic images showing docking of the K-wire on the facet complex (***a***), first dilator (***b***), second dilator after K-wire is removed (***c***), third dilator (***d***), fourth dilator (***e***), and tubular retractor in place with curette-identifying facet (***f***).

soft tissue dilators. It is important to remove the K-wire after the initial dilator is passed. A series of dilators are then sequentially inserted using a gentle downward rotating maneuver through the posterior neck musculature, over which an 18-mm tubular retractor was inserted. Real-time lateral fluoroscopic images were obtained throughout the above procedure to insure proper docking of the sequential dilators and tubular retractors on the facet complex (fig. 6a–f). The working channel (tubular retractor) is then attached to a flexible arm affixed to the operating table side rail and locked in position. The retractor arm is positioned to avoid obscuring the lateral fluoroscopic image. The endoscope is then attached to the tubular retractor via a circular plastic friction couple. Additionally, the endoscopic camera used today has far superior resolution and clarity than the cameras used during our previous cadaveric studies and initial operative cases. Further modifications of the instruments are ongoing to improve the safety, efficacy, and ease of this procedure.

Once the tubular retractor is set in the desired position, a Bovey cautery with a long insulated tip is used to remove the remaining muscle and soft tissue overlying the facet complex. A small straight or up-going curette in conjunction with lateral fluoroscopic imaging can further define the bone anatomy and localization of surgical anatomy (fig. 6f). The dissection is initially started laterally where the bone is easily palpated with the Bovey tip. Once the bone of the lateral facet complex in exposed, the dissection of muscle off the facet complex continues medial to expose the laminofacet junction with care not to enter the interlaminar space with the Bovey tip. To prevent Bovey cautery smoke from obscuring the endoscopic image during this procedure a frequent on/off technique is used that allows smoke to clear from the tube before proceeding. A suction tubing is also attached to the endoscopic device. If the tubular retractor is properly placed initially only a small piece of muscle tissue needs be removed to expose the facet complex. Often the ligamentum flavum is thinned or altogether absent near the lateral edge of the interlaminar space thereby placing the dura and spinal cord at higher risk. With the bone well visualized the inferior edge of the superior lamina and the medial edge of the lateral mass-facet complex are identified with a small straight or up-going endoscopic curette. The facet complex at the proper level is clearly identified before proceeding. Bleeding from epidural veins is controlled using a long tipped endoscopic bipolar cautery. For bleeding underneath the edge of the lamina, angled bipolar forceps with a 45° angle are often useful. After the medial facet plane has been clearly defined, a small angled 1- or 2-mm Kerrison rongeur is used to begin the foraminotomy (fig. 7a). Periosteal and bone bleeding is addressed with bone wax and cautery. In cases of marked facet arthropathy and enlargement, a drill with a long endoscopic bit (e.g. AM-8 bit with Midas Rex or TAC bit with MEDNext drill) can be used to further thin the medial facet and lateral mass.

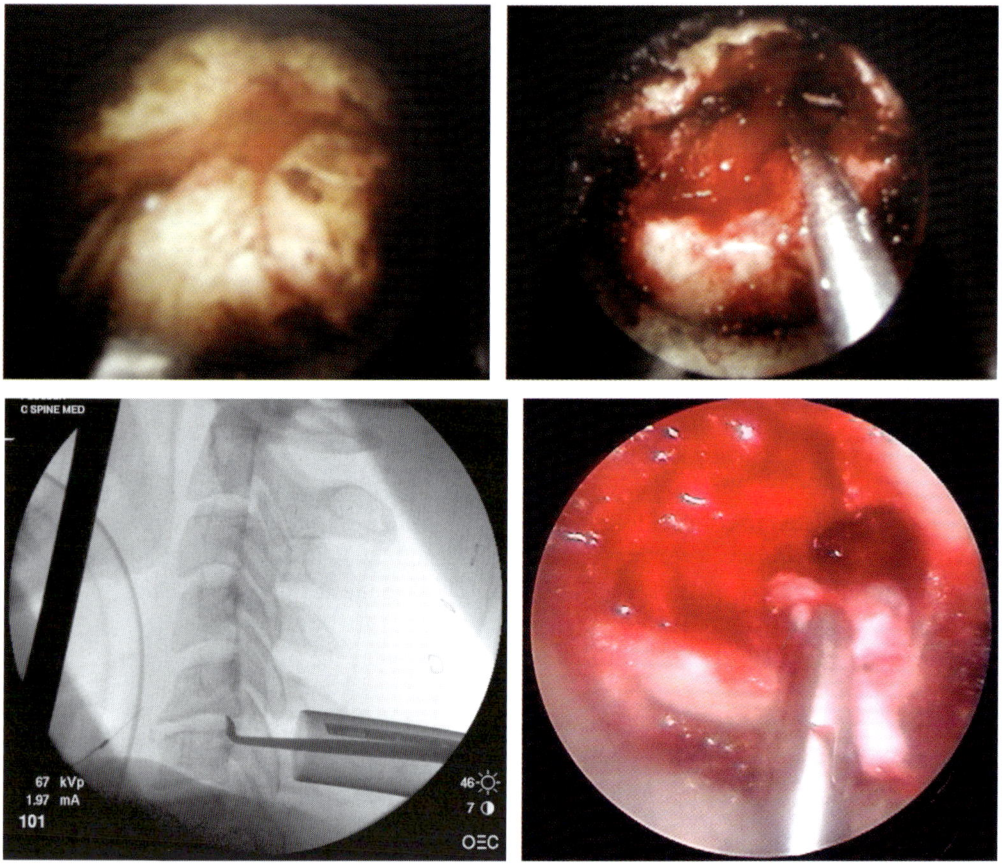

Fig. 7. Intraoperative images showing Kerrison punch initiating medial facet removal (***a***), nerve probe passing out of the foramen once foraminotomy is performed with underlying nerve root exposed (***b***), lateral fluoroscopic image with down-going curette on disc under nerve root (***c***), and endoscopic image showing removal of disc fragment (***d***).

Frequent dissection of the soft tissue off the bone with an angled curette facilitates safe use of the Kerrison rongeur. In this fashion, the decompression is carefully continued inferiorly and laterally along the course of the neural foramen. The laminoforaminotomy is completed when the nerve root had been well exposed along its proximal foraminal course. The adequacy of the decompression should be confirmed by palpating the root along its course with a small nerve hook (fig. 7b).

In cases where a herniated cervical disk or free disc fragment is present, additional exposure is obtained by drilling a small portion of the superomedial pedicle directly below the exiting nerve root. As the nerve root lies directly against this portion of the pedicle, removing a small portion of the pedicle will create enough space for passing a down-going curette (fig. 7c) under the nerve root to remove a disc fragment without traumatizing the nerve root (fig. 7d). Additionally osteophytes encountered in this region can also be drilled or curetted as needed. Prior to closure the nerve root is palpated along its anterior surface to ensure that no residual compression exists along its course.

Far lateral foraminal stenosis or disc herniations can also be decompressed through this approach. As the nerve root often passes in close proximity to the vertebral artery laterally, particular attention should be paid during decompression in this area. Inadvertent passage of instruments beyond the bone defining the posterior margin of the foramen transversarium should be avoided. Brisk dark bleeding is often encountered from the rich venous plexus, which typically surrounds the space around the vertebral artery. When encountered, such bleeding should serve as a useful warning to limit further dissection and thus prevent inadvertent arterial injury. Unnecessary excessive decompression of the facet should be avoided to prevent iatrogenic instability of the cervical motion segment. Raynor et al. [15] concluded that the integrity of the majority of the facet joint is essential for stability and that no more than 50% of the facet should be removed to maintain its integrity.

Wound Closure

After inspection of the nerve root, meticulous hemostasis should be obtained by a combination of bipolar cautery and gentle tamponade with thrombin-soaked gel-foam pledgets. The area is then copiously irrigated with lactated ringers impregnated with bacitracin antibiotics. Although optional, we have usually placed a small piece of gel-foam soaked with Solumedrol gently over the laminoforaminotomy defect. Use of epidural morphine paste or similar cocktails is reasonable if there is no evidence of dural erosion or tear. Alternatively, Marcaine (0.25%) can be injected around the incision. Such agents may help to reduce postoperative pain and allow for more rapid recovery and ambulation. The tubular retractor and endoscope are then removed and a routine closure of the fascia and skin performed. As the defect is typically quite small, only a limited amount of closure need be performed and a drain is not needed. A 0-Vicryl-type reabsorbable stitch is used to close the lumbodorsal fascia in a figure of 8. Inverted 2-0 Vicryl stitches are used to reapproximate the subcutaneous layer. Dermabond is used to reapproximate the skin edges and no dressing is applied as the Dermabond will adhere to it. Dermabond is attractive as it keeps the skin edges closely approximated for a 7- to 10-day period as well as providing a waterproof barrier. The patient can thus shower almost immediately after surgery.

Postoperative Care

The patient was then awakened from anesthesia and taken to the postanesthesia recovery unit. Most patients have the procedure on an ambulatory basis; therefore, long-acting inhalational and intravenous agents should be avoided to allow for rapid awakening of the patient postoperatively. Additionally, use of only short-acting muscle relaxants for initial induction will allow for better monitoring of nerve root function as well as quicker extubation of the patient after surgery. This procedure performed on an outpatient basis requires thorough perioperative patient education [14].

Once in the postanesthesia recovery area, the patients are allowed to rapidly mobilize and ambulate as tolerated. Arterial and intravenous lines are removed early on. If a Foley catheter was placed it is generally removed before the patient leaves the operative suite. Done correctly, this procedure does not result in either instability or fusion of the operated cervical motion segment. Therefore no cervical collar is required. Soft collars and other comfortable semirigid collars can be given to patients for their comfort if desired. It is important to emphasize to patients, however, that chronic dependence on such orthosis will only lead to further deconditioning of the cervical musculature. Depending on their preoperative medications, patients are typically discharged on a combination of muscle relaxants (e.g. baclofen or Flexeril), nonsteroidal anti-inflammatories (e.g. Toradol, Vioxx, or Celebrex), and an oral opioid for breakthrough pain (i.e. Vicodin or Darvocet). When we compared our patients with patients treated via open cervical foraminotomy, we found that the microendoscopic foraminotomy (MEF) group used significantly less pain medications postoperatively than did the open group [11]. Patients undergoing this procedure typically recovered rapidly with only mild to moderate discomfort upon discharge. Of our last 30 cases, the majority of patients were discharged in 6 h or less.

Complication Avoidance

Complications can be avoided by having a thorough understanding of cervical anatomy, proper training in endoscopic spinal techniques and a knowledge of possible complications. Adamson [1] retrospectively reviewed 100 cases of patients undergoing endoscopic posterior cervical laminoforaminotomy

(MEF) and reported complications in 3 patients; 2 cases of dural puncture required no intervention other than gel-foam and 1 case of superficial wound infection was reported. In a series by Khoo et al. [11] three complications occurred in 25 patients and were attributable to surgical technique. These included two small cerebral spinal fluid (CSF) leaks and 1 case of partial-thickness dural violation. For the 2 cases where a CSF leak occurred, no direct repair was required as the durotomy was very small. After 2–3 days of routine lumbar drainage for patients with CSF leaks, none of these patients went on to have long-term clinical sequelae of chronic CSF leak or symptomatic pseudomeningocele. Thus we have routinely employed a lumbar drain for 2–3 days postoperatively to help closure of the small dural tear. Additional adjuncts such as fibrin glue, fat or muscle grafts can also be used. Spinal headaches and nausea associated with the lumbar drainage were treated symptomatically with nonsteroidal anti-inflammatory medications and bed rest. If a large durotomy occurs, direct dural repair can be attempted if specialized instruments are available for use through the endoscopic tube. Castro-Viejo-type needle holders and long forceps are particularly useful in this regard. In rare instances, conversion to an open procedure may be necessary to close large dural violations. To date, we have not had problems with delayed pseudomeningoceles or continued CSF leaks. The risk of dural injury can be reduced with experience in performing this technique with most durotomies occurring on initial patients undergoing this procedure. Patients should be advised of this potential complication and informed that with appropriate management durotomy results in no adverse clinical result.

A potential complication, which has not been reported, is iatrogenic injury during the surgical approach and muscle dilatation portion of this operation. Unlike the thoracodorsal fascia, the posterior cervical fascia is very thick and must be cut under direct visualization to prevent hyperextension of the neck during insertion of the dilators. The initial K-wire or smaller dilators can be inadvertently pushed between the cervical lamina resulting in nerve root or spinal cord injury; therefore, this portion of the procedure is performed under lateral fluoroscopic guidance. An anteroposterior fluoroscopic image can also help in safely docking the K-wire and subsequent dilators on the facet complex. Additionally, lateral displacement of the K-wire or dilators can result in nerve root or vertebral artery injury. Brisk venous bleeding can also result if the dilators inadvertently slip lateral to the facet complex during placement. This is controlled with gentle gel-foam packing and/or bipolar cautery. The K-wire is removed after the first dilator is passed and subsequent dilators securely docked onto the laminar facet junction.

To help reduce intraoperative bleeding the CMED procedure is performed in the semisitting position (fig. 4). A series of patients comparing cervical laminoforaminotomy performed in the open prone position, microendoscopic prone position, or microendoscopic sitting position revealed reduced operative times, estimated blood loss, postoperative length of stay, and pain medication requirements in the microendoscopic sitting position group [11]. The sitting position significantly reduces epidural venous engorgement, thus decreasing blood loss. In addition, this position allows blood to flow out of the tubular retractor, rather than accumulating and obscuring the endoscopic view of the operative field. Although none of the sitting position patients experienced an air embolism the potential increased risk for air embolism precludes the use of a pericardial Doppler even though the incidence of clinically significant embolic event remains extremely low.

Conclusion

The endoscopic posterior cervical laminoforaminotomy and discectomy technique is a safe and effectively treatment of posterior lateral cervical disc herniation and/or foraminal stenosis. The learning curve associated with this technique requires additional training and we recommend that this training be performed under the guidance of an experienced endoscopic minimally invasive spine surgeon. Cadaveric training can further familiarize the surgeon with this technique. The clinical results are very satisfying since patients experience less postoperative pain and can be discharged on the same operative day.

References

1 Adamson TE: Microendoscopic posterior cervical laminoforaminotomy for unilateral radiculopathy: Results of a new technique in 100 cases. J Neurosurg 2001;95(1 suppl):51–57.
2 Aldrich F: Posterolateral microdiscectomy for cervical monoradiculopathy caused by posterolateral soft cervical disc sequestration. J Neurosurg 1990;72:370–377.
3 Baba G, Furusawa N, Imura S, et al: Late radiographic findings after anterior cervical fusion for spondylotic myeloradiculopathy. Spine 1993;18:2167–2173.
4 Brayda-Bruno M, Cinnella P: Posterior endoscopic discectomy (and other procedures). Eur Spine J 2000;9:S24–S29.
5 Fager CA: Posterolateral approach to ruptured median and paramedian cervical disc. Surg Neurol 1983;20:443–452.
6 Foley KT, Smith MM: Microendoscopic discectomy. Tech Neurosurg 1997;3:301–307.
7 Henderson CM, Henney RG, Shuey HM, et al: Posterolateral foraminotomy as an exclusive operative technique for cervical radiculopathy: A review of 846 consecutively operated cases. Neurosurgery 1983;13:504–512.
8 Herkowitz HN, Kurz LT: Surgical management of cervical soft disc herniation: A comparison between the anterior and posterior approach. Spine 1990;15:1026–1030.
9 Hilibrand AS, Yoo JU, Carlson GD, et al: The success of anterior cervical arthrodesis adjacent to a previous fusion. Spine 1997;22:1574–1579.

10 Hunter LY, Braunstein EM, Bailey RR: Radiographic changes following anterior cervical fusion. Spine 1980;5:399–401.
11 Khoo LT, Perez-Cruet MJ, Laich DT, Fessler RG: Posterior cervical microendoscopic foraminotomy; in Perez-Cruet MJ, Fessler RG (eds): Outpatient Spinal Surgery. St. Louis, Quality Medical Publishing, 2002, pp 71–93.
12 Krupp W, Muke R: Clinical results of the foraminotomy as described by Fryholm for the treatment of lateral cervical disc herniation. Acta Neurochir (Wien) 1990;107:22–29.
13 Perez-Cruet MJ, Smith M, Foley K: Microendoscopic lumbar discectomy; in Perez-Cruet MJ, Fessler RG (eds): Outpatient Spinal Surgery. St. Louis, Quality Medical Publishing, 2002, pp 171–183.
14 Perez-Cruet MJ, Rice-Wyllie L, Pieper DR: Patient education; in Perez-Cruet MJ, Fessler RG (eds): Outpatient Spinal Surgery. St. Louis, Quality Medical Publishing, 2002, pp 35–47.
15 Raynor RB, Pugh J, Shapiro I: Cervical facetectomy and its effect of spine strength. J Neurosurg 1985;63:278–282.
16 Roh SW, Kim DH, Cardoso AC, Fessler RG: Endoscopic foraminotomy using microendoscopic discectomy system in cadaveric specimens. Spine 2000;25:260–264.
17 Simeone F, Dillin W: Treatment of cervical disc disease: Selection of operative approach. Contemp Neurosurg 1986;8:1–6.
18 Tomaras CR, Blacklock JB, Parker WD, Harper RL: Outpatient surgical treatment of cervical radiculopathy. J Neurosurg 1997;87:41–43.
19 Williams RW: Microcervical foraminotomy. A surgical alternative for intractable radicular pain. Spine 1983;8:708–716.

Mick J. Perez-Cruet, MD, MS
Institute for Spine Care, Department of Neurosurgery
Chicago Institute of Neurosurgery and Neuroresearch,
Rush-Presbyterian-St. Luke's Medical Center, 1725 West Harrison Street
Suite 970, Chicago, IL 60612 (USA)
Tel. +1 708 250 3194, Fax +1 312 942 2176, E-Mail perezcruet@yahoo.com

Haid RW Jr, Subach BR, Rodts GE Jr (eds): Advances in Spinal Stabilization.
Prog Neurol Surg. Basel, Karger, 2003, vol 16, pp 266–276

An Update on Endoscopic Thoracic Spinal Surgery: Thoracic Microendoscopic Discectomy

Mick J. Perez-Cruet[a], *Bong-Soo Kim*[b], *Faheem Sandhu*[b], *Richard G. Fessler*[b]

[a] Directory of Minimally Invasive Spine Surgery, Department of Neurosurgery, Chicago Institute of Neurosurgery and Neuroresearch, Rush-Presbyterian St. Luke's Medical Center and
[b] Division of Neurosurgery, University of Chicago, Chicago, Ill., USA

Clinically significant thoracic disc herniation is a relatively rare condition with an estimated annual incidence of approximately one per million. Surgical management of thoracic disc herniation comprises between 0.15 and 4% of all operations for herniated discs including those of the cervical and lumbar spine [3, 40, 41].

Several surgical techniques have been developed to approach the thoracic spine including costotransversectomy, lateral extracavitary, lateral parascapular extrapleural, transfacet, transpedicular, and transthoracic approaches [1, 17, 41]. Although all of these approaches have been successful in reaching thoracic pathology, each procedure requires a relatively large skin incision and extensive bony work that subsequently may lead to considerable postoperative morbidity [4, 12, 37, 41].

Outcomes from the traditional posterior approach, thoracic laminectomy, to treat thoracic disc herniation are especially poor with large percentages of patients failing to improve or, more significantly, deteriorating further. Although anterior approaches facilitate exposure to the ventral aspect of the thecal sac, they require entry into the pleural cavity and place the intrathoracic contents at risk. Posterolateral approaches, especially the lateral extracavitary one, provide many of the benefits of an anterior approach without the additional risks of entering the thoracic cavity. Unfortunately, the exposure for this approach requires extensive muscle dissection that adds to the postoperative morbidity.

Perot and Munro [33] and Ransohoff et al. [34] performed the initial transthoracic approach to thoracic disc herniation after which the transthoracic approach became a standard procedure to manage thoracic disc herniations. This approach provides excellent visualization of the ventral aspect of the thoracic spine without the risk of spinal cord manipulation. However, the thoracotomy used in this approach requires a large skin incision, extensive lung and rib retraction, and muscle dissection, all of which can contribute to postoperative pulmonary dysfunction, pain and increased morbidity.

To reduce the morbidity associated with the thoracotomy technique and other approaches previously mentioned, less invasive thoracoscopic techniques have been developed and more recently refined for the treatment of herniated thoracic disc [1, 8, 9, 35, 36]. Thoracoscopy is capable of producing the same exposure as the transthoracic route without the need for a large thoracotomy incision. Thoracoscopy was introduced by Jacobeus in 1910 [19]. However, this technique was not widely adopted at that time due to poor illumination of intrathoracic structures and other technical limitations. It was not until the 1970s that the modern era of surgical endoscopy began following a number of technical advancements such as fiberoptics, and the operating endoscopes. Introduction of the video camera into thoracoscopic surgery was the next major advance leading to the introduction of the video-assisted thoracoscopic surgery technique [14, 18, 19, 35]. Thoracoscopic discectomy is an effective alternative to traditional open thoracotomy techniques that has been found to reduce the incidence of pulmonary morbidity [11, 13], intercostal neuralgia, and shoulder girdle dysfunction [13, 20]. Although the incidence thoracoscopic complications may vary they are similar to those encountered with open thoracotomy [16, 30].

Although the procedure-associated morbidity is much less than with thoracotomy, the prevalence of pulmonary complications such as postoperative atelectasis, pneumothorax, pleural effusion, and hemothorax is considerable [7, 10, 22, 37, 39]. In addition, thoracoscopic surgery is technically demanding and requires attainment of new surgical skills. Therefore, it is advised that surgeons perform the thoracoscopic procedures only after pursuing appropriate training that includes extensive practice of this skill in a surgical laboratory [4]. Even today the use of video-assisted thoracoscopic surgery techniques to treat thoracic disc herniation have not been widely adopted due to the steep learning curve which requires specialized training to master.

The primary indication for thoracoscopic spinal surgery is management of herniated discs that compress the spinal cord and/or nerve root. Severe or progressive myelopathy from spinal cord compression caused by disc herniation is an absolute indication for surgery [19, 27]. In addition to thoracic discectomy, current indications for thoracoscopic spine surgery include tissue biopsies, thoracic paravertebral abscess drainage and debridement, anterior spinal release and/or fusion for spinal deformity, stabilization and fusion of thoracic and thoracolumbar fractures, corpectomy for vertebral tumors and placement of anterior spinal instrumentation for fusion [2, 5–8, 23–26, 29, 36].

We have developed a novel posterolateral, minimally invasive thoracic microendoscopic discectomy (TMED) technique that potentially provides a less morbid approach to the treatment of thoracic disc herniation. The procedure is performed via a posterolateral approach with the patient in the prone position (fig. 1a) and therefore avoids entry into the thoracic cavity. A number of studies have shown that minimally invasive spine surgery is associated with less disruption of normal tissue, less blood loss, and less procedure time than traditional open procedures, which translates to patients experiencing reduced postoperative pain, reduced hospitalization, and reduced recovery time [1, 4, 15, 32]. Based on our validation data from cadaveric studies we have demonstrated that this technique could be safely implemented into clinical use. The technique is a modification of the lateral extracavitary approach, which was a further modification of the lateral rachiotomy initially performed in 1961 for the treatment of Pott's disease by Larson et al. [21]. Unlike the traditional lateral extracavitary approach which requires significant muscle, rib head and transverse process excision to reach the thoracic disc, the TMED approach avoids much of this dissection. It uses a series of muscle dilators, a tubular retractor and endoscope that was initially developed to approach lumbar herniated disc pathology [31]. Herein we report this novel minimally invasive technique to treat herniated thoracic disc pathology.

Indication

The clear indication to perform the TMED procedure is in patients with thoracic disc herniation causing myelopathy in order to improve neurological function and prevent further injury to the spinal cord. However, the longer the myelopathy has been present the less likely is restoration of normal neurological function. Severe and refractory radiculopathy is another indication for surgery. Thoracic radicular pain from disc herniation is typically sharp, lancinating pain that radiates unilaterally from posterior to anterior around the chest wall in its dermatomal distribution correlating to the herniated thoracic disc. Radiculopathy can develop without loss of neurological function because of the overlap of innervation of adjacent intercostal nerves. Radiculopathy may be present without myelopathic manifestations. Isolated thoracic radiculopathy often responds to conservative management such as nonsteroidal anti-inflammatory medications, oral steroids, epidural injection, intercostal nerve injection, activity modification, and hyperextension brace [41]. Pain relief after thoracic discectomy is usually favorable in patients with radiculopathy, even for those with long-standing radiculopathy. Although it is controversial whether patients with localized back pain and axial pain without myelopathy require surgery or not, most surgeons do not recommend thoracic discectomy for isolated back pain unless it is associated with a neurological deficit [28, 29, 37, 38, 40]. This technique is not recommended for a large calcified midline thoracic disc that may require an anterior approach.

Technique

Posterolateral Microendoscopic Discectomy

We have developed a novel posterolateral, minimally invasive TMED technique that potentially provides a less morbid treatment for thoracic disc herniation compared to traditional techniques. This method has been used successfully to treat lateralized and central thoracic disc herniations causing radicular and myelopathic symptoms. This technique was developed with similar instruments used to perform a microendoscopic lumbar discectomy using the METRx system of tubular dilators and retractor initially developed by Smith and Foley, see Perez-Cruet et al. [31]. The procedure is performed as follows.

Patient Positioning and Operative Setup

After general endotracheal induction and placement of a Foley catheter, the patient is positioned prone on a radiolucent Wilson frame. All pressure points are padded adequately and the arms are placed above the patient making sure not to overextend at the shoulder beyond 90° (fig. 1a). Somatosensory evoked potentials are measured throughout the procedure. Any change in somatosensory evoked potentials during the procedure warrants investigation as to the probable cause. The fluoroscopic C-arm is positioned to allow for a lateral x-ray image of the operative area. A video monitor is placed opposite the surgeon to allow for a clear field of view of the monitor. The back is shaved and prepped in a routine surgical fashion.

Under fluoroscopic guidance a spinal needle was used to locate the level of the herniated thoracic disc. The exact location of the thoracic disc herniation was confirmed by counting from the sacrum below and/or from the occiput above. Once the correct location was identified, a Steinmann pin was placed at the medial aspect of the transverse process at the level of the thoracic disc herniation. An incision of approximately 2 cm was made 3–4 cm lateral to the midline, depending on the size of the patient, through which a series of tubular muscle dilators was placed (fig. 1b, c). A tubular retractor was placed over the final muscle dilator and then affixed to a flexible arm secured firmly to the operative table (fig. 1d). The endoscopic assembly was then focused, white balanced, and passed down the center of the tubular retractor (fig. 1e). Once the endoscope was in place the orientation of the endoscopic image seen on the monitor was adjusted so that medial anatomy was at the top of the monitor screen, lateral anatomy at the bottom, and rostral and caudal anatomy was in the same orientation as the patient on the operative table. This greatly facilitated the procedure and aided in orienting the surgeon throughout the procedure. Surgical orientation throughout the case is of upmost importance to prevent inadvertent entrance into the spinal canal and this is facilitated by lateral and AP fluoroscopic images to help confirm the location of dissection. The proper level was then reconfirmed using lateral fluoroscopy and the TMED procedure was performed under endoscopic visualization. The muscle and soft tissue overlying the proximal portion of the transverse process and lateral facet complex were removed using an insulated Bovey cautery. Careful probing with a ball-ended probe helps in defining the bone margins and liberal use of fluoroscope imaging also helps to orient the surgeon thoroughout the procedure. The approach is similar to that of a transforaminal approach and adequate laterality of the approach reduces any manipulation of the spinal cord during disc removal. Access to the disc space required removal of a small amount of bone. This is facilitated by the use of a long tapered high-speed drill. Once the bone architecture is defined a small portion of the proximal rib head and transverse process and a portion of the lateral aspect of the facet complex are removed. This procedure facilitated widening of the neural foramen. The thoracic pedicle of the more caudal vertebral body was identified and followed to the appropriate disc level. The disc annulus was identified and the epidural veins coagulated with a bipolar cautery. The annulus was cut with a thin anulotomy knife and the discectomy was performed. The lateral projectory of the tubular retractor through a transforaminal type approach allowed for extensive disc removal under the thoracic spinal cord and dura enabling even midline placed thoracic disc herniations to be removed (fig. 2a, b). Following complete discectomy further inspection underneath the dura and spinal cord using a Woodson elevator or similar instrument assured complete decompression (fig. 1f). The tubular retractor was removed and a suture was placed in the thoracodorsal fascia. Interrupted subcuticular sutures were placed and the skin closed with Dermabond.

This technique has a number of advantages over other traditional techniques used to perform thoracic discectomy and includes the following: avoidance of traversing through the thoracic cavity, maintaining the integrity of the disc, avoidance of the need for thoracic fusion, and avoidance of extensive

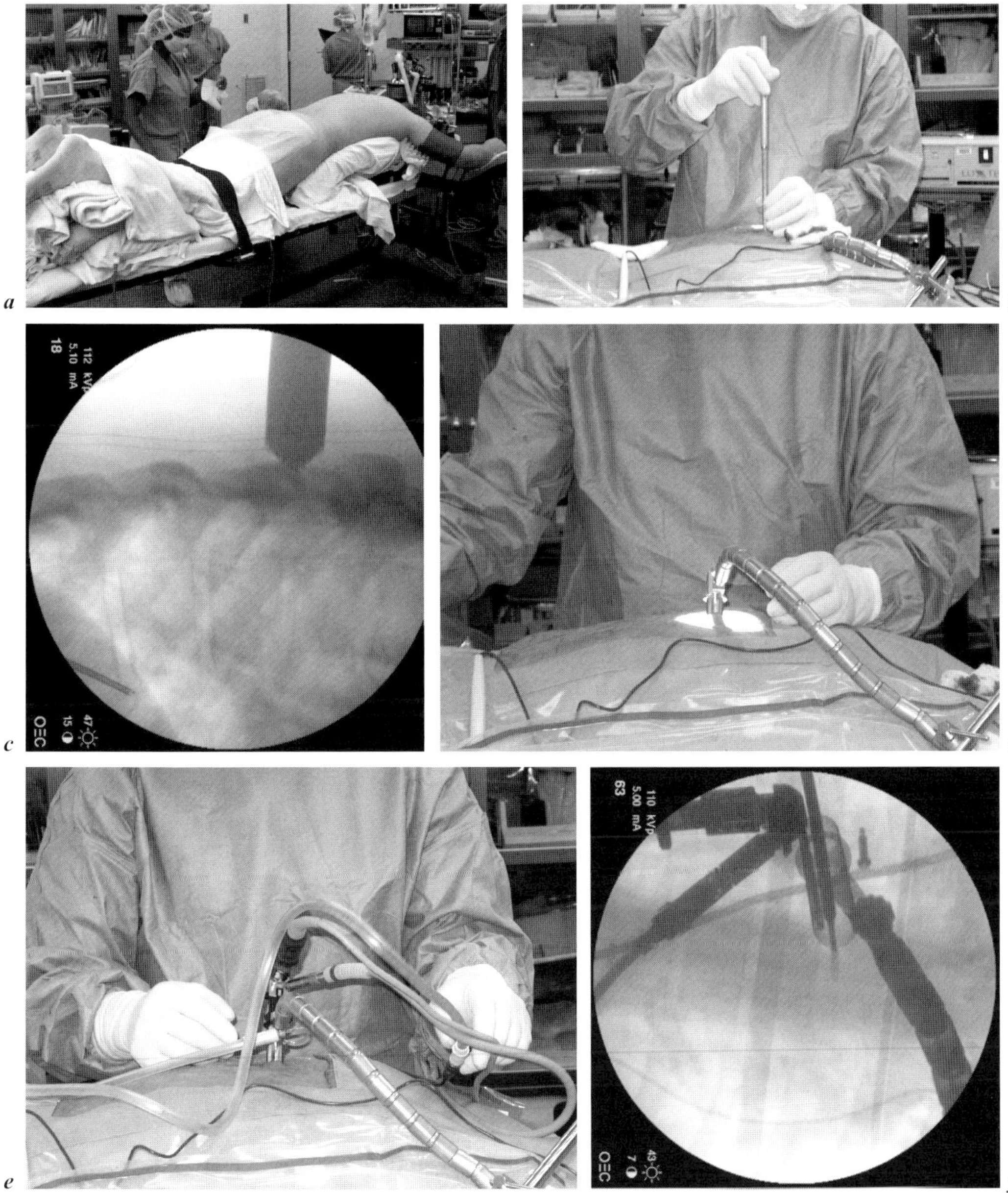

Fig. 1. ***a*** Positioning of the patient in the prone position on a radiolucent frame with lateral fluoroscopy for performing TMED procedure. After placing a K wire on the transverse process (***b, c***) a series of muscle dilators are used over which a tubular retractor is placed (***d***). ***e*** The operation is then performed under endoscopic visualization. ***f*** A Woodson elevator instrument is useful in removing a central disc herniation.

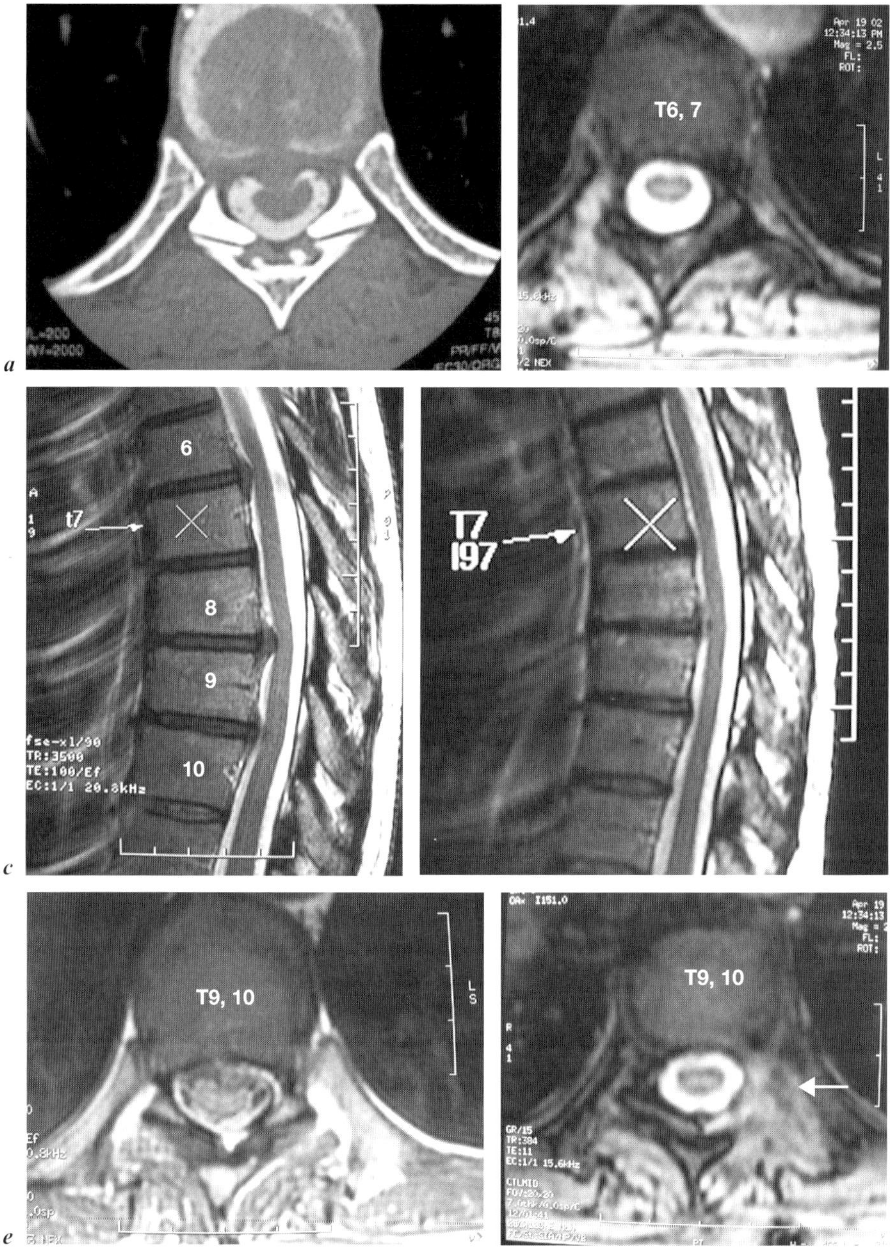

Fig. 2. Pre (***a, c, e***)- and respective post (***b, d, f***)-operative images showing decompression of the spinal cord following a three-level (T6, 7; T8, 9, and T9, 10) TMED.

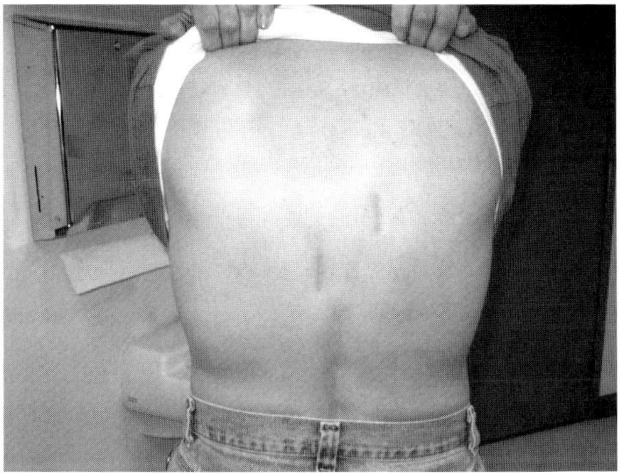

Fig. 3. Postoperative scar after three-level TMED procedure. Of note, no fusion was required nor entry into the thoracic cavity for performing a multilevel thoracic discectomy.

posterior muscle dissection. As a result, patient stays are brief with the majority of patients being discharge the following morning.

Illustrative Case

A 45-year-old female presented with polyradiculopathy and myelopathy from three thoracic disc herniations one at T6, 7, another at T8, 9 and another at T9, 10. The patient underwent a right-sided T6, 7 TMED and a left-sided T8, 9 and T9, 10 TMED. Pre- and postoperative sagittal and axial MRI images show the extent of disc removal (fig. 2c–f) with final decompression of the spinal cord. The patient went on to make a full recovery with minimal postoperative wound scar (fig. 3) and returned to work. In a series of 5 patients treated in this manner, aged 23–54 years, operative times averaged 1.8 h per level and blood loss was approximately 113 ml per level. No cases required conversion to an open procedure and all patients showed improvement in functional outcome as measured by visual pain analog, Oswestry scores, and SF-36.

Discussion

The natural history of thoracic disc herniation is not well delineated. Currently, the only absolute indication for surgery is myelopathy. Surgery for thoracic disc herniation for controlling radicular thoracic pain is controversial as is the role of fusion. A number of approaches currently exist for the treatment of this condition including the posterior (laminectomy, transpedicular, transfacet pedicle-sparing), anterolateral (transthroacic, thoracoscopic), anterior (transsternal), and lateral (costotransversectomy, lateral rachiotomy, lateral extracavitary). Though many of these approaches are effective, they require significant dissection and retraction of normal anatomic structures, which can increase patient morbidity. The novel approach described above which uses a series of muscle dilators, tubular retractor, and endoscopic visualization can reduce much of the morbidity associated with this procedure and avoids the need for fusion and entrance into the thoracic cavity. By using a tubular retractor and endoscope, less muscle, rib and transverse process resection is required. The 30° angle endoscope allows for visualization under the dural sack to reduce any spinal cord manipulation during the procedure and facilitate removal of the herniated thoracic disc. Since the majority of the functioning disc is left in place, no iatrogenic instability is created from extensive disc removal that would require bone fusion. Although the series presented is small, the technique is promising as a new minimally invasive approach to thoracic spine pathology that can lead to reduced operative times, less blood loss, and quicker patient recoveries.

References

1 Anand N, Regan JJ: Video-assisted thoracoscopic surgery for thoracic disc disease: Classification and outcome study of 100 consecutive cases with a 2-year minimum follow-up period. Spine 2002;27:871–879.

2 Arlet V: Anterior thoracoscopic spine release in deformity surgery: A meta-analysis and review. Eur Spine J 2000;9(suppl 1):S17–S23.

3 Awwad EE, Martin DS, et al: Asymptomatic versus symptomatic herniated thoracic disc: Their frequency and characteristics as detected by computed tomography after myelography. Neurosurgery 1991;28:180–186.

4 Birch BD, Desai RD, et al: Surgical approaches to the thoracolumbar spine. Neurosurg Clin N Am 1997;8:471–485.

5 Burgos J, Rapariz JM, et al: Anterior endoscopic approach to the thoracolumbar spine. Spine 1998;23:2427–2431.

6 Cunningham BW, Kotani Y, et al: Video-assisted thoracoscopic surgery versus open thoracotomy for anterior thoracic spinal fusion. A comparative radiographic, biomechanical, and histologic analysis in a sheep model. Spine 1998;23:1333–1340.

7 Dickman CA, Mican CA: Multilevel anterior thoracic discectomies and anterior interbody fusion using a microsurgical thoracoscopic approach. J Neurosurg 1996;84:104–109.

8 Dickman CA, Rosenthal D, et al: Thoracic vertebrectomy and reconstruction using a microsurgical thoracoscopic approach. Neurosurgery 1996;38:279–293.

9 Dickman CA, Rosenthal D, et al: Reoperation for herniated thoracic discs. J Neurosurg 1999;91(suppl 2):157–162.

10 Faciszewski T, Winter RB, et al: The surgical and medical perioperative complications of anterior spinal fusion surgery in the thoracic and lumbar spine in adults. Spine 1995;20:1592–1599.

11 Ferson PF, Landreneau RJ, Dowling RD, Hazelrigg SR, Ritter P, Nunchuck S, Perrino MK, Bowers CM, Mack MJ, Magee MJ: Comparison of open versus thoracoscopic lung biopsy for diffuse infiltrative pulmonary disease. J Thorac Cardiovasc Surg 1993;106:194–199.

12 Fessler RG, Sturgill M: Review: Complications of surgery for thoracic disc disease. Surg Neurol 1998;49:609–618.

13 Hazelrigg SR, Landreneau RJ, Boley TM, Priesmeyer M, Schmaltz RA, Nawarawong W, Johnson JA, Walls JT, Curtis JJ: The effect of muscle-sparing versus standard posterolateral thoracotomy on pulmonary function, muscle strength, and postoperative pain. J Thorac Cardiovasc Surg 1991;101:394–401.

14 Horowirz BH, Moossy JJ, et al: Thoracic discectomy using video assisted thoracoscopy. Spine 1994;19:1082–1086.

15 Huang TJ, Hsu RW, et al: Video-assisted thoracoscopic treatment of spinal lesions in the thoracolumbar junction. Surg Endosc 1997;11:1189–1193.

16 Huang TJ, Hsu RW, et al: Complications in thoracoscopic spinal surgery: A study of 90 consecutive patients. Surg Endosc 1999;13:346–350.

17 Huntington CF, Murrell WD, et al: Comparison of thoracoscopic and open thoracic discectomy in a live ovine model for anterior spinal fusion. Spine 1998;23:1699–1702.

18 Karahalios DG, Apostolides PJ, et al: Thoracoscopic spinal surgery. Treatment of thoracic instability. Neurosurg Clin N Am 1997;8:555–573.

19 Kuklo TR, Lenke LG: Thoracoscopic spine surgery: Current indications and techniques. Orthop Nurs 2000;19/6:15–22.

20 Landreneau RJ, Hazelrigg SR, Mack MJ, Dowling RD, Burke D, Gavlick J, Perrino MK, Ritter PS, Bowers CM, DeFino J: Postoperative pain-related morbidity: Video-assisted thoracic surgery versus thoracotomy. Ann Thorac Surg 1993;56:1285–1289.

21 Larson SJ, Holst RA, Hemmy DC, Sances A: Lateral extracavitary approach to traumatic lesions of the thoracic and lumbar spine. J Neurosurg 1976;45:628–637.

22 McAfee PC, Regan JR, et al: The incidence of complication in endoscopic anterior thoracolumbar spinal reconstructive surgery. Spine 1995;20:1624–1632.

23 Newton PO, Shea KG, et al: Defining the pediatric spinal thoracoscopy learning curve: Sixty-five consecutive cases. Spine 2000;25:1028–1035.

24 Newton PO, Wenger DR, et al: Anterior release and fusion in pediatric spinal deformity. A comparison of early outcome and cost of thoracoscopic and open thoracotomy approaches. Spine 1997;22:1398–1406.

25 Niemeyer T, Freeman BJ, et al: Anterior thoracoscopic surgery followed by posterior instrumentation and fusion in spinal deformity. Eur Spine J 2000;9:499–504.

26 Nymberg SM, Crawford AH: Video-assisted thoracoscopic releases of scoliotic anterior spines. AORN J 1996;63:561–562, 565–569, 571–575; quiz 576, pass.

27 Oskouian RJ Jr, Johnson JP, et al: Thoracoscopic microdiscectomy. Neurosurgery 2002;50/1: 103–109.

28 Otani K, Yoshida M, et al: Thoracic disc herniation. Surgical treatment in 23 patients. Spine 1988;13:1262–1267.

29 Peker S, Akkurt C, et al: Multiple thoracic disc herniations. Acta Neurochir (Wien) 1990; 107/3–4:167–170.

30 Perez-Cruet MJ, Fessler RG, Noel PI: Review: Complications of minimally invasive spinal surgery. Neurosurgery 2002;51(suppl 2):26–36.

31 Perez-Cruet MJ, Foley KT, Isaacs RE, Rice-Wyllie L, Wellington R, Smith MM, Fessler RG: Microendoscopic lumbar discectomy: Technical note. Neurosurgery 2002;51(suppl 2):129–136.

32 Perez-Cruet MJ, Smith MM, Foley KT: Microendoscopic lumbar discectomy; in Perez-Cruet MJ, Fessler RG (eds): Outpatient Spinal Surgery. St Louis, Quality Medical Publishing, 2002, pp 171–183.

33 Perot PL, Munro DD: Transthoracic removal of midline thoracic disc protrusions causing spinal cord compression. J Neurosurg 1969;31:458.

34 Ransohoff J, Spencer F, et al: Transthoracic removal of thoracic discs: Case reports and technical notes. J Neurosurg 1969;31:459–461.

35 Regan JJ: Percutaneous endoscopic thoracic discectomy. Neurosurg Clin N Am 1996;7/1:87–98.

36 Regan JJ, Guyer RD: Endoscopic techniques in spinal surgery. Clin Orthop 1997;335:122–139.

37 Rosenthal D, Dickman CA: Thoracoscopic microsurgical excision of herniated thoracic discs. J Neurosurg 1998;89/2:224–235.

38 Rosenthal D, Rosenthal R, et al: Removal of a protruded thoracic disc using microsurgical endoscopy. A new technique. Spine 1994;19:1087–1091.
39 Roush TF, Crawford AH, et al: Tension pneumothorax as a complication of video-assisted thoracoscopic surgery for anterior correction of idiopathic scoliosis in an adolescent female. Spine 2001;26:448–450.
40 Stillerman CB, Chen TC, et al: Experience in the surgical management of 82 symptomatic herniated thoracic discs and review of the literature. J Neurosurg 1998;88:623–633.
41 Stillerman CB, Chen TC, et al: The transfacet pedicle-sparing approach for thoracic disc removal: Cadaveric morphometric analysis and preliminary clinical experience. J Neurosurg 1995;83: 971–976.

Mick J. Perez-Cruet, MD, MS
Institute for Spine Care, Department of Neurosurgery
Chicago Institute of Neurosurgery and Neuroresearch,
Rush-Presbyterian-St. Luke's Medical Center, 1725 West Harrison Street
Suite 970, Chicago, IL 60612 (USA)
Tel. +1 708 250 3194, Fax +1 312 942 2176, E-Mail perezcruet@yahoo.com

Haid RW Jr, Subach BR, Rodts GE Jr (eds): Advances in Spinal Stabilization.
Prog Neurol Surg. Basel, Karger, 2003, vol 16, pp 277–289

Laparoscopic versus 'Mini-Open' Anterior Lumbar Interbody Fusion

Michael G. Kaiser, Regis W. Haid, Jr., Brian R. Subach, Gerald E. Rodts, Jr.

Department of Neurosurgery, Emory Clinic, Atlanta, Ga., USA

The anterior approach for a lumbar interbody fusion was originally designed to treat Pott's disease [1]. Since that time, the anterior lumbar interbody fusion (ALIF) has evolved into an effective and popular alternative in the treatment of a variety of lumbar degenerative disorders, including degenerative disc disease, low-grade spondylolisthesis, and posterior pseudoarthrosis. Compared to traditional posterior fusion techniques, the ALIF operation is associated with shorter operative times, decreased blood loss, less postoperative pain, reduced hospital stay, and shorter recovery periods [2–5].

Supporters of the ALIF argue that reconstruction of the anterior column is biomechanically superior, avoids paraspinal muscle trauma and denervation, indirectly decompresses the intervertebral foramen, improves sagittal balance, and allows a more efficient restoration of disc interspace height compared to posterior fusion techniques [6–8]. The anterior position of the interbody graft increases the likelihood of fusion by exposing the graft to fusion-promoting forces in accordance with Wolff's law [9]. The interbody space also provides an increased surface area for fusion formation and robust blood supply following decortication of the vertebral endplates [10].

Early in the development of the ALIF technique, open approaches, such as the transperitoneal or retroperitoneal approach, were utilized to expose the anterior lumbar spine. Although providing adequate visualization, these more extensive exposures were associated with increased postoperative morbidity. As the ALIF technique evolved, emphasis was placed on exposing the spine through less invasive approaches. These minimally invasive techniques are intended to decrease postoperative morbidity, reduce hospitalization time, and shorten the recovery period with comparable or superior treatment outcomes compared to more traditional techniques.

Laparoscopic ALIF

Today's spine surgeon has two such options for approaching an ALIF: the laparoscopic approach and the 'mini-open' laparotomy. Zucherman et al. [11] were the first to report the use of the laparoscopic approach for an anterior interbody fusion. This technique is considered by many as the least invasive approach to the ventral lumbar spine and in many centers has become the standard technique when performing an ALIF, particularly at the L5/S1 disc interspace. The safety and efficacy of an anterior laparoscopic fusion have been reported in numerous reports [2, 3, 12–16].

The small incisions required for insertion of the laparoscopic working channels reduce the extent of abdominal wall muscle dissection and blood loss, both contributing to a decrease in postoperative pain. The laparoscopic approach is also associated with less direct manipulation of the abdominal contents, resulting in a decreased incidence of postoperative ileus. These characteristics are thought to reduce postoperative morbidity and contribute to a shorter length of hospitalization.

Mini-Open ALIF

More recently the traditional open transperitoneal approach has been modified into a mini-open technique that incorporates similar principles as the anterior cervical exposure. Originally reported by Mayer [17] in 1997, the mini-open technique reduces the degree of postoperative morbidity associated with the traditional open laparotomy by utilizing a smaller incision combined with a muscle splitting exposure, dividing the abdominal muscles in the direction of the fiber orientation. In this initial report, a total of 25 patients underwent an ALIF across various lumbar levels utilizing the mini-open laparotomy. It was the authors' belief that this technique was associated with negligible surgical trauma, decreased operative time and blood loss, decreased postoperative morbidity, and a shorter recovery time. The authors concluded that this approach could be employed for a variety of lumbar spinal disorders and fusion techniques. The mini-open approach has been described with both a transperitoneal and retroperitoneal route to the anterior lumbar spine [6, 17, 18]. Recently there has been evidence to suggest that the laparoscopic approach does not offer a significant advantage over the mini-open approach when performing an ALIF at the L4/5 interspace [5].

The mini-open approach provides direct access to the disc interspace and allows easier identification of the anatomical midline. The open technique allows complete disc removal, resection of any herniated fragments, and increased endplate exposure, improving the preparation of the disc interspace for fusion formation compared to the trephine technique used with the laparoscopic approach. The mini-open laparotomy is less technically demanding, contributing to a shorter preparation and operative time. The reduced incidence of retrograde ejaculation has also been observed with the mini-open laparotomy [4].

Surgical Technique

Patient Positioning

There are a number of previously published reports describing the details of both the laparoscopic and mini-open techniques [3, 6, 14, 18]. For both approaches the assistance of either a general or vascular surgeon, familiar with laparoscopic techniques when indicated, is advised. This team approach will optimize the speed and safety of the procedure, providing the patient with maximal benefit.

Patient positioning is essentially identical for each approach, however accommodations for the video monitor are required with the laparoscopic exposure. The patient is positioned supine on a radiolucent operative table with a pillow or bolster placed under the patient's hips to accentuate the natural lumbar lordosis and under the knees to avoid hyperextension. The patient is securely strapped to the operative table. This is particularly necessary for the laparoscopic approach due to the steep Trendelenburg position required to allow the abdominal viscera to move rostrally out of the pelvis. Fluoroscopic imaging is used with both techniques during positioning of the implants.

Laparoscopic Technique

The patient is prepared and draped under sterile conditions in the usual fashion. The fluoroscopic equipment is brought into the operative field to confirm the midline prior to any incisions. For the laparoscopic approach, intra-abdominal access is obtained through four small incisions in the anterior abdominal wall (fig. 1). The viewing camera is inserted through a curvilinear umbilical incision and two lower paramedian incisions provide portals for the

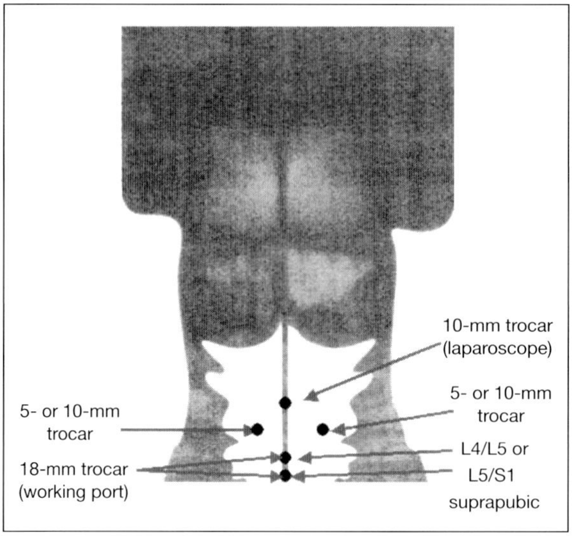

Fig. 1. Diagram demonstrating the trocar placement for laparoscopic ALIF. The channels for working instruments are provided through two paramedian incisions. The laparoscope is inserted through an umbilical incision and the instrumentation portal through a suprapubic incision.

working instruments. The channel for interbody implant insertion is passed through a midline suprapubic incision and measures approximately 2–4 cm in length (fig. 2).

Harvesting of the bone graft is performed at the beginning of the procedure. During this period the laparoscopic surgeon obtains access and insufflates the abdominal cavity. At this point the operative table is placed in a steep Trendelenburg position to assist in mobilizing the abdominal viscera out of the pelvis inlet.

Adequate exposure of the disc is critical. It is essential to identify the appropriate anatomical landmarks and midline (fig. 3). The sacral promontory is identified by palpation and the midline determined with fluoroscopic imaging. The posterior peritoneum is opened sharply. In an attempt to avoid retrograde ejaculation in male patients the presacral sympathetic plexus is mobilized through blunt dissection and the use of monopolar cautery avoided at the disc interspace. More liberal use of the monopolar cautery is allowed with female patients. The middle sacral artery and vein are then identified, ligated, and divided.

The insertion of interbody implants is performed only after confirmation of the midline is repeated. The implants are inserted through a trephine

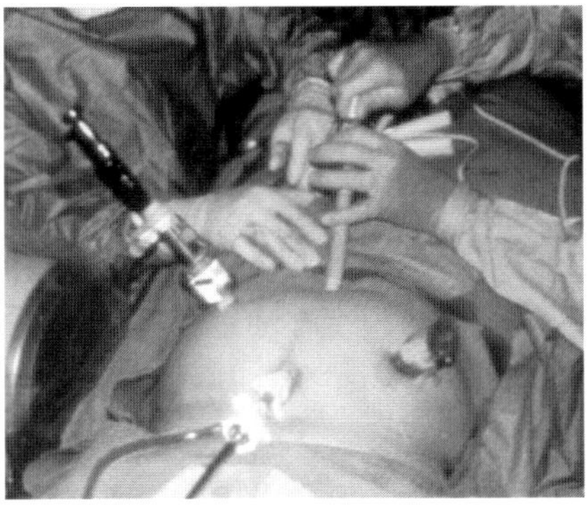

Fig. 2. Final placement of abdominal trocars following insufflation of the abdomen. The instrumentation trocar is positioned toward the top and the laparoscope toward the bottom of the photograph.

3 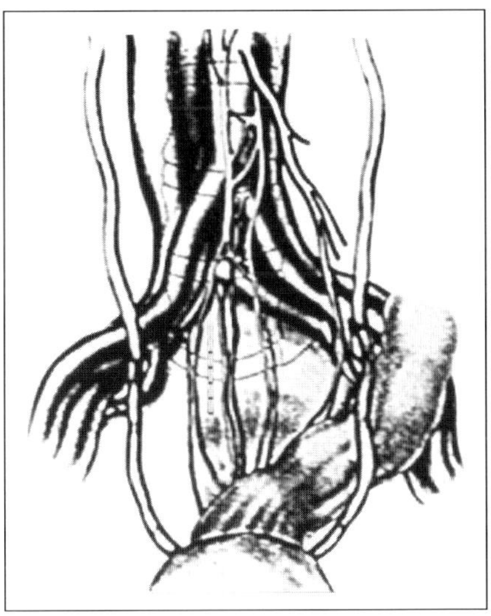

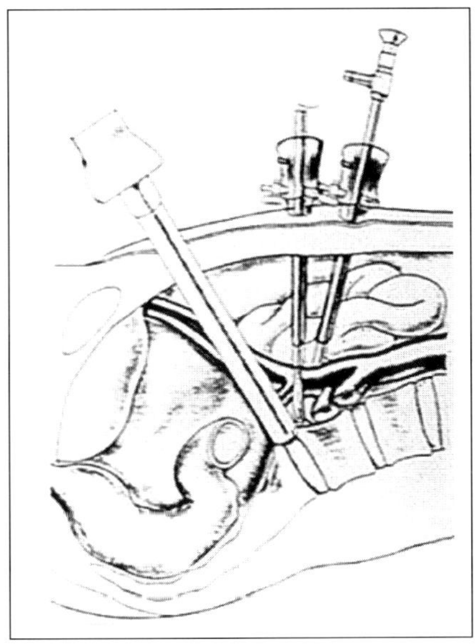 *4*

Fig. 3. Anterior view of the lumbosacral spine prior to retroperitoneal exposure. The dotted line indicates a possible peritoneal incision to access the retroperitoneum and anterior disc space.

Fig. 4. Lateral view of the instrumentation port positioned within the disc interspace for trephination of the disc material and insertion of implant.

technique according to the guidelines specific for the implant chosen (fig. 4). Following radiographic confirmation of implant position, the posterior peritoneum is closed using clip ligation. The abdominal incisions are closed with interrupted absorbable sutures and Steri-Strips.

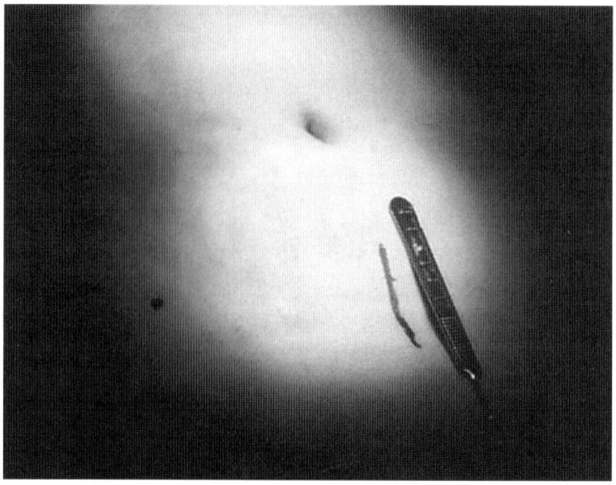

Fig. 5. Typically a transverse incision is used for single level exposure for cosmesis, however a longitudinal incision can be used for obese patients, history of prior abdominal surgery, or if more than one level is addressed. The incision is usually 4–6 cm in length.

Mini-Open Technique

Excluding the equipment required for a laparoscopic approach, the operative setup is identical. The level of incision is determined with fluoroscopic imaging, with a bias toward the caudal border of the level of arthrodesis. This bias will provide a more tangent approach into the disc space and avoid excessive reaming into the inferior vertebral body. A longitudinal or transverse incision approximately 4–6 cm in length is made in the suprapubic region. A longitudinal incision is reserved for two-level ALIF procedures or for obese patients (fig. 5). After the skin incision is made, monopolar cautery is used to dissect down to the rectus abdominus muscle that is split in a longitudinal fashion parallel to the muscle fiber plane. The posterior rectus sheath and transversalis fascia are divided to expose the underlying peritoneum. The peritoneum is incised and the abdominal contents packed superiorly held in position with a table-mounted retractor (fig. 6). Although the anterior lumbar spine can be approached through either a transperitoneal or retroperitoneal exposure, our preference has been the transperitoneal route since a more direct anterior trajectory is obtained.

The posterior peritoneum overlying the disc interspace is identified and sharply divided. Exposure of the L5/S1 interspace is usually easier due to the more rostral bifurcation of the great vessels. In order to expose L4/5 interspace the left iliac artery and vein are mobilized. It is imperative that the iliolumbar vein be identified and ligated. Transection of this vein without adequate control can

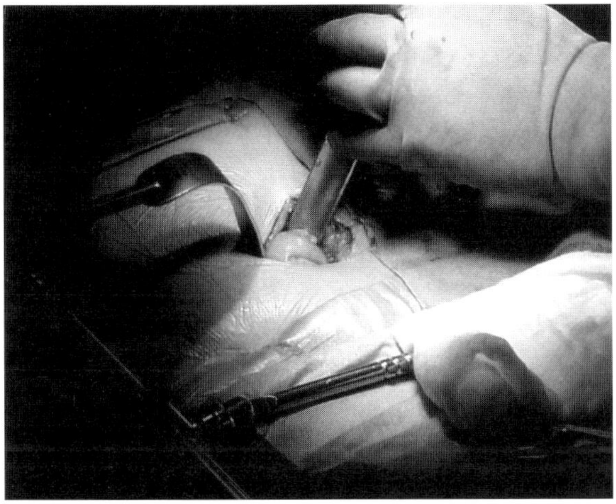

Fig. 6. A table-mounted retractor system is placed to optimize exposure and retract the abdominal contents rostrally.

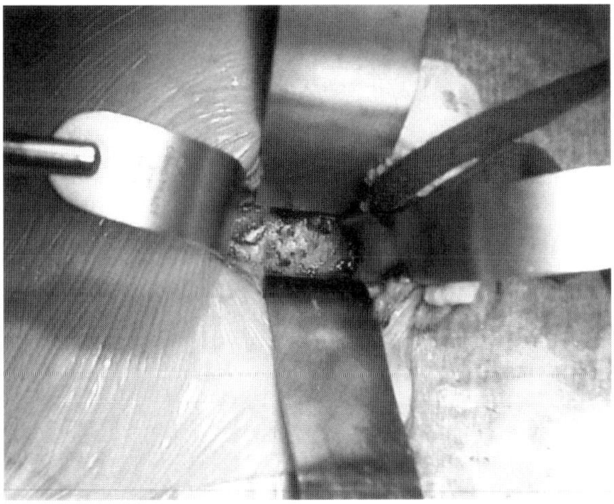

Fig. 7. Once the retractor blades are positioned and the posterior peritoneum opened the anterior surface of the disc is easily identified.

lead to catastrophic blood loss. Mobilizing the presacral sympathetic plexus in male patients is performed with blunt dissection, avoiding the use of monopolar cautery. In females monopolar cautery may be used more liberally to expose the anterior surface of the vertebral bodies and disc space (fig. 7). Midline identification is made through direct visualization and fluoroscopic imaging.

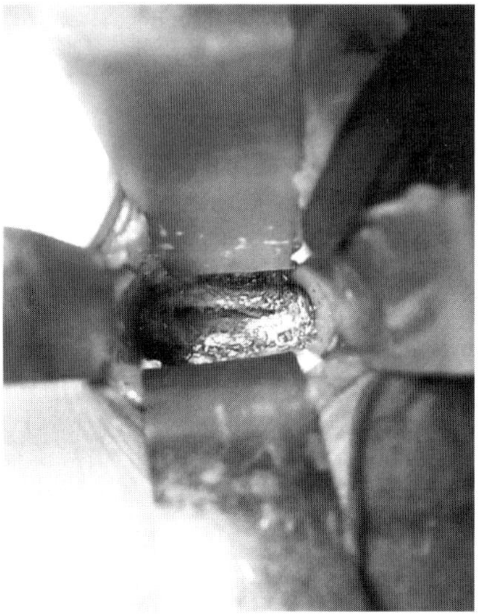

Fig. 8. Intraoperative photograph demonstrated the generous discectomy, with preservation of the lateral annulus, required for adequate endplate exposure prior to implant insertion.

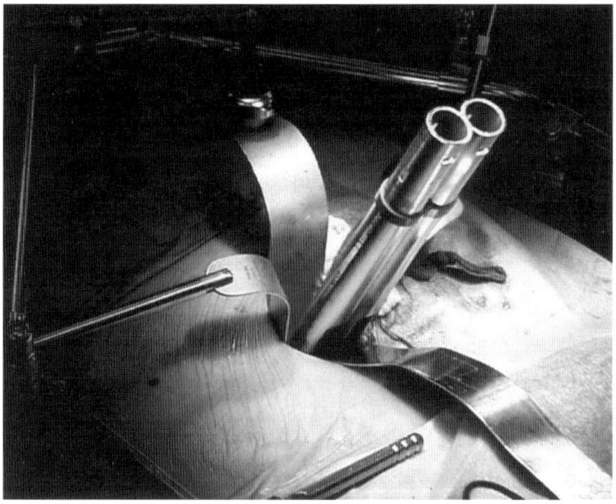

Fig. 9. Intraoperative view of the double-barrel channel in position for implant insertion.

A complete removal of the disc is performed and the entire endplate prepared for graft insertion (fig. 8). The interbody implant is then inserted according to manufacturers' guidelines along with additional autologous bone (fig. 9). Once the appropriate implant position is verified with intraoperative fluoroscopic images, the posterior peritoneum is primarily closed with a running absorbable suture. The anterior peritoneum, transversalis fascia, and rectus sheath are closed with interrupted absorbable sutures and the skin closed with staples.

Postoperative Care

The postoperative course for both the laparoscopic and mini-open groups is essentially identical. Mobilization occurs early, typically on the first postoperative day, and their diet advanced with the initiation of bowel sounds. Patients are generally discharged once they are able to tolerate an oral diet, able to ambulate, and voiding without difficulty. Occasionally this may be as early as the 2nd day following surgery. Radiographic images, to determine implant position, are obtained prior to discharge and during scheduled follow-up visits, at approximately 6 weeks, 3, 6, 9, 12 and 24 months postoperatively.

Laparoscopic versus Mini-Open ALIF

There have been few studies that directly compared the mini-open laparotomy to the laparoscopic ALIF. Regan et al. [19] compared their experience of 65 laparoscopic fusions to a large number of both anterior and posterior open interbody fusions. The mean operative time was significantly shorter for the mini-open ALIF compared to the laparoscopic approach, 149 compared to 207 min. The average blood loss during the mini-open procedure was 224 ml (range 20–2,000 ml) and for the laparoscopic approach 176 ml (range 10–2,200 ml). The trend for decreased blood loss with the laparoscopic approach did not prove statistically significant. The mean length of hospitalization was essentially the same for both groups, approximately 3.9 days for the laparoscopic group and 4.0 days following the mini-open approach. There were several technical complications associated with the laparoscopic approach that occurred early in the surgeon's operative experience. Nine attempts at a laparoscopic fusion were aborted and converted to an open approach, 3 secondary to laceration of the iliac vein. In 2 cases a herniated disc was noted to impinge upon a nerve root requiring a second operation for removal of the herniated fragment.

More recently Zdeblick and David [5] presented their experience with both the mini-open and laparoscopic approaches. Over a 3-year period data was prospectively collected on 50 patients who underwent an ALIF involving the L4/5 disc interspace, with an equal number of laparoscopic and mini-open laparotomy procedures. The authors found no statistical difference in operating time, intraoperative blood loss, or length of hospital stay between the two groups. When two-level procedures were considered separately, a significant increase in the mean operative time was noted with the laparoscopic approach, 185 versus 160 min. The laparoscopic group demonstrated a significantly higher complication rate, 20 versus 4%. Based on these observations, the authors concluded that the laparoscopic approach offered no advantage over the mini-open laparotomy when performing an ALIF involving the L4/5 level.

Table 1. Comparison of operative variables for all ALIF procedures

	Laparoscopic	Mini-open
Preparation time, min	50.8	26.2
Surgical time, min	185.0	171.9
Operative blood loss, ml	188.2	231.3
Hospitalization, days	2.9	3.7

Table 2. Comparison of operative variables for L5/S1 ALIF

	Laparoscopic	Mini-open
Preparation time, min	50.2	24.8
Surgical time, min	173.6	145.1
Operative blood loss, ml	178.3	160.1
Hospitalization, days	2.8	3.5

Complications associated with an ALIF approach can be categorized as either major or minor and divided into visceral, vascular, neural, and fusion-related complications. Rajaraman et al. [20] recently reported the complications recorded in their series of 60 patients undergoing open anterior lumbar surgery. A total of 24 complications were noted in 23 patients (38.3%), including sympathetic dysfunction in 6, vascular injury in 4, somatic nerve injury in 3, sexual dysfunction in 3, prolonged ileus in 3, wound incompetence in 2, and bowel injury, deep venous thrombosis, and acute pancreatitis in 1 patient. The majority of complications were only transient in nature.

In a study focusing on the complications associated with endoscopic spinal surgery, McAfee et al. [16] included 22 patients that underwent a laparoscopic ALIF at either L4/5 or L5/S1. One approach-related complication was noted, a tear in the left common iliac vein that required conversion to an open procedure. The authors concluded that a laparoscopic fusion was a safe and effective procedure compared to traditional open techniques.

Over the past 5 years our group has gained extensive experience with both the laparoscopic and mini-open ALIF procedures [3, 6, 14, 18]. Between 1996 and 2001 a total of 98 ALIF procedures were performed at our institution, equally distributed between a laparoscopic and mini-open approach. Recently we performed a retrospective review of our ALIF experience, comparing data regarding operative parameters, length of hospital

Table 3. Intraoperative complications

Laparoscopic
Bladder perforation
Iliac vein laceration
Conversion to open procedure (n = 2)
Mini-open
Iliac vein laceration (n = 2)

Table 4. Postoperative complications

Laparoscopic
UTI
New onset radiculopathy
Mini-open
Transient ileus (n = 5)
Retroperitoneal hematoma
UTI
Wound infection
Worsened radiculopathy

UTI = Urinary tract infection.

stay, and approach-associated complications (tables 1–4). Comparisons were made for the entire series as well as for patients undergoing an L5/S1 ALIF [21].

One of the more striking differences observed between the two approaches was the time required to organize the operating room. This interval was estimated from the time of anesthesia induction to the point of surgical incision. The operative preparation time was significantly shorter for the mini-open laparotomy. For the entire patient series as well as patients undergoing an L5/S1 ALIF the operative organization time was reduced by approximately 50% during a mini-open approach. Although this time interval is an arbitrary measurement, the increased preparation time is directly related to the technically demanding equipment required for the laparoscopic approach.

The procedure time was also reduced following a mini-open laparotomy, although the decrease only proved statistically significant for patients undergoing an L5/S1 ALIF. The lack of significance observed for the entire series is likely the result of a selection bias for two-level and L4/5 interspace procedures performed with the mini-open approach. As with the operative preparation interval, we concluded that the increased procedure time was related to the equipment required for the laparoscopic approach.

No significant differences, for the entire series or the L5/S1 cohort, were observed regarding the degree of intraoperative blood loss or intraoperative complications. Vascular and visceral injuries occurred following both approaches. A clear advantage of the mini-open approach is the immediate and direct access provided in the event of such an injury.

An increased incidence of immediate postoperative complications was noted with the mini-open laparotomy. The majority of these complications consisted of a transient ileus that resolved by the 5th postoperative day. A retroperitoneal hematoma was the only additional complication directly related to the mini-open approach and required observation only.

Retrograde ejaculation resulting from injury to the superior hypogastric plexus has a reported incidence of up to 22% in men undergoing an open anterior lumbar fusion [4, 5, 20, 22] and up to 20% following a laparoscopic fusion [3–5, 12]. Up to one third to half of these patients will return to normal function within 2 years [22]. In our entire series of male patients a significantly higher incidence of retrograde ejaculation occurred following the laparoscopic ALIF, 45.4 versus 6.0%. The percent of men suffering an episode of retrograde ejaculation following a laparoscopic L5/S1 ALIF was unchanged, however following a mini-open laparotomy the incidence decreased to 0%. Although an exact explanation for the increased incidence observed in the laparoscopic group is lacking, we speculate that sweeping the neural plexus off the midline using the laparoscope instead of a cotton sponge is more difficult and damaging. It is unclear why our observed incidence was so high; however, as with previous reports the majority of these cases were transient in nature.

Conclusions

Based on the theoretical considerations described, previous published series, and our own operative experience, we have developed a bias toward the mini-open laparotomy when performing an ALIF at either the L4/5 or L5/S1 level. It is our contention that the mini-open ALIF is technically less demanding, allows for a shorter operative time, provides the access necessary for complete disc removal, allows for resection of a herniated fragment, and provides direct visualization of the disc interspace for optimal interbody graft insertion. In addition the incidence of retrograde ejaculation is significantly reduced with the mini-open laparotomy. Both the mini-open and laparoscopic techniques, however, are effective and safe and ultimately surgeon preference will dictate the choice of approach utilized when performing an ALIF.

References

1 Ito H, Tsuchiya J, Asami G: A new radical operation for Pott's disease. J Bone Joint Surg Br 1934;16:499–515.

2 Dickman C, Sonntag V, Russell J: The laparoscopic approach for instrumentation and fusion of the lumbar spine. BNI Q 1997;13:26–36.

3 McLaughlin M, Zhang J, Subach B, Haid R, Rodts G: Laparoscopic anterior lumbar interbody fusion: Technical note. Neurosurg Focus 1999;7:1–6.

4 Reagan J, Yuan H, McAfee P: Laparoscopic fusion of the lumbar spine: Minimally invasive spine surgery. A prospective multicenter study evaluating open and laparoscopic lumbar fusion. Spine 1999;24:402–411.
5 Zdeblick T, David S: A prospective comparison of surgical approach for anterior L4–L5 fusion: Lapàroscopic versus mini anterior lumbar interbody fusion. Spine 2000;25:2682–2687.
6 McLaughlin M, Haid R, Rodts G, Miller J: Current role of anterior lumbar interbody fusion in lumbar spine disorders. Semin Neurosurg 2000;11:221–229.
7 Voor MJ, Mehta S, Wang M, Zhang YM, Mahan J, Johnson JR: Biomechanical evaluation of posterior and anterior lumbar interbody fusion techniques. J Spinal Disord 1998;11:328–334.
8 Greenough CG, Peterson MD, Hadlow S, Fraser RD: Instrumented posterolateral lumbar fusion. Results and comparison with anterior interbody fusion. Spine 1998;23:479–486.
9 Egger E, Gottsauner-Wolf F, Palmer J, et al: Effects of axial dynamization on bone healing. J Trauma 1993;34:185–192.
10 Lin P: Posterior lumbar interbody fusion; in Cauthen J (ed): Lumbar Spine Surgery. Indications, Techniques, Failures, and Alternatives, ed 2. Baltimore, Williams & Wilkins, 1988, pp 228–247.
11 Zucherman JF, Zdeblick TA, Bailey SA, Mahvi D, Hsu KY, Kohrs D: Instrumented laparoscopic spinal fusion. Preliminary results. Spine 1995;20:2029–2035.
12 Zdeblick TA: Laparoscopic spinal fusion. Orthop Clin North Am 1998;29:635–645.
13 Mahvi DM, Zdeblick TA: A prospective study of laparoscopic spinal fusion. Technique and operative complications. Ann Surg 1996;224:85–90.
14 McLaughlin M, Comey C, Haid R: Laparoscopic anterior lumbar interbody fusion. Cont Neurosurg 1998;20:1–9.
15 Bhatnagar MK, Mathur SK, Mess CF: Laparoscopic spinal fusion. Md Med J 1999;48:161–164.
16 McAfee PC, Regan JR, Zdeblick T, Zuckerman J, Picetti GD 3rd, Heim S, Geis WP, Fedder IL: The incidence of complications in endoscopic anterior thoracolumbar spinal reconstructive surgery. A prospective multicenter study comprising the first 100 consecutive cases. Spine 1995;20:1624–1632.
17 Mayer HM: A new microsurgical technique for minimally invasive anterior lumbar interbody fusion. Spine 1997;22:691–700.
18 McLaughlin M, Haid R, Rodts G, Miller J: Open anterior lumbar interbody fusion. Tech Neurosurg 2001;7:140–151.
19 Regan J, Zdeblick T, Zucherman J: Comparison of open versus laparoscopic fusion of the lumbar spine using the BAK threaded fusion cage. 10th Annual Meeting, North American Spine Society, Washington, 1995, p 131.
20 Rajaraman V, Vingan R, Roth P, Heary RF, Conklin L, Jacobs GB: Visceral and vascular complications resulting from anterior lumbar interbody fusion. J Neurosurg 1999;91:60–64.
21 Kaiser M, Haid R, Subach B, Miller J, Smith C, Rodts G: Comparison of the mini-open versus laparoscopic approach for anterior lumbar interbody fusion: A retrospective review. Neurosurgery, in press.
22 Flynn JC, Price CT: Sexual complications of anterior fusion of the lumbar spine. Spine 1984;9: 489–492.

Regis W. Haid, Jr., MD
Department of Neurosurgery, The Emory Clinic,
1365B Clifton Road, Atlanta, GA 30322 (USA)
Tel. +1 404 778 5770, Fax +1 404 778 4472, E-Mail regis_haid@emoryhealthcare.org

Haid RW Jr, Subach BR, Rodts GE Jr (eds): Advances in Spinal Stabilization.
Prog Neurol Surg. Basel, Karger, 2003, vol 16, pp 290–301

Epidemiology and Variations in Care of Spine Disease

James P. Burke, Peter C. Gerszten

Department of Neurological Surgery, University of Pittsburgh Medical Center, Pittsburgh, Pa., USA

Spine disease, with associated neck, back, and radicular pain, is common and costly. In the current American health care environment, many types of practitioners (primary care physicians, spine surgeons, physical therapists, chiropractors, and others) are involved in managing patients with spine disease, often with very different approaches. The varied nature and economic costs of spine disease are driving a growing interest in research. The coming years may reveal the fundamental aspects of this problem, as well as standardized treatment regimens, in more detail.

Epidemiology of Spine Disease

Degenerative spine disease is extremely common in our society. It is well accepted that the vast majority of the population will develop degenerative spinal abnormalities; some form of spondylosis is present radiographically in more than 80% of males and females older than 55 years [1]. In the more mobile cervical and lumbar spinal segments, the development of bony and ligamentous hypertrophy, along with facet arthropathy, is expected. While spinal degeneration may develop at an earlier age in some patients, these asymptomatic degenerative changes are almost universal in the elderly, active individual. The patient with a congenitally narrow spinal canal may present at a young age with symptomatic spinal stenosis [2].

Age-related spinal disease typically presents in the 6th through 8th decades. Patients may complain of nonspecific neck pain, low back pain (LBP), or both. Radicular complaints in the upper extremities or symptoms suggestive of neurogenic claudication are common. Typical age-related changes may be expected on plain radiographs of the spine. These degenerative changes include some minimal interspace collapse, moderate osteophyte formation with associated foraminal encroachment, small ventral traction spurs, minimal vertebral body compression or collapse in the osteoporotic patient, and moderate spinal canal stenosis, without evidence of fracture, instability, or subluxation [2].

The true incidence of symptomatic cervical spondylosis is difficult to assess because minor cervical discomfort or neck stiffness often goes unreported. Teresi et al. [3] reviewed cases in which cervical MRIs had been obtained from patients with no subjective complaint or objective physical finding of degenerative spinal disease. They noted disc space narrowing in 67% of patients older than 64 years, compared with a 24% occurrence rate for those aged 45–64 years. Patients with degenerative spinal disease in the cervical region may present with a myriad of signs and symptoms. The mean age of onset of symptoms ranges from 60 to 69 years, with men affected slightly more than women [4]. The natural history of myelopathy has been well described, with progression usually during a prolonged period. Spontaneous improvement is uncommon [4, 5]. The natural history of radiculopathy and discogenic neck pain is less well defined. It is believed that many patients with radiculopathy improve with time; however, some patients will fail to improve, particularly those with a soft disc herniation [6]. Up to 80% of patients with neck pain will improve with time.

While the thoracic spine is much less mobile than either the cervical or the lumbar spine and degenerative disease is less common, the thoracic spine is not exempt from the effects of aging and degeneration. Kyphosis occurs commonly among elderly women. Although symptomatic degeneration in the thoracic spine is uncommon, relatively less compromise of the thoracic spine may result in neurological deficits for two reasons. First, the spinal cord occupies a relatively larger percentage of the canal throughout the thoracic spine, and compression may occur from relatively smaller osteophytes. Second, the vascular supply to the thoracic spinal cord comes primarily from segmental or radicular arteries. This supply places the thoracic cord at an even greater risk of ischemia from compression.

Symptomatic herniation of thoracic discs is uncommon. While early studies reported that surgery for thoracic disc herniation accounted for only 3–5 of every 1,000 disc operations [7], the true incidence of symptomatic thoracic disc herniation probably is higher. MRI of the spine has allowed diagnosis of the problem in many patients before neurological signs develop. Thoracic disc herniations occur most commonly in adults aged 30–60 years, although these lesions may occur in children [8], and are equally common in men and women. Approximately two thirds of thoracic disc herniations occur below the level of

T8, presumably because of the greater forces acting on the lower thoracic spine. Midline herniations are several times more common than those that are laterally placed [7, 9].

In general, degenerative disease of the lumbar spine is clinically stable, with relatively few minor symptoms and signs. The progression of symptoms is often slow, and the patient usually describes a history of steady worsening of symptoms and signs over years or even decades. Given the varied descriptions and definitions of lumbar spondylosis, it is not surprising that the prevalence varies widely depending upon the reporting authority. In one series of 850 myelograms, researchers noted a 6% occurrence of 'stenosis of the thecal sac' [10]; however, there was no mention as to why the myelograms were performed nor how many of these patients were symptomatic. On the other hand, Roberson et al. [11] reported a 1.7% occurrence of lumbar stenosis in a series of 2,000 lumbar myelograms. Because a certain percentage of patients have lumbar stenosis secondary to degenerative disease, the absolute prevalence of stenosis varies according to the age and sex of the population studied. The prevalence in the general population remains unknown.

The patient's age at the onset of symptoms also varies with the criteria used to define lumbar spondylosis. In a study by Paine [12] that included conditions with or without disc herniation, the mean age of onset was 30 years in patients with preexisting stenosis. The age of onset in patients with congenital or developmental stenosis (such as achondroplasia) is similar. Most studies evaluating acquired lumbar stenosis place the average age of onset of symptoms in the late 5th to early 7th decades [13]. Symptomatic degenerative spondylolisthesis is infrequent in patients younger than 50 years of age [14].

Currently, there is some controversy in the literature regarding the sexual preponderance of lumbar spondylosis. Both the developmental and acquired forms of lumbar stenosis have shown a male preponderance in most early studies [12, 15]. However, in more recent studies noting the increased recognition of this disease process, the ratio appears to favor women over men by as much as 5 to 1 [16, 17]. Symptomatic degenerative spondylolisthesis has been reported to occur 4–6 times as frequently in women as in men, perhaps because of hormonal factors leading to ligamentous laxity of the motion segment [18].

In contrast to degenerative spine disease, there are approximately 11,000 new cases of acute spinal cord injuries per year or 4 per 100,000 persons. The estimated prevalence of persons living with spinal cord injuries is between 300,000 and 500,000 cases. An increased prevalence during the past decade has been mainly attributed to enhanced longevity of spine-injured patients. Increased survivorship, as well as improvements in neurological outcome, has been attributed to enhanced medical, surgical, and prehospital care. Spinal cord

Table 1. Incidence of several neurosurgical disease states

Diagnosis	Incidence per 100,000 persons
LBP	30,000
Carpal tunnel syndrome	2,800
Traumatic brain injury	150
Occlusive cerebral vascular disease	96
Intracerebral/intracranial hemorrhage	30
Malignant neoplasm of the brain	12
Subarachnoid hemorrhage (nontraumatic)	8
Traumatic spinal cord injury	4

injury is most common in young adult men. It is estimated that 63% of new traumatic injuries occur in individuals between the ages of 16 and 30 years, with a 4:1 male:female ratio [19].

Epidemiology of LBP

LBP is a very common health problem in western industrialized countries. Up to 80% of Americans report having LBP at some point in their lives, most often between the ages of 30 and 50 years. To put this in perspective, table 1 lists the incidence of LBP compared to a variety of other neurosurgical disease states. In addition, clinically significant sciatica is seen in 5% of the US population. Recurrent episodes of LBP occur very frequently, and a considerable number of people have permanent discomfort from LBP. Chronic LBP is present in 3–7% of the population in western industrialized countries [20–22]. In the USA, back pain is the most common cause of activity limitation in people younger than 45 years [23], the second most frequent reason for visits to the physician, the fifth-ranking cause of admission to the hospital, and the third most common cause of surgical procedures [21]. About 2% of the US workforce are compensated for back injuries each year [21]. In 1988, the annual combined cost of back pain-related medical care and disability compensation in the United States was estimated to be between USD 26 and USD 56 billion [24].

LBP affects men and women equally, with onset most often between the ages of 30 and 50 years. It is the most expensive cause of work-related disability in terms of workers' compensation and medical expenses. Risk factors for chronic LBP include heavy lifting and twisting, bodily vibration, obesity, and poor conditioning, although LBP is common even in people without these risk factors [21, 22].

Recovery from nonspecific LBP is generally rapid. One study reported that 90% of patients seen within 3 days of LBP onset recovered within 20 weeks [25]. However, in cross-sectional studies, which oversample patients with multiple visits, the prognosis is less favorable. These studies may best reflect the experience of primary care physicians, and suggest that one third of patients are substantially improved at 1 week, with two thirds improved at 7 weeks [26, 27]. Recurrences are common, affecting 40% of patients within 6 months. Most recurrences are not disabling, but the emerging picture is that of a chronic problem with intermittent exacerbations, analogous to asthma, rather than an acute disease that can be cured [22].

LBP is second only to upper respiratory problems as a symptom-related reason for visits to a physician [20, 21]. Unfortunately, there are wide variations in care, a fact that suggests there is uncertainty about the optimal approach to management. In addition, there is evidence of excessive imaging and surgery for LBP in the United States, and many experts believe the problem has been 'overmedicalized' [22].

The association between clinical symptoms and radiographic imaging shows little correlation. Most diagnostic evaluations focus on exclusion of herniated discs, stenosis, infection, neoplasms, and trauma. However, up to 85% of patients with isolated LBP cannot be given a precise pathoanatomical diagnosis, with nonspecific terms, such as 'strain', 'sprain', or 'degenerative process', commonly used [20]. Strain and sprain have never been anatomically or histologically characterized, and patients given these diagnoses might accurately be said to have 'idiopathic LBP' [22].

Patients with chronic LBP (i.e., pain duration more than 3 months) use health services more often than most other patient groups [20]. Spontaneous recovery in these patients is slow and unpredictable, and the return-to-work rate after 2 years absence from work due to LBP has been shown to be exceedingly low. At any given time, about 1% of the work force is chronically disabled because of back problems [28].

In contrast, the natural history of herniated discs is more favorable. Improvement is the norm, although it is often slower than improvement in LBP alone. Only about 10% of patients have sufficient pain after 6 weeks that surgical intervention is considered. Sequential MRI studies reveal that the herniated portion of the disk tends to regress with time, with partial or complete resolution in two thirds of cases after 6 months [29]. Patients with herniated discs who undergo surgery do not return to work earlier than those who receive nonsurgical therapy, although they have better symptomatic and functional outcomes [30].

A paradox exists in that the American economy has become increasingly postindustrial, with less heavy labor and more automation and more robotics, while medical advances in spine treatment with diagnostic imaging and new forms of surgical and nonsurgical therapy have developed. At the same time, however, work disability caused by back pain has steadily risen! The positive aspect is that most back pain patients will substantially and rapidly recover, even when their pain is severe. This prognosis holds true regardless of treatment method or even without treatment. Only a minority of patients with back pain will miss work because of it. Most patients who do leave work return within 6 weeks, and only a small percentage never return to their jobs.

Variations in Treatment for Spinal Disorders

Patients with neck and back pain seek care from general practitioners, chiropractors, orthopedists, neurosurgeons, rheumatologists, and others. There is a wide variation in how doctors care for patients with neck and back pain, with evidence of excessive imaging and surgery for the problem. In most cases of LBP, patients recover within a few weeks of the onset of symptoms. The fact that LBP often resolves spontaneously may partially explain the proliferation of unproven treatments that may seem to be effective. When patient descriptions are standardized, physician recommendations for neck and back pain evaluations vary enormously. Rheumatologists are twice as likely to order blood work to rule-out arthritic conditions. Neurosurgeons are twice as likely to order imaging studies. Neurologists are 3 times more likely to order EMGs [28].

Surgical procedures for herniated discs and spinal stenosis accounted for 83% of the more than 188,000 spine surgeries done in Medicare patients in 1996–1997. There were approximately 39,000 discectomies, 90,000 lumbar decompressions, and 27,000 cervical spine procedures. The remaining 32,000 procedures were for other spinal conditions. Overall, spine surgery rates increased by 57% over the 10-year period from 1988 to 1996, from 2.1 to 3.4 per 1,000 Medicare enrollees (fig. 1) [31].

There remains significant variation within the United States in the use of surgery for many spine-related problems. Rates of spine surgery vary more than any other common inpatient procedure. In 1996–1997, rates of spine surgery varied by a factor of 6, from 1.4 per 1,000 Medicare enrollees in the Bronx, N.Y. hospital referral region to 8.6 per 1,000 Medicare residents in Bend, Oreg. Cervical spine procedures accounted for 14% of the spine surgery performed in the Medicare population in 1996–1997; rates of cervical spine surgery varied by a factor of more than 10, ranging from 0.16 to 1.72 per 1,000 Medicare enrollees in the different hospital referral regions [31].

The use of spinal fusion displays a wide variation among geographic areas, as well as varying from 0.3 to 3.0 per 1,000 Medicare enrollees (fig. 2).

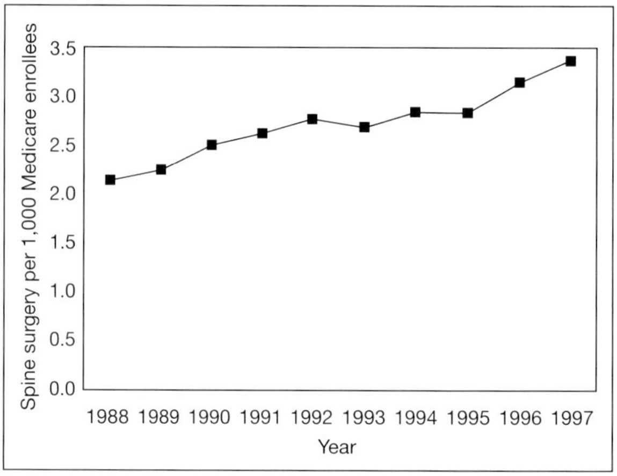

Fig. 1. Increase in rates of spine surgery among Medicare enrollees (1988–1997). Overall surgery rates increased by 57% between 1988 and 1997 [from 31, p. 29].

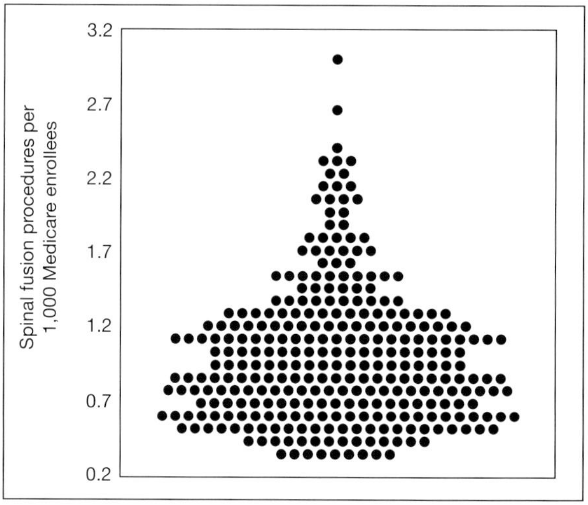

Fig. 2. Rates of spinal fusion varied by a factor of almost 10, from 0.3 to 3.0 per 1,000 Medicare enrollees, after adjustment for differences in population age, sex and race (1996–1997). Each point represents 1 of 306 hospital referral regions in the United States [from 31, p. 38].

The proportion of patients undergoing spine surgery who received a spinal fusion increased from 23% in 1993 to 29% in 1997. During the same period, the proportion of patients undergoing fusion who received hardware fixation devices rose from 50 to 60%. Among Medicare patients undergoing laminectomy for

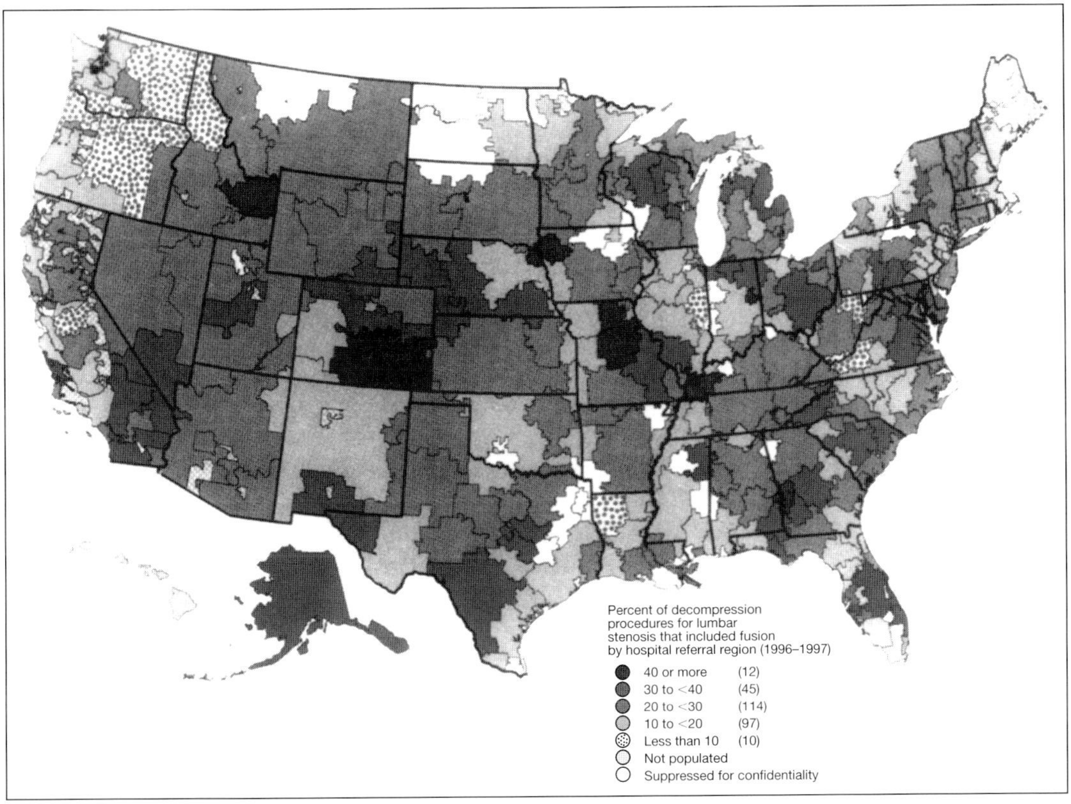

Fig. 3. Use of fusion with surgery for lumbar spinal stenosis (1996–1997). Fusion was used in at least 40% of lumbar decompression procedures in 12 hospital referral regions. In 10 regions, fusion was used in less than 10% of operations [from 31, p. 41].

lumbar spinal stenosis, the use of fusion varied from 4% of the operations to 56%. Figure 3 shows the variation across the United States in the use of fusion with surgery for lumbar spinal stenosis [31].

It is unlikely that the large degree of regional variation in the use of spine surgery reflects regional differences in the incidence of disease. Instead, regional variation in surgery reflects differences in physician practice style – physicians in some regions of the United States are simply more inclined to recommend surgery in patients with surgically treatable conditions of the spine. The likelihood that patients will undergo particular surgical procedures of the spine is remarkably variable. This is apparent on a local level, as well as with 'surgical signatures' reflecting the practice patterns of individual physicians and the local medical culture. Neighboring regions with similar demographics

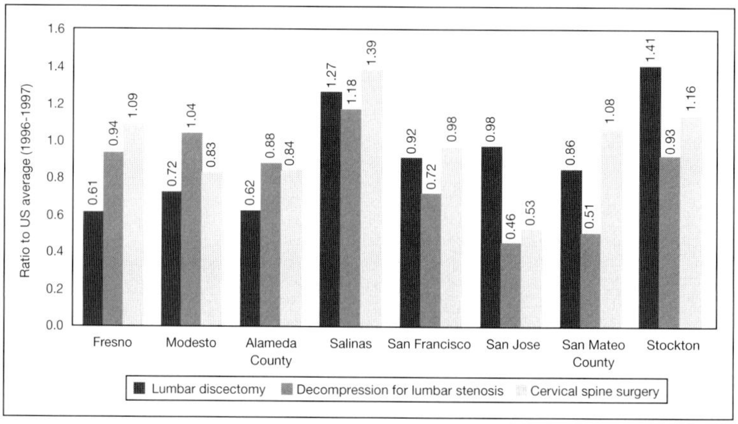

Fig. 4. The surgical signature of spine surgery in 8 California hospital referral regions (1996–1997). Patterns of spine surgery – the 'surgical signatures' of hospital referral regions – varied in idiosyncratic ways. This graph compares rates of three kinds of spine surgery in 8 California hospital referral regions to the national average [from 31, p. 44].

and about the same per capita numbers of spine surgeons can have very different signatures for spine surgery. Figure 4 shows the variation in spine surgery in eight different hospital referral regions. The rate of lumbar discectomy was 41% higher than the national average in the Stockton, Calif. hospital referral region, but the rate of decompression for lumbar stenosis was 7% lower than the average. By contrast, the rate of lumbar discectomy in Fresno, Calif. was 39% below the average, but the rate of cervical spine surgery was 9% higher than the national average. In San Jose, Calif. the rate of decompression was 54% below the average, but the rate of lumbar discectomy was only 2% below the average [31].

Among the surgeons who performed spine surgery in Medicare enrollees in 1996, 3,011 were orthopedic surgeons and 2,934 were neurosurgeons. Overall, neurosurgeons performed 64% of all spine surgery among Medicare enrollees, compared to 36% by orthopedists. The proportion of spine surgery performed by either neurosurgeons varied markedly among hospital referral regions, from 19% in Akron, Ohio to 99% in Rapid City, S.D. The relative contributions of orthopedists and neurosurgeons also varied widely according to the kind of procedure. While neurosurgeons performed 85% of surgical procedures on the cervical spine, they performed only 59% of decompressions for lumbar stenosis. Neurosurgeons and orthopedic surgeons were quite different in their use of fusion for some types of spine surgery. While both performed noninstrumented fusions in about one third of cervical procedures, orthopedic surgeons were much more likely to

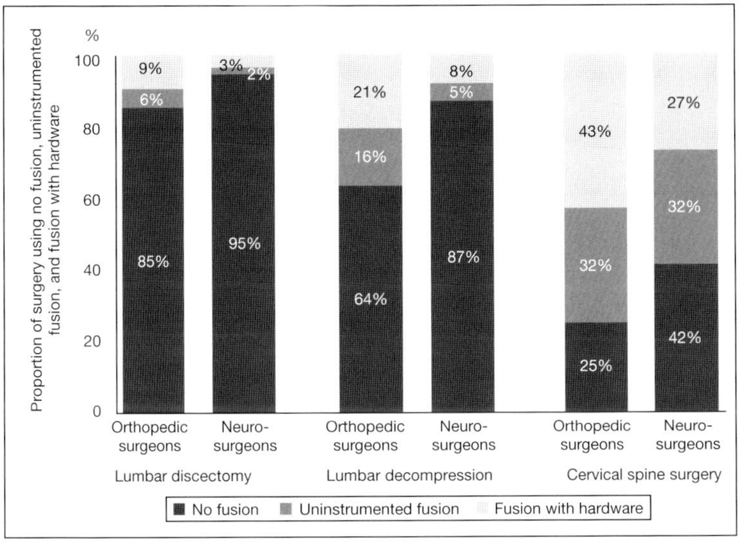

Fig. 5. Use of fusion (uninstrumented and with hardware) by orthopedists and neurosurgeons in spine surgery, by indication (1996) [from 31, p. 49].

perform a fusion during lumbar procedures and were much more likely to perform an instrumented fusion during both cervical and lumbar procedures (fig. 5) [31].

The Cost of Spine Disease

It has been said that next to the common cold, no condition afflicts the American population with greater incidence and prevalence than LBP. Back pain affects about 31 million people annually, and over 10 million people are disabled because of back pain, with upwards of 250 million workdays lost per year. Over USD 50 billion is expended on the management of back pain each year, with approximately USD 11 billion of that in the worker's compensation system. Two thirds of Americans suffer an incapacitating episode of back pain at least once in their lives, one third are suffering at any one time, and over one tenth are seeking medical care [19]. An estimated 25% of American workers will experience some back pain each year, with 50–60% experiencing some disabling pain during their working career [32]. While the annual rate for compensable back pain is approximately 2%, this varies with occupation: less than 1% for administrative and clerical personnel, and 1–15% for industrial workers [19].

Of the total money spent annually for the management of back pain, the distribution of total direct costs is 45% for permanent disability payments,

22% for temporary disability payments, and 33% for medical expenses. The medical expenses are distributed with 33% to physicians, 33% for hospital bills, 7% for medication, 5% for appliances, 9% for physical therapy, and 12% for diagnostic tests [32]. Surgical intervention represents only a small fraction of the total socioeconomic impact of this disease process, with less than 0.5% of patients with back pain undergoing surgery [33].

Spinal cord injuries also represent a significant cost to our society. There are very few accurate data on the total cost of spinal cord injuries. The estimated annual cost to support and treat all patients with a spinal cord injury is over USD 4 billion [34]. As expected, the initial hospitalization costs (including acute care and rehabilitation) and the annual follow-up expenses vary tremendously depending on the level of the injury. In one study, researchers found that costs of acute and rehabilitation care vary from USD 67,950 in the low-level paraplegic patient to USD 426,592 in the respirator-dependent, high-quadriplegic patient. Similarly, these researchers noted that annual follow-up expenses for the low-level paraplegic patient were USD 10,109 compared with USD 141,238 for the respirator-dependent, high quadriplegic patient [32]. Regarding economic opportunities lost, foregone lifetime earnings vary from USD 141,253 in the patient who is incompletely paraplegic to USD 308,054 in the completely quadriplegic patient [35]. Swift diagnosis and treatment that result in a rapid return to a premorbid level of activity would greatly reduce costs to the patient and to society.

References

1 Lawrence JS, Bremmer JN, Bier F: Osteoarthrosis: Prevalence in the population and relationship between symptoms and x-ray changes. Ann Rheum Dis 1966;25:1–24.
2 Hadley MN, Robinson RD: Clinical assessment of degenerative disorders of the spine; in Tindall GT, Cooper PR, Barrow DL (eds): The Practice of Neurosurgery. Philadelphia, Williams & Wilkins, 1996, pp 2367–2375.
3 Teresi LM, Lufkin RB, Reicher MA, Moffit BJ, Vinuela FV, Wilson GM, Bentson JR, Hanafee WN: Asymptomatic degenerative disk disease and spondylosis of the cervical spine: MR imaging. Radiology 1987;164:83–88.
4 Clarke E, Robinson P: Cervical myelopathy: A complication of cervical spondylosis. Brain 1956; 79:483–510.
5 Wilberger JE Jr, Chedid MK: Acute cervical spondylotic myelopathy. Neurosurgery 1988;22: 145–146.
6 Zeidman SM, Ducker TB: Cervical disc disease. Neurosurg Q 1992;2:116–163.
7 Love JG, Schorn VG: Thoracic disc protrusions. J Am Med Assoc 1965;191:91–95.
8 Brennan M, Perrin JCS, Canady A, Wesolowski D: Paraparesis in a child with a herniated thoracic disc. Arch Phys Med Rehabil 1987;68:806–808.
9 Arce CA, Dohrmann GJ: Herniated thoracic disks. Neurol Clin 1985;3:383–392.
10 De Villiers PD, Booysen EL: Fibrous spinal stenosis: A report on 850 myelograms with a water-soluble contrast medium. Clin Orthop 1976;115:140–144.
11 Roberson GH, Llewellyn HJ, Tavenas JM: The narrow lumbar spinal canal syndrome. Radiology 1973;107:89–97.
12 Paine KWE: Clinical features of lumbar spinal stenosis. Clin Orthop 1976;115:77–82.

13 Getty CJM: Lumbar spinal stenosis: The clinical spectrum and the results of operation. J Bone Joint Surg Br 1980;62:481–485.
14 Epstein JA, Epstein BS, Lavine LS, Carras R, Rosenthal AD: Degenerative lumbar spondylolisthesis with an intact neural arch (pseudospondylolisthesis). J Neurosurg 1976;44:139–147.
15 Verbeist H: Pathomorphologic aspects of developmental lumbar stenosis. Orthop Clin North Am 1975;6:177–196.
16 Hall S, Bartleson JD, Onofrio BM, Baker HL Jr, Okazaki H, O'Duffy JD: Lumbar spinal stenosis. Clinical features, diagnostic procedures, and results of surgical treatment in 68 patients. Ann Intern Med 1985;103:271–275.
17 Spengler DM: Degenerative stenosis of the lumbar spine. J Bone Joint Surg Am 1987;69:305–308.
18 Rosenberg NJ: Degenerative spondylolisthesis. Predisposing factors. J Bone Joint Surg Am 1975; 57:467–474.
19 Gerszten PG: The socioeconomic implications of neurosurgical disease; in Linskey ME, Rutigliano MJ (eds): Quality & Costs in Neurological Surgery. Philadelphia, Lippincott, Williams & Wilkins, 2001, pp 295–302.
20 Hart LG, Deyo RA, Cherkin DC: Physician office visits for low back pain: Frequency, clinical evaluation, and treatment patterns from a U.S. national survey. Spine 1995;20:11–19.
21 Andersson GBJ: Epidemiological features of chronic low-back pain. Lancet 1999;354:581–585.
22 Deyo RA, Weistein JN: Low back pain. N Engl J Med 2001;344:363–370.
23 Kelsey JL, White AA: Epidemiology of low back pain. Spine 1980;6:133–142.
24 Mitchell LV, Lawler FH, Bowen D, Mote W, Asundi P, Purswell J: Effectiveness and cost-effectiveness of employer-issued back belts in areas of high risk for back injury. J Occup Med 1994;36:90–94.
25 Coste J, Delecoeuillerie G, Cohen de Lara A, Le Parc JM, Paolaggi JB: Clinical course and prognostic factors in acute low back pain: An inception cohort study in primary care practice. BMJ 1994;308:577–580.
26 Cherkin DC, Deyo RA, Street JH, Barlow W: Predicting poor outcomes for back pain seen in primary care using patients' own criteria. Spine 1996;21:2900–2907.
27 Croft PR, Macfarlane GJ, Papageorgiou AC, Thomas E, Silman AJ: Outcome of low back pain in general practice: A prospective study. Br Med J 1998;316:1356–1359.
28 Deyo RA: Low-back pain. Sci Am 1998;279:48–53.
29 Bozzao A, Gallucci M, Masciocchi C, Aprile I, Barile A, Passariello R: Lumbar disk herniation: MR imaging assessment of natural history in patients treated without surgery. Radiology 1992;185:135–141.
30 Atlas SJ, Chang Y, Kammann E, Keller RB, Deyo RA, Singer DE: Long-term disability and return to work among patients who have a herniated lumbar disc: The effect of disability compensation. J Bone Joint Surg Am 2000;82:4–15.
31 Weinstein JN, Birkmeyer JD: The Dartmouth Atlas of Musculoskeletal Health Care. The Trustees of Dartmouth College, Dartmouth Medical School, 2000.
32 Watts C, Esser GB 3rd: Economic overview of spinal disorders; in Menezes AH, Sonntag VK (eds): Principles of Spinal Surgery. New York, McGraw-Hill, 1996, pp 25–36.
33 Conrad DA: Low back pain: Economic analysis of its impact on the U.S. non-elderly population; in Bigos S (ed): Report of the Low Back Pain Guidelines Panel to the Office of the Forum of the Agency for Health Care Policy and Research. Washington, Department of Health and Human Services, 1993.
34 Stripling TE: The cost of economic consequences of traumatic spinal cord injury. Paraplegia News, August 1990, pp 50–54.
35 DeVivo MJ: The cost of spinal cord injury: A growing national dilemma; in Apple DF Jr, Hydson LM (eds): The Spinal Cord Injury Model: Proceedings of the National Consensus Conference on Catastrophic Illness and Injury. Atlanta, 1989, pp 109–113.

Peter C. Gerszten, MD, MPH
Department of Neurological Surgery, University of Pittsburgh Medical Center
200 Lothrop Street, Suite B-400, Pittsburgh, PA 15213 (USA)
Tel. +1 412 647 3685, Fax +1 412 647 0989, E-Mail gerszten@neuronet.pitt.edu

Haid RW Jr, Subach BR, Rodts GE Jr (eds): Advances in Spinal Stabilization.
Prog Neurol Surg. Basel, Karger, 2003, vol 16, pp 302–313

The Changing Economics of Spine Surgery

Gregory J. Przybylski

Seton Hall University, Orange, N.J., USA

Advances in minimally invasive as well as complex spinal surgery during the past decade have been revolutionary. The practical application of molecular, biomechanical and computer engineering have enabled the spinal surgeon to have more options available in treating patients with a variety of simple and complex spinal disorders. However, the contraction of health care dollars available to pay for this wonderful growth of technology has begun to limit the choices available to the physician that hospitals are willing to purchase and maintain. This chapter will examine the separate issues facing spinal surgeons in their personal practice as well as the problems that hospitals face in managing the ever-changing and concurrently more expensive technological innovations brought to us.

The complexity of managing the spinal physician's practice has faced similar dramatic change, requiring increasing direct physician involvement to reduce the risk of fraud and abuse accusations and even prosecution. Accurate use of current procedural terminology (CPT) coding and application of a resource-based relative value system (RBRVS) methodology for physician payment and practice expense accounting have been the hallmarks of this change. In order to better adapt to these changes, it is important for the spinal practitioner to understand the methodology behind CPT coding as it applies to spinal surgery, as well as the use of RBRVS to the fee schedule and cost accounting of a practice.

CPT remains the standard method by which physicians communicate to the payer the services that were provided to their patients. This method for compiling and communicating physician procedural services was standardized and developed by the American Medical Association (AMA) in 1966 as current procedural terminology (CPT) [1]. Although initially reflecting predominantly surgical procedures, the second version 4 years later expanded the description of medical services using a five-digit coding system. The current fourth edition was completed in 1977 and contained substantial revisions to include improvements in medical technology. Each year, the book is updated to reflect the elimination of older procedures that are no longer performed as well as the addition of new procedures that reflect improvements in technology. The Health Care Finance Administration (HCFA, now renamed CMS for the Centers for Medicare and Medicaid Services) did not adopt CPT as part of their Common Procedure Coding System (HCPCS) until 1983, after which it mandated use of this system to report services for payment under Part B of the Medicare program. Three years later, HCFA also required Medicaid agencies to use the method.

The CPT system undergoes annual revision under the direction of the CPT Editorial Panel. This 16-member panel meets quarterly and is comprised of 11 AMA-appointed physicians that serve 4-year terms. Four of these seats rotate among specialists to allow a multidisciplinary influence. The other members of the panel include the co-chairman of the Health Care Professionals Advisory Committee (HCPAC), a representative from CMS, and appointees from the Blue Cross and Blue Shield Association, the Health Insurance Association of America, and the American Hospital Association. The panel is assisted by AMA staff as well as the CPT Advisory Committee, which is comprised predominantly of physicians selected by national medical specialty societies.

The largest change in CPT affecting the spine practitioner has been in the reporting of anterior thoracolumbar spinal surgery performed by more than one physician. With improvements in anesthetic technique and available instrumentation, greater attention had been drawn to anterior surgical approaches to spinal diseases. Although some spinal surgeons perform their own thoracolumbar exposures, many utilize the expertise of other surgeons to perform the initial approach to the anterolateral spinal column. Over several years, the American College of Surgeons and Society of Thoracic Surgeons in cooperation with orthopedists and neurosurgeons from 5 additional specialty societies worked to develop a consensus proposal to describe the approach component of anterior thoracolumbar spine surgery. Using the model of skull base surgery that separated the approach from the definitive procedure, emphasis was placed upon creating a scheme that would allow separate coding of the surgical exposure and closure from the spinal decompression or reconstruction. After several years of committee and work-group discussions and multiple presentations before the CPT Editorial Panel, the surgical representatives concluded that the substantial variability in physician practice made such a proposed system excessively complicated. Consequently, a consensus proposal was presented to the CPT Editorial Panel in February of 2001 requesting an expanded application of the –62 co-surgery modifier.

For several years previously, the –62 co-surgery modifier could only be used once per operative session. Since the approach has been considered included in the work value of the decompression and arthrodesis codes by the Relative Value Update Committee (RUC) and by CMS, it was proposed that the additional level codes describing adjacent segment decompression and/or arthrodesis must also contain a component representing the additional work of exposing the additional level(s). Concerned about the potential financial impact of expanding the use of the –62 co-surgery modifier, representatives from CMS presented data regarding the current usage of –62 as well as a summary of actual claims data in which anterior thoracolumbar surgery was performed by more than one surgeon. Several interesting observations made included less frequent usage of –62 to describe this work than was expected, but more importantly, serious concerns were raised about actual payments made on claims. For example, the correct method for reporting co-surgery requires both the approach surgeon and the spinal surgeon to submit the same code (though not necessarily the same charge) appended with the –62 modifier. However, CMS identified claims in which one surgeon used the modifier, whereas the other did not. Rather than paying both surgeons 62.5% of the Medicare allowable, only the surgeon coding correctly with the modifier was paid 62.5% of the allowable. In contrast, the other surgeon was paid 100% of the allowable, raising the vigilance of CMS in scrutinizing past and future claims regarding anterior thoracolumbar spine surgery. The CPT Editorial Panel accepted the consensus proposal to expand the use of the –62 modifier to allow reporting of the additional physician work involved in approaching adjacent segments for decompression or arthrodesis. The modifier will not be applicable to instrumentation or bone graft harvest codes, as specific language will be provided listing codes excluded from use of the modifier. These changes were implemented for January 2002.

With changes in the structure and management of CMS, an effort has been made to improve the transparency of certain activities, one of which is the correct coding initiative (CCI). Despite the large number of codes available to describe spinal procedures, the work included in many of these codes overlaps. The process of unbundling, which involves description of a larger procedure with several codes that contain overlapping work, resulted in significant increases in health care expenditures. On January 1, 1996, Medicare initiated the CCI to reduce unbundling and inappropriate reporting of CPT codes. At that time, HCFA contracted with Administar Federal, an Indiana Medicare carrier, to create and maintain a nationally used computer software program to preclude payment of otherwise bundled services. Despite the USD 700,000 development cost, Medicare reported savings in excess of USD 700 million since the program's inception. Most of the edits represented payment policies in which a comprehensive code would be paid while the component code would be disallowed, whereas a small percentage of edits identified mutually exclusive codes which would not be performed concurrently.

An example of the limitations of CCI placed on spinal surgery can be found in posterior lumbar interbody fusion (PLIF, CPT code 22630). The service description of posterior interbody fusion includes laminectomy, facetectomy, and discectomy to approach and prepare the endplates for the interbody arthrodesis. Consequently, CCI includes edits that preclude coding PLIF with many decompression procedures. However, this does not account for circumstances in which decompression is performed beyond the typically bony removal required to perform a PLIF. An editorial revision to 22630 was instituted in 2001 that included only the laminar, facet and disk removal required for performance of the PLIF, thereby allowing for coding of additional decompressive work if performed and medically indicated. The CCI process prevents payment for these additional physician services for the most part, unless a –59 modifier is also appended to identify the code as a distinct procedural service from the PLIF. This example distinguishes the differences between coding rules (developed and maintained by the AMA) and reimbursement rules (developed individually by CMS and third party payers).

However, the development of RBRVS has had the greatest impact upon the billing practices of physicians this past decade after its full implementation on January 1, 1996. The impetus to revise the Medicare payment system arose from the rapidly increasing expenditures for payment of physician and hospital services by Medicare. Since hospital services accounted for more than two thirds of Medicare expenditures, cost containment efforts were naturally directed at hospitals first. In 1983, a prospective pricing system (PPS) for hospital services using a diagnosis-related group (DRG) payment was developed for approximately 500 diseases. Using the national average cost of hospital care for that particular illness, it was assumed that the average cost for providing care for patients with a range of illness severity would equal the calculated DRG payment. Additional payments were also authorized to account for unusually severe illnesses requiring prolonged hospital stays. Since the payment was identical regardless of the hospital cost, the PPS provided a strong incentive for hospitals to improve cost-efficiency. Not surprisingly, the annual growth of Medicare expenditures was reduced by more than half between 1975 and 1990.

In 1994, physician payments on behalf of Medicare beneficiaries represented more than three quarters of the expenditures from Medicare Part B [2]. The original method for determining the physician payment schedule was based on customary, prevailing and reasonable (CPR) charges. This resembled the usual, customary, and reasonable (UCR) charge system utilized by private insurers to pay for physician's services based upon their actual fees, but included some adjustments to keep government costs predictable. However, the wide variation in the amount Medicare paid for physician services both among physician specialties as well as among geographical regions caused dissatisfaction within the medical profession [3]. Although costs were initially controlled by reducing payments from the 90th to the 75th percentile prevailing charge, Medicare later introduced a temporary price freeze on physician's services. In 1976, this was replaced by linking increases in prevailing charges to the Medicare Economic Index (MEI). As a result, Medicare payments were based upon prevailing charges in 1971 and remained nearly unchanged until 1992.

After a second freeze on payment levels in the 1980s and reduced payments for 'overpriced' surgical procedures, several payment reform proposals were suggested by the government. Although additional modifications to CPR were considered, it seemed that this method evolved into a complex system that no longer reflected physician fee schedules. Consideration was given toward developing a DRG system similar to that developed for hospital payments under Medicare Part A [4]. Another option was to create a managed care or capitation model of payment. Finally, a proposal was offered for replacing the CPR method with a payment schedule based on a relative value scale.

The concept of a relative value system (RVS) was not new. In fact, the California Medical Association developed an RVS in 1956, with regular updates for nearly two decades. Although this method still represented a CPR charge system, physicians used the RVS to determine fee schedules, whereas government and private insurers used the system to establish payment rates. However, the Federal Trade Commission raised concerns regarding the possible antitrust violations from price fixing, prompting the California Medical Association to discontinue updating the charge data collected.

Rather than using a charge-based RVS, a resource-based RVS was adopted in which physician services were valued based upon the relative costs incurred in providing them. Since antitrust concerns precluded direct physician involvement in the development of RBRVS, the AMA accepted a proposal submitted by the Harvard University School of Public Health to perform a national study of resource-based relative value scales (RBRVS) for physician services.

On July 1, 1986, the Consolidated Omnibus Budget Reconciliation Act mandated that the department of Health and Human Services develop an RBRVS to be submitted to Congress. In addition, the law created the Physician Payment Review Commission (PPRC) to study a variety of additional options for Medicare payment reform including changing CPR, capitation, and physician DRG [5]. The PPRC recommended development of a payment schedule linked to an RBRVS [6].

Six months earlier, the Harvard study, under the direction of William Hsiao, PhD and Peter Braun, MD, began with funding from HCFA. The first phase of the national study supported development of an RBRVS for 12 physician specialties. In addition, independent funding was obtained for the study of 6 additional specialties. Not only were specialty-specific scales developed, but also a method for creating cross-specialty links allowed integration of a single cross-specialty RBRVS. The Omnibus Budget Reconciliation Act of 1986 provided a 2-year extension for submission of RBRVS to Congress as well as mandated inclusion of 15 additional specialties during the second phase of the study [7–10]. Although the AMA adopted in principle the results of the Harvard study, they also recommended that the new Medicare payment system include geographical differences in practice costs and professional liability as well as a transition period to prevent disruptive changes between the CPR and RBRVS systems. The PPRC likewise endorsed the study and supported these AMA recommendations.

In December of 1989, Congress enacted the Omnibus Budget Reconciliation Act (OBRA 89) that mandated a Medicare payment schedule based on RBRVS from the Harvard study with inclusion of physician work, practice expense, and professional liability costs. Geographical adjustments to all three components were included. Calculation of a relative value unit (RVU) of a physician's service under RBRVS is as follows:

$$\mathrm{MFS} = [(\mathrm{RVUw} \times \mathrm{GPCIw}) + (\mathrm{RVUpe} \times \mathrm{GPCIpe}) + (\mathrm{RVUm} \times \mathrm{GPCIm})] \times \mathrm{CF}$$

where MFS = Medicare fee schedule, GPCI = geographical practice cost index, w = work, pe = practice expense, m = malpractice and CF = conversion factor.

The conversion factor for the calculated RVU was based on keeping the overall Medicare expenditure the same as the cost using the CPR system. A process was created to annually adjust the conversion factor, maintaining a 'budget-neutral' value, which limited increases in expenditures to USD 20 million annually. The final comprehensive RBRVS for physician services was published in the November 25, 1992 Federal Register.

After implementation of the RBRVS fee schedule by Medicare, additional health insurers have gradually implemented an RVS as well. Although RBRVS is the method most commonly used, an alternative RVS called St. Anthony's is also used in certain regions. This privately maintained system, formerly known as McGraw-Hill, utilizes RVUs based upon the time, risk, and complexity of the physician service. In contrast, the RBRVS uses physician work, practice expense, and malpractice expense as the components for determining the relative value of a particular physician service. The physician work component comprises approximately 55% of the total relative value of the service, whereas practice expense comprises 42%. In addition, a geographic practice cost index is

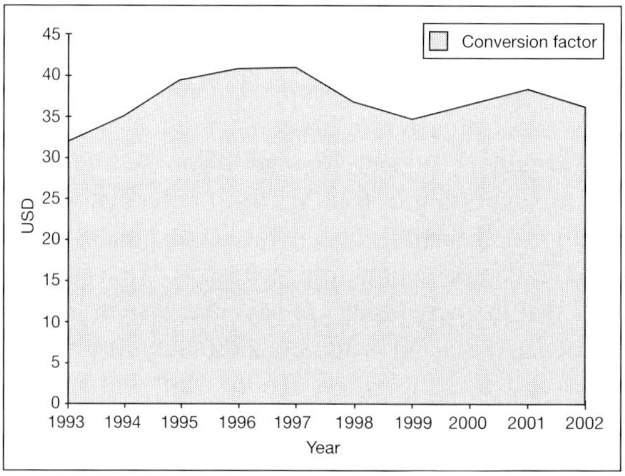

Fig. 1. Change in Medicare's surgical conversion factor over the past decade.

incorporated to adjust for geographical differences. Consequently, conversion factors between RBRVS and St. Anthony's RVS are different. Based upon the congressional mandate to maintain budget neutrality, CMS adjusts the conversion factor annually to assure budgetary control of expenditures for physician services (fig. 1). The recent 5.4% reduction in the conversion factor has prompted multitudes of physician organizations to petition Congress for legislation to reform the method for tying Medicare expenses to the gross domestic product. Growing evidence of reduced access for Medicare patients, including an American Academy of Family Physicians survey finding 17% of the respondents are no longer accepting new Medicare patients and a similar survey by the North American Spine Society showing a greater proportion of spine practitioners limiting access to Medicare patients, may prompt change in the continued contraction of reimbursement.

In order to coordinate changes in CPT with assignment of RVU by CMS, the AMA/Specialty Relative Value Update Committee (RUC) was created in 1991. Twenty-three of the twenty-eight members are appointed by major national medical specialty societies. The other five panelists include the RUC chair, the co-chair of HCPAC, and members of the AMA, American Osteopathic Association, and CPT Editorial Panel. A RUC Advisory Committee composed of members appointed by 94 specialty societies develop and suggest RVU for new codes to the RUC. Specialty society representatives are responsible for compiling physician survey data to determine the time spent in performing the medical service and ranking the service relative to existing services. Subsequently, consensus recommendations are forwarded to HCFA for annual consideration. During the 5-year period ending in 1998, nearly 2,300 relative value recommendations were made to HCFA with a recent acceptance rate of more than 90%.

The spine practitioner can take advantage of the RBRVS system in determining the cost required to provide physician services and thereby in developing a fee schedule that reflects these costs. Although practice costs are not linearly related to physician work, the RVU can serve as a surrogate. Consequently, a fee schedule can be constructed based on a 'conversion' factor determined by the practice and applied to the RVU assigned by Medicare to procedural codes. However, the appropriate conversion factor is influenced by many factors including personnel, equipment, and insurance (disability, health, malpractice) costs among others. The practice manager should determine the average annual RVU performed for the entire practice as well as stratified by individual physician. As a result, simply dividing the total practice (or individual physician) costs by the RVU performed during the same period provides a cost/RVU figure that reflects the expense to provide physician services.

Determination of cost/RVU is essential in negotiating contracts with third-party payers. Since many third-party payers have adopted fee schedules based on RBRVS, it is to your advantage to determine your costs on a similar scale. First of all, your analysis of the payment schedule is much more meaningful once you have determined your practice cost to provide the service. Secondly, the cost analysis allows the physician to focus on elements of the practice in which costs can be reduced. Finally, one can assess the time required to perform particular services. Certain services may be more economical than others, thereby allowing the physicians to focus efforts on their most efficient services.

Although work values are resource-based, practice expense was based upon the AMA's Socioeconomic Monitoring System 1989 Core Survey (SMS). While overall practice costs including office rent, wages of nonphysician personnel, equipment and supplies were measured, costs specific to a given single procedural service were unknown. Moreover, practice expenses varied among specialties. For example, these expenses represented 52.2% of family physicians' practice costs but only 38.9% of neurosurgeons' costs. In contrast, the average neurosurgical professional liability component of practice cost was 7.6%, compared with a 3.9% proportion for the family physician. The method enacted by OBRA 89 involved multiplying the specialty-specific practice expense factor by the average Medicare payment of the service in 1991. Similarly, professional liability was calculated based upon the proportion of cost multiplied by the Medicare payment.

The Omnibus Budget Reconciliation Act of 1993 mandated reductions in the practice expense of 'overvalued' services. Over a 3-year period, the practice expense was reduced annually by 25% of the amount that the value exceeded the physician work RVU until it was no greater than 128% of the work component.

However, concerns over the non-resource-based OBRA 89 method of calculating practice expense as well as a 1994 Social Security Act amendment mandating resource-based practice expense calculations prompted HCFA to contract with Abt Associates, to perform a national study of physician's practice expense. Fifteen Clinical Practice Expert Panels (CPEPs) were formed from nominations by medical associations to develop a list of direct cost components of a selected group of reference codes. In addition, a national mail survey of 5,000 practices was performed to obtain a sample of practice costs and service mix to validate the CPEP estimates. However, poor response rates from physicians led HCFA to abandon efforts at obtaining actual survey data. In order to meet the deadline of January 1998 set by Congress, HCFA planned to implement new practice expense values based on CPEP data. Lack of validation of the CPEP data with actual practice expense information as well as failures to account for actual differences in practice cost among all specialties prompted the AMA to urge Congress to extend the deadline for implementation of new practice expense values. As a result, Congress not only delayed implementation until 1999, but also directed the General Accounting Office (GAO) to review HCFA's methodology and make recommendations for a valid resource-based model. The GAO report supported the concerns raised by the AMA.

Beginning in January 1999, HCFA initiated a transition to a resource-based practice expense valuation that differs based on the site of the service. If a medical service can be performed either in an office or a hospital, then both a nonfacility and facility practice expense value will be assigned. Whereas locations assigned nonfacility practice expense include physician offices and independent imaging or laboratory centers, facility practice expense is attributed to hospitals, surgical centers, and nursing homes. The method for estimating practice costs is based upon the AMA's SMS data. Since the SMS data came from small sample sizes with sufficient variability to introduce sampling bias, there continues to be concern regarding this methodology. The transition to a resource-based method for calculating practice expense has been largely responsible for gradual decline in RVU assigned to spinal and other surgical codes.

More recently, rapidly escalating professional liability costs have had a substantial impact on the spinal surgeon's practice. A combination of a decade of underestimating the underwriting costs of these policies by insurers and increasingly frequent large judgments has resulted in a national professional liability crisis. For example, it has been estimated that USD 1 in premiums have been collected for every USD 1.36 in claims paid [11]. At the same time, the average medical liability award increased from USD 1.95 million to USD 3.5 million between 1993 and 1999 [12]. The Pennsylvania Medical Society has found that liability insurance charges were hiked 21–91% in 2001 alone. Similarly, a recent survey presented at the Council of State Neurosurgical

Societies meeting in 2001 revealed substantial increases in insurance costs in the past year, which have led some physicians to curb practice or move to more favorable geographical regions. For example, Indiana and California have adopted tort reform legislation that includes caps on noneconomic damages that have helped in reducing the unreasonable judgments awarded by some juries. Unfortunately, CMS does not update the professional liability component of the RVU on an annual basis, leading to a significant underestimation of these costs for certain specialties including orthopedic and neurological surgery.

The AMA estimates that 12 states are currently experiencing a medical liability crisis, whereas 30 additional states are on the verge of similar problems. For example, the closure of a level 1 University Trauma Center in Las Vegas, Nev. prompted the state legislature to temporarily give the physicians 'state employee status', thereby limiting their liability to USD 50,000. The growing liability crisis has prompted a bipartisan bill termed the 'Health Act' that seeks to institute national tort reform and includes limits on noneconomic damages modeled after California and Indiana.

Finally, the increasing influence of governmental regulation on the practice of medicine will continue to have a significant influence upon the manner in which spinal surgeons provide health care. For example, the Kennedy-Kassebaum Health Insurance Portability and Accountability Act 1996 (HIPAA) changed the US Government's Fraud and Abuse regulations by increasing civil monetary damages from USD 2,000 to USD 10,000 and by applying fraud and abuse laws to the private as well as the public sector, by permitting confiscation of personal property for health care fraud convictions, and by changing health care frauds from misdemeanors to federal felonies with mandatory prison sentences. Surgeons are liable for fraud and abuse violations in the documentation, coding and billing tasks of their practice. Compliance plans and programs are aimed at satisfying the Office of the Inspector General's requirements for the constant surveillance of these responsibilities. The requirement to comply with the complex regulations that have evolved from the law begins next year and poses a significant economic burden for smaller practices in developing and maintaining compliance programs.

Similarly, the regulations that have arisen from the Emergency Medical Treatment and Labor Act (EMTALA) of 1986 apply to physicians providing on-call services to emergency departments. The requirements that have evolved from the expanded interpretation of EMTALA include the need for the on-call physician to arrive to the emergency department within 30 min of notification of a true emergency. Possible violations of the act include inability to see a patient at a second hospital if call is simultaneously taken at two hospitals and both require concurrent patient evaluation and inability to leave an elective procedure if a patient arrives in the emergency room requiring attention by the operating surgeon. Both hospitals and physicians can be fined up to USD 50,000 for each violation, in addition to the damages allowed by state law for injury sustained by the patient from an EMTALA violation.

Although the changing economic environment for the physician has been quite dramatic over the past decade, hospitals have faced similar issues that have resulted in more frequent closures secondary to bankruptcy. With increasing granularity of actual hospital costs to provide patient services, administrators have identified areas that are being targeted for cost containment. For example, the cost of spinal implants has had a significant impact upon the hospitals' expense in treating spine patients. In the absence of 'carve-outs' that exclude implant cost from the DRG, much if not all of the hospital reimbursement for a patient's particular diagnosis is needed for purchase of the implants, thereby creating a shortfall in accounting for the nursing, medication, imaging, and facility costs of the procedure.

As a result, hospital administrators are becoming increasingly influential in determining the types and source of implants available for the spinal surgeon to use. With many manufacturers vying for an opportunity to provide implants and services, increasing price competitiveness may result in single-source purchase of equipment and implants that may be different from the physician's preference. Efforts at proactive cost containment by the physicians may help the hospital while simultaneously allowing the physician to participate in the decision-making process. For example, the Lahey Clinic implemented a system by which the equipment vendors supplied all of the implants as well as the disposable and nondisposable instruments to perform a particular procedure (termed single price/single case purchasing). As a result, costs were reduced by 23–45% [13]. Although some savings required a change of vendors, some of the equipment savings were achieved with maintenance of the same provider.

Another area of increasing scrutiny involves outpatient surgery. Although there have been efforts in place for some time now to reduce length of hospital stay (and therefore cost) for patients recovering after spinal procedures, some procedures like lumbar discectomy are now performed on an outpatient basis. However, CMS has suggested that the costs to provide an outpatient procedure are typically less than the cost to provide the service to an inpatient. Consequently, CMS has identified a group of 'outpatient' procedures with a different payment schedule. As a result, the hospital may not receive sufficient payment for procedures performed on an outpatient basis that are identified as inpatient procedures. This policy may curtail efforts at cost containment, as procedures are not approved by the hospital unless the patient is kept overnight.

In conclusion, the dramatic improvements in technology that have allowed the spinal surgeon a vastly greater armamentarium for the management of spinal disorders have been mirrored by an increasingly complex socioeconomic environment that has both directly and indirectly affected the daily practice of the spinal surgeon. An awareness of and adaptation to this changing environment should help the spinal surgeon in meeting both the clinical demands of treating patients with the economic constraints that may limit options going forward. Increasing individual as well as professional societal involvement in the legislative process is imperative to shaping a more favorable landscape for practicing spinal surgery.

References

1 Gordon BL: Current Procedural Terminology. Chicago, American Medical Association, 1973.
2 Committee on Ways and Means: Overview of entitlement programs: 1994 Green Book. Washington, Committee on Ways and Means, 1994, p 1075.
3 Burney IL, Schreiber GJ, Blaxall MO, Gabel JR: Geographic variation in physician's fees. JAMA 1978;240:1368–1371.
4 Mitchell JB: Physician DRG's. N Engl J Med 1985;313:670–675.
5 Physician Payment Review Commission: Medicare physician payment: An agenda for reform; in Annual Report to Congress No 68-227. Washington, US Government Printing Office, 1987.
6 Physician Payment Review Commission: Medicare physician payment; in Annual Report to Congress. Washington, US Government Printing Office, 1988.
7 Hsiao WC, Braun P, Becker ER, Thomas SR: The resource based relative value scale. JAMA 1987;258:799–802.
8 Hsiao WC, Braun P, Dunn D, Becker ER: Resource based relative values: An overview. JAMA 1988;260:2347–2353.
9 Hsiao WC, Braun P, Dunn D, Becker ER: Results and policy implications of the resource based relative value study. N Engl J Med 1988;319:881–888.
10 Hsiao WC, Braun P, Yntema D, Becker ER: Estimating physicians' work for a resource-based relative value scale. N Engl J Med 1988;319:835–841.
11 Zimmerman R, Oster C: Insurers' price wars contributed to doctors facing soaring costs. Wall Street Journal, June 24, 2002.
12 Marcus MB: Healthcare's 'perfect storm'; soaring malpractice costs are causing critical shortages of doctors. US News and World Report, July 1, 2002.
13 Healy WL, Iorio R, Lemos MJ, Patch DA, Pfeifer BA, Smiley PM, Wilk RM: Single price/case price purchasing in orthopaedic surgery. Experience at the Lahey Clinic. J Bone Joint Surg Am 2000;82:607–612.

Gregory J. Przybylski, MD
The New Jersey Neuroscience Institute at JFK,
Seton Hall University, 65 James Street, Edison, NJ 08818 (USA)
Tel. +1 732 632 1624, Fax +1 732 632 1584, E-Mail gprzybylski@solarishs.org

Author Index

Subject Index